IRIDOLOGY

*A complete guide to diagnosing through the iris
and to related forms of treatment*

IRIDOLOGY

A complete guide to diagnosing through the iris and to related forms of treatment

Farida Sharan MD MA MH ND FBRI

Thorsons
An Imprint of HarperCollinsPublishers

Thorsons
An Imprint of HarperCollins*Publishers*
77–85 Fulham Palace Road,
Hammersmith, London W6 8JB

Published in hard cover by Thorsons 1989
Paperback edition 1992
1 3 5 7 9 10 8 6 4 2

© Farida Sharan 1989, 1992

Farida Sharan asserts the moral right to
be identified as the author of this work

A catalogue record for this book
is available from the British Library

ISBN 0 7225 1645 2 (hardback)
ISBN 0 7225 2778 0 (paperback)

Iridology chart on jacket reproduced
by permission of Dr Bernard Jensen

Printed in Great Britain by
The Bath Press, Bath, Avon

Contents

Dedication

"The Lord has given eyes with which to see Him."
                                        Saint Paltu

To my Beloved Spiritual Teacher,
who opened my eyes, and who continues
to remove the veils of illusion that
separate me from Him. I offer this
work entirely in His service, knowing
that everything comes from Him, and that
I am only an instrument in His hands.

IRIDOLOGY

*A complete guide to diagnosing through the iris
and to related forms of treatment*

Introduction

The Eyes of the World

We live in this life within a sea of energy, the life of each person streaming communication from the eyes, the light of each person's innermost self radiating outward, connecting and exchanging with that of other living creatures. This exchange of spirit shining from life to life represents the closest communication we experience with each other.

We also receive light from the world which we take into our being, as our view of the world happens before our eyes, moment to moment, every second. This pageant of light and colour floods us, bathing every cell of our being with energy and vitality. Life dances in front of us, constantly enchanting us with its kaleidoscopic flow. Eighty-five per cent of what we experience is taken in through the major sense organs, the eyes, into the discriminatory brain centres. How we live our life in response to this information is our own individual life story.

The eye is a two-way threshold, energy moving inward and outward. How open is this gateway? Do we welcome the light and energy from the world? Do we radiate warmth and love from our spirit and heart to those we meet? Do the veils of fear, selfishness, shyness, disinterest, greed or anger inhibit this flow of spirit to the world, and to other living beings? When we radiate warmth and nurturing, life meets life in loving communion.

Eyes tell us many things. We have all experienced the flash of anger, the ice cold scornful look of disapproval or rejection, or the bored indifferent stare. It is as though the thought and heart of each person speaks through their eyes. Eyes can dance. They can sparkle with joy and leap with merry laughter. They can also look tired and drained. We can be drawn towards someone's eyes, wanting to look into them more and more, yet other eyes make us turn away in fear or discomfort. Often, women turn their eyes away when men stare at them. We can feel scorned, welcomed or totally blessed by the glance from someone's eyes.

Think of the eyes of someone you love. You are drawn to them as if by an irresistible magnet. Their love touches you, stirs your innermost heart and you long for more. You can speak so many deep feelings without words. Whether it is an infant, child, sister, brother, mother, friend or lover, your closest relationships will always include this language of the eyes.

An ancient Chinese text says: 'The liver opens into the eyes', 'when the liver receives blood the eyes can see', or 'when the liver is harmonized, the eyes can distinguish the five colours'. All the organs contribute their purest energy to the eyes, giving the bright awareness that characterizes harmonious spirit. A healthy liver contributes a relaxed, easy-going internal environment and an even disposition, all of which shine out of the eyes.

When we are afraid or shy, and we do not want to be known, we hide our eyes. We turn away from the light in other peoples' eyes. We may speak to each other but we do not connect with the radiating life stream unless we look into their eyes.

When people pass on the street, they often avoid each other's eyes, or turn away after catching the other's eye. Consider how different it is if a person turns to you and flashes a welcoming glance. No words are needed. The person has greeted you from their spirit and you feel the effect of that in your heart and mind. There is a world behind each person's eyes, a world that can be shared or hidden away. We can hold our loving energy back and cut off from giving it to others or we can let it flow, bathing those around us with the spirit we nourish inside. If we have something special to give it will show in our eyes. Think back and remember the times when the language of the eyes meant something special to you. You will always find that memories of those you love will include the light and the love that shone from their eyes. We are irresistibly drawn to eyes because of our inherent seeking after light and spirit.

Babies stare intently into the eyes of those around them. Their pure new natures, actively involved in learning about the world around them, find a deep clear reality in the life of the eyes that surround them, as though eyes were the centre of the dance of life. Children seek interaction with the world with open faces and wide eyes.

Different cultures have their own unique manners regarding eye contact. For example, some cultures look with direct eyes that pierce deeply, curiosity flashing. When shyness overtakes them they hide their eyes behind their hands, as if that makes them invisible. In India, your presence on a beach will attract crowds of onlookers whose only purpose is to stare at you. Yet, in the West, if someone stares at you, you think they want to start a fight or that they have an ulterior motive. In commuter trains, if you should happen to catch someone's eye, they shut off. Muslim women are hidden behind the dark veils, yet their eyes reveal the strong quality of the women underneath, their longing, their fearful shyness, as well as their courage and their strength.

And, in old age, when poor health dims the vision, the pupils contract, and the elderly drift inward into dreams and memories, loosening their connection with the outside world. Just as they shut down their ability to receive, they also shut out the expression of their own love and light. When you see an older person still alive and vibrant with life, the sparkle of wisdom and enjoyment in their eyes is bright and satisfying.

Eyes surround us everywhere we look. Even if we disdain the company of fellow human beings we still meet the eyes of animals or birds. You must be able to remember a time when you have looked out on a garden, meadow or mountain and suddenly see the shining eye of a living creature among the leaves or trees. The glowing eyes of owls, or a dog caught in the light of the fire or the moon reveal their living spirit. This conscious recognition and the spark of the exchange is experienced by both the creature and the human being.

The seductive displays of advertising and media presentations are abundant with eyes that gaze at us from every magazine, newspaper, television and movie screen. Every season new colours and makeup techniques draw attention to the lure of the eyes. Women in every country and culture enhance their beauty with eye makeup, from the black kohl of the Egyptians, to Moroccan henna painting, African tattoos and North American clay markings. 'Look at my eyes', they say, 'Look at me. Love me. Desire me.'

Eyes can have a transforming power. In the East, the disciple sits at the feet of the teacher and even a look can communicate 'darshan'—the special spiritual consciousness that comes from the master. One look is said to burn off the karmas of 10,000 lives, and uplift the devotee into a cool, blissful radiance and a perfect peace. Now we can travel to that level of consciousness where we close our eyes, and the seemingly real world dissolves.

Many forms of religious art attempt to portray the longing devotion of the disciple and the radiant grace bestowing glance of the saint. Because the saint's consciousness abides in divine union, this radiance is expressed through their eyes into the world and into the eyes of those who look with searching devotion.

Our eyes radiate what we are at every moment. This dynamic process changes according to our vitality, emotions and attitudes. When we are clear and balanced we radiate warmth and love, but when we are tired and depleted or have a headache, we find the light we transmit is diminished. Because the source of the saint's nourishment is infinite and unchangeable, their light transcends these earthly mutable moods, overcoming even the darkest persecutions and difficulties.

We look outward into the world with our eyes. This uniquely personal view of the world has been gathered by the sum total of what we have seen and experienced. By far the largest share of information is taken in through the eyes. This vast storehouse of accumulated vision has been discriminated upon in the brain centres and stored for reference. The child forms its concepts of reality in this way. However, the views of perception are infinite. We may all see the landscape in front of us, but according to our perception we will organize, select and interpret what we see. An old woman looking out over an estuary might be noting the subtle shifts of cloud, water and colours. Her neighbour may be naming plants and recognizing birds. The child may only see a big red ball, two spaniel puppies, and the warm sun as she plays happily with her sandcastle. So the eyes filter information in through the mind which builds up our everyday reality. Our spirit radiating outwards is likewise filtered by the thoughts and emotions of the moment. What we have seen and experienced makes us what we are and what we are is what we radiate through our eyes, our personality and our life.

We look out of our eyes and organize our pattern of reality by interpreting what we see according to our personality, interests and experience. Is it not possible then that we could look into the eyes and see the interior world reflected in the iris patterns?

Let us look closer now. Add the lens of the magnifying glass and discover the meaning of the iris fibres, colours and markings of each person's own unique irisprint. We will learn how our interior life affects the iris patterns, and thus our view of the world, life, and how we live it.

Chapter 1

The Transparent Body

Iridology enhances our ability to visualize and understand our inner world. Because our intention has been focused outwards into the world for so long we often do not feel or understand the body in which we live. We need to flood our body with the light of conscious awareness and rediscover feeling and attention. Our body speaks to us. It tells us what is happening all the time if we will but tune in to its messages.

We live in a soft, vulnerable, transparent body. Although our outer eyes look at the body and see only the outer envelope, our inner eye of conscious awareness can visualize the streams of energy, colour and light that energize our body during the living interplay of body systems and organs. This expanded imaginative perception makes anatomy and physiology come alive.

The world within, in all its pulsing, vibrant tapestry of dynamic action, the living, chemistry in motion, the miraculous processes of cellular metabolism, and the waves of absorption and elimination, harbours so much life, so much energy and so much power. This body that we live in is a miracle. It is the temple of our life and our spirit, our home while we are in this world. It is truly the crown of creation.

We have this incredible opportunity to discover the world within the body in which we live. We can understand it. We can listen to it. We can give it what it needs. We can work with it instead of against it. We can treasure and protect our inheritance, making the most of what we have, instead of wasting it and waking up to the cold realities of ill health and weakness only when it is too late. This heightened consciousness and respect will not only help us to appreciate the body we have been given, but it will encourage respect and responsibility towards the world of nature in which we live and the forces which nourish and protect us.

When veils of ignorance and fear inhibit our natural wisdom and self awareness, our body is a mystery. Symptoms and illness force us to desperate measures, to relieve not only our own suffering but that of our loved ones. Throughout the ages men and women have been held in fear and ignorance about their bodies and the cause of disease, and they have had to endure even worse suffering from treatment, which often proved to no avail.

Iridology breaks the chain of ignorance and dependence. It gives the opportunity to those who seek enlightenment to take a higher responsibility for their own bodies and how they live their life. Iridology gives you the opportunity to understand your individual body, its strengths and weaknesses, what you have inherited and how your body has been affected by how you have lived in this world. It guides you to make the most of what you have. Like a guardian on the path, it points the way to truth. It is then up to us to follow that guidance, through the ups and downs of life. This enlightenment is an essential wisdom which allows us to live in our body with faith, respect and understanding. Just as we take care of cars, houses and other possessions iridology will help us attain the objective discrimination needed to be able to live consciously.

Let us learn to look at our body in new ways, to see our transparent body. I once asked my teacher, Dr John Christopher, 'What is our main purpose as an iridologist?' He replied with a loving light in his eyes, 'It is my sincere belief that we prepare our patients for better things to come.' I have held this inspiration at the very heart of my practice, and I have always observed this to be true.

Treatment proceeds like the opening of a flower within the patient's life, melting the mental and physical crystallization which forced the individual into a disease pattern. As the body is relieved emotional energies are released. Problems are solved. They may get promotion or change jobs. Relationships improve. It is as though their outside world was a reflection of their inner world, and when the interior world changed, their life reflected that change. Transformation.

This knowledge is light upon the way, illumination, wisdom that releases us from darkness and disease, a gift that transforms our life and gives us the opportunity to attain clearer, higher ways of being. Instead of being at the mercy of forces we do not understand, we are given the grace of understanding and the choice to live from that new understanding. Discrimination is the quality which separates us from other living creatures, and when we can make choices based on an iridology analysis, we can be sure we are on a path leading to health and a fuller life.

Iridology is a universal language, true for all ages, cultures and races. The iris reveals its mysteries to those who learn the language and observe the markings in relation to the person. One soon observes that every case of arthritis is different, because iridology shows the cause of illness within each unique person. Treatment is especially effective as the iridology interpretation guides the practitioner to prescribe exactly what each person needs. The right thing at the right time is a very powerful medicine.

As well as revealing deep knowledge of physical conditions, the iris teaches us about mental attitudes, masculine/feminine balances, attitudes towards the mother and father, relationship of mind and body, personality, heredity, constitutional types and much more. The frontiers are wide open for exploration and discovery. We are building on the foundation of the early iridologists, most of whom were medical doctors. They observed iris markings as they went about their work in private practice, before and after surgery, with terminal patients and in institutions for the mentally ill, and the deaf, dumb and blind. This is how they were able to create the first iris charts. We follow in their footsteps, adding our observations and experience.

Ancient medicine contains references to iris markings, from the earliest days of Chaldean and Egyptian history. The Cairo museum contains a display case that is full of ceramic eyes covered with hand painted iris markings, obvious proof that they were aware of their significance. In fact the iris is as personal as a handprint or fingerprint. It is a distinctly unique representation of who and what we are, and that is, of course, different for each person, as are the blade of grass, the grain of sand or the snowflake.

Animal and bird irides also reveal invaluable information about their condition. The earliest written records contain references of horse and sheep traders looking into their animals' eyes for signs of inherent strength or weakness. Pigeon breeders also look into their birds' eyes to determine whether they will be a good investment.

The modern interest in iridology was sparked off in Hungary when a young boy, later known as Dr Ignatz von Peczeley observed that a dark mark appeared in an owl's eye immediately after its leg was broken. When he saw the black mark heal and weave together as the leg healed, his interest was captured. Years later, when he became a doctor he observed iris markings until he was able to design one of the first iridology charts.

In Russia today the government is very enthusiastic about the results doctors are achieving with iridology in mental institutions. Their patients not only become well, but they stay well, saving the government considerable expense.

Once the vocabulary and methods of interpretation are grasped Iridology can be integrated with any method of treatment, whether orthodox or alternative, and to any condition. It is a truth of living bodies. We need only turn our attention to observing the truth the irides reveal. For those who discover the hidden worlds of the iris, the knowledge and wisdom gained will be off untold value in any healing work.

Iridology — Pathway to transformation

Iridology transforms the way we feel about our bodies. When we actually see the effects of how we live reflected in the iris and realize the changes that drugs and chemicals inflict upon our body tissue, we can no longer live unconsciously. The veil of ignorance is lifted. When the early pioneer doctors discovered iridology, they were inspired to stop the use of chemical medicines. They became natural physicians who learned to understand the causes of disease and how to work with the body to restore function, balance and health. As the eyes teach us about the interior world, we learn to see at a deeper level and to take responsibility for how we create illness. We also learn to respect the body and to refrain from administering harmful medicines.

When a patient consults a trained iridologist they are shown their strengths and weaknesses, given understanding of their constitutional type and how their body proceeds towards disease. They are also guided to change their living habits. Natural medicines and therapies are given to assist the body to return to vitality so that it will be able to throw off the disease condition. Early signs of chronic disease can be recognized so the condition can be treated before manifestation of an incurable condition.

The foundation level of treatment should activate all the eliminative channels (bowel, lymph, skin, lungs and kidneys) so that toxins, acids, chemicals and inorganics can leave the body without creating a strong healing crisis. This, together with constitutional treatment and the strengthening of any weak systems or organs, will support the body until it reaches a healthy state. Then its own inherent vitality and power will overcome the disease condition. Once patients have gone through a course of treatment in which they have been actively involved, they develop a greater independence. They are now more able to take care of themselves. They know what diet suits them best and which natural medicines and therapies are helpful. Then patients only need occasional advice from the practitioner. Instead of developing a practice based on dependency and return visits as patients progress towards illness, the iridologist's practice grows by referrals from satisfied patients.

We need to know how to keep ourselves well, and to have the knowledge to take this responsibility on our own shoulders. Then our overworked doctors can concentrate on cases of strongest need. Alternative and orthodox practitioners can work together. As more people learn how to keep themselves well, health budgets and taxation will be less. In this day and age the body does not need to be a mystery. Enlightenment is all around us, waiting to be found. We can live in our body with consciousness and take care of it with respect. It is the temple for our life; the only body that we have. Iridology can provide the key so that we can not only prevent the development of chronic disease, but also achieve higher levels of health and well being.

The microcosm holds the macrocosm

The idea of the microcosm and the macrocosm and how they interrelate is an ancient one, but now global consciousness and the realization of how the part affects the whole is a concept to be found in all fields of science, medicine, psychology, ecology and religion; indeed, such an idea is necessary if we are to survive. We are all interdependent and the nature that we are a part of is an intricate, interwoven system that moves in constant response and reaction.

The crust that supports life on this planet is thin and fragile. Modern man seeks now out of necessity, as well as a more sensitive responsible global consciousness, to preserve the balance of nature so that not only can catastrophe be avoided but also quality of life can be maintained.

Just as these attitudes for the preservation of life and our world need to be nurtured, we can also learn to appreciate the needs of our inner world.

Every cell and part of our inner world affects the function of the whole. Treatment may proceed from any part towards the whole. Everything affects everything else. Instead of treating a disease, we evaluate each body organ, system and area and their relationship to each other, treating what shows up as weak, deficient, inflammatory, etc. As the body regains balanced function it also regains its own inherent healing powers. Optimum function of all the working parts does not tolerate disease, which comes as a result of breakdown in function. Our approach to health and the prevention of disease also needs to consider each 24 hour cycle in all its aspects, physical, mental, emotional and spiritual. One's total life must be brought into harmony with one's inner and outer worlds.

Man is the microcosm in the universal macrocosm. As part of nature man vibrates with or against the laws of harmony and love. Even modern science has had to move into mystical spheres to explain and order the phenomena of nature. Dr Henry Lindlahr's Vol. 1 of *Natural Therapeutics* describes this concept:

'If there is to be health, the vibratory conditions of the organism must be in harmony with nature's established harmonic relations in the physical, mental and psychical realms of human life and action. Everthing that is to be normal, natural, healthy, good, beautiful, must vibrate in unison with its correlated harmonics in nature'.

We are each responsible for the attunement of our being to this divine harmony.

Once we accept the relationship of the individual to creation as a whole, and seek to understand the laws of nature, we will know what is right. Then we can strive to uphold these truths through personal effort, discipline and a loving desire for obedience. When this is achieved and maintained man reaches the peak of fulfilment. Lindlahr describes this state thus,

'These highest and purest attainments of the human soul are not the results of mere physical well being, but of the peace and harmony which come only through obedience to natural law'.

The natural healer recognizes the necessity of the harmonic relationship between man and nature, and seeks attunement to its melodious rhythms. This attitude is taught gradually during the healing process to patients, by example, direct instruction and personal experience. Naturopathy means nature's path.

The iris is a perfect microcosmic screen displaying symbolically the microcosmic realities of constitutional inherited strengths, weaknesses, pathways to disease, toxic accumulations, inflammatory and exudative conditions, personality, the emotional life, as well as revealing data on

The iris — brain tissue that meets the outside world

body systems and organs and their interrelated function. How can we explain this?

The eye emerges out of the forebrain of the human embryo as it reaches 6 mm in size. By the time it is 13 mm the eye has separated forward and is now connected to the brain by the optic nerve. The pupillary ruff is an extension of the central nervous system.

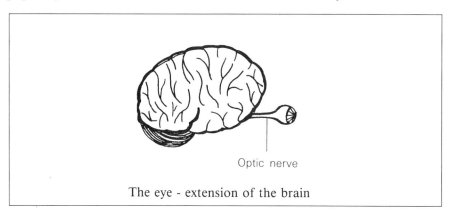

Optic nerve

The eye - extension of the brain

Imagine that the eye is a screen on which the central and autonomic nervous systems project information about what is happening all over the body. If man creates a control panel in order to monitor what is happening in the various parts of the machines he makes, why would our Creator leave out such an important detail? Now that the increasing popularity of alternative medicine is making available understanding of body patterns through therapies like reflexology and acupuncture we can see how different parts of the body reflect the whole. The same is true with iridology.

Although anatomy and physiology books do not give explanations as to why there are over 28,000 nerve fibres in the iris, iridology proves that information gathered from all areas of the body is being transmitted. Although iridology is a science, it is in its pioneer days. The reason it is not more widely accepted is that there are many attitudes which prevent the medical profession from exploring and observing iridology. This is an era when doctors prefer to rely on expensive machines, even though the body could tell them what they wish to know. And yet, there are professionals from both orthodox and alternative medicine who respond immediately to iridology knowing instantly and intuitively that it is true.

However it is a study that proves itself. We are not asking you to believe anything. Learn the language. Observe a few hundred eyes in relation to their symptoms and diseases and then make up your own mind. It simply works. The fact that orthodox medicine has so far turned a blind eye to research, or the fact that perhaps we do not yet have sensitive enough technology to explain or measure according to scientific protocol, does not alter the fact that if you look, observe and follow up, iridology will prove itself.

Our body is like a chameleon. It is a constantly changing and adjusting **The mutable body** transformer which works at all times to maintain balance between its various parts and the inner and outer worlds. Everything we do at every moment is creating our future, and yet we still carry the effects of our past with us. This concept is symbolized by the lotus flower, an ancient symbol for spirituality. It is the only plant which contains both the seed and the fruit at the same time. At every moment of our life we carry the fruit of our past actions and the seeds of our future. And yet, all we really have is the ever changing present.

When we are ill, in pain or discomfort, we need to remember that the cause of what we are experiencing was in the past and that every moment we have the opportunity to create a new and a better future. As disease crystallizes, we believe in it more and more, eventually becoming completely identified with it. What is needed is to break that identification and to remember that our body is a continuum of past, present and future. We have the opportunity to transform the present by clearing the past and creating new causes for the future.

Iridology evaluates the causes of illness at a very deep level, and guides the practitioner to recommend specific focused treatment to manifest change in the quickest way possible, in harmony with natural processes. This does not mean the radical and somewhat dangerous use of drugs, lasers and other modern medicinal warfare, but gentle non-invasive purification and regeneration. The assistance of non-toxic non-habit forming herbal foods and other naturopathic and complementary therapies, combined with diet and advice on living habits will work harmoniously to restore balanced function to body systems and organs.

The foundation level of treatment, based on the activation, clearing and stimulation of the elimination channels is essential if treatment of symptoms, body symptoms and organs is to be effective. This is the first step. We must clear obstructions to function. Once the eliminative channels are doing their work, the crystallization and identification with the disease pattern begins to disintegrate, and the person is able to create a healthier pattern.

In this life, two things are certain. Both change and death are inevitable. Nothing lasts forever. Just because we have created disease does not mean it is solid or permanent. We can evolve out of that disease pattern. We can take charge of the present and direct change for the future. We can learn to make the most of what we have and to achieve maximum performance. Once the work is done we will be able to continue maintenance care and enjoy a full life in a body that serves us well.

Health is not static. Neither is it an achievement. Think of health by imagining a surfer riding the waves, adjusting every second to the power and beauty of the waves in order to enjoy skimming over the sea. We are always adjusting to life. No matter how well we plan our life, stress, stimulation, conflict, shocks, responsibilities keep coming at us. Whatever we can learn to help us become a surfer in life, to give us that free joyful ride is worth knowing about. Coming to terms with your own body by understanding your iris markings is a significant factor in helping the vehicle that carries you through life achieve maximum performance.

Ecological iridology

The iris tells us what is happening within the body interior. Just as we can look out on the world and see that there are droughts in Africa and floods in India, we can also determine excess and deficiency in body function in the iris. When one organ has ceased to work properly, another or others take up part of the load. When toxins collect because of constipation the liver, lymph and kidneys have to work harder to purify the blood. If the skin is not functioning the kidneys and respiratory system have to eliminate the excess water.

Every part affects every other part. Every part needs to do its job, to contribute its influence to the harmony of the whole. So many students ask me how I work with patients, and I always say, 'I am an interior ecologist.' I look to see what isn't working properly and take steps with natural means to restore proper levels of function. Once all the systems and organs of the body are working efficiently the body itself will take care of illness.

This may seem simple. It is simple. Health and disease are very simple. We look for complexities because we have moved from simplicity, yet the simplicity is always there to be found. If people understood the natural laws of living and didn't let health imbalances go untreated for too long, we could live healthier lives.

If any part of your body is not working or any part of your body is drawing your attention to it, stop, look and listen. Just as children are instructed how to cross roads, we need to be reminded how to live in our body. Stop, look and listen. If you have been through a period of stress, take time to unwind and restore yourself. Don't keep yourself wound up with stimulants or dulled with alcohol. If you have a problem, face it. If you feel pain listen for its message. Escape never solves the problem. It only delays it until it becomes larger and more insistent. By the time it can't be avoided it may be too late.

This is all simple advice, but it works. We create our problems and we can de-create them. This is what my work is about. In ten years of practice I have treated a never ending stream of patients. If I ask them how they came to hear of my work the answer usually is that another patient recommended them. Why? Because the treatment works. The principles prove themselves in practice.

Psychological iridology

The iris of the eye is the only brain tissue to meet the outside world. The iris, therefore, reflects the one brain, both right and left hemispheres, and the entire life of the person, body, mind and spirit. Iridology resonates in harmony with the principles of holistic, alternative, complementary natural medicine.

While early iridology concentrated primarily in verifying physical readings, there has also been attention to the psychological correspondences from the early part of this century when Dr Lindlahr and Dr Kritzer mapped out the brain areas while they were observing and treating patients in mental homes.

It is also important to realize that they recognized variations in right and left irides and their psychological counterparts. Dr Kritzer defined the Apprehension mental zone in the right iris and the Introspection mental zone in the left iris. Dr Jensen later renamed these zones as the Inherent Mental brain zone, which I call the Anxiety zone. We see that Kritzer already had a grasp of the more interior quality of the left side. Also, the Mental Ability Brain Zone was named Will in the right iris by Lindlahr and Ideation by Kritzer. The left iris zone was named Imagination and Vision by Lindlahr and Intellect by Kritzer, who both recognized the left iris reflecting that which was not so involved in outward manifestation.

In my own research since 1980, I began observing that when nerve rings are more intense on the right iris, the issues are connected with the father and their ability to deal with the world, and on the left iris with the mother and their relationship to their inner life. Whether there are differences in nerve rings, lacunae, lymphatic tophi or psora, these correlate to the mental and emotional life as well as revealing information about the physical body.

As I was aware of the correspondences of body organs, parts, and systems in such healing methods as acupuncture and polarity therapy I began to consider the emotional issues whenever a patient manifested strong markings on organs such as heart, kidney, or liver, and later found that I had discovered the same correspondences. Lindlahr said

'That the ancients understood the connection between diseases of the liver and spleen and emotional conditions is proved by the fact that the word "melancholia" means "black gall". Obstruction of the gall duct is frequently caused by the accumulation of colloid materials in the form of black, tarry accretions in the gall bladder. This interferes with the flow of the bile through the gall duct into the intestine which in turn causes the surging back of the bile into the blood stream. The absence of bile in the intestines results in constipation. Bile in the blood stream irritates brain and nerve matter, causing depression, melancholia or hysteria. Engorgement of the spleen and of the lymph nodes results in an excess of pathogenic materials in the circulation. These benumb brain and nerve matter, causing physical and mental lassitude, melancholia, insanity, or, in acute disease, mental depression, coma and death.'

It is quite obvious to all that body and mind affect each other, and it is a small step to correlate iris readings to the appropriate corresponding mental or emotional state.

I was very pleased to hear of the Rayid Method in 1985 and to meet its creator, Denny Johnson, in 1987. Because he started from the point of view of the spiritual and psychological life as observed in the iris, without knowing about iridology, his research over ten years gives us more valuable information. He goes much further with left and right iris differences, correlating them to right and left brain psychology.

The main foundation of his work centres on his structural types, so named after patterns in nature, the jewel, flower, stream and shaker or mixed type. He presents a thorough psychology of each type, considering how each type learns, communicates what their lessons are, and what they need to achieve wholeness.

He also considers introversion/extroversion tendencies and how certain iris signs reveal these tendencies. Johnson renames the Lymphatic Rosary as the Ring of Harmony, the Hypercholesterol Ring as the Ring of Decisiveness, the Anaemia Ring as the Ring of Purpose and the Stomach Ring as the Ring of Perception. Nerve Rings are renamed Sensitivity Rings. His chart reveals correspondences of body areas and organs to mental and emotional states. For example, liver and spleen areas relate to emotional issues of anger and jealousy, the heart to issues of love and nurturing, and the kidneys to problems with creativity.

He believes that medial iris areas, those closest to the nose, display information about our relationship to our self, and lateral areas, about our relationship to others. He also considers differences in the top or bottom of the iris and the movement of ascending and descending energies.

Current Rayid research focuses on treatment recommendations for each iris type and the search for key fibres or traits in the iris that give the key to the structure.

Regenerative iridology

Now that our consciousness of constitution and structure gives us valuable information to consider heredity and its implications in childbirth and the inheritance of chronic disease patterns, we can use iridology as a guide to prevent illness by reading infant irides, and to guide treatment in preparation for conception and childbirth. Perhaps we can observe the positive changes in iris structure over generations and prove that correct living creates stronger constitutions, and that we can overcome the inherited tendencies to manifest the diseases of our ancestors.

Chapter 2

The Fabric of Life

IMAGO IRIDIS—IMAGO HOMINIS. The iris is the man. (Deck)

No knowledge is perfect unless it includes an understanding of the origin—that is, the beginning; and as all man's diseases originate in his constitution, it is necessary that his constitution should be known if we wish to know his diseases. (Paracelsus)

The understanding of our inherited constitution, the stuff from which we are made, our strengths and weaknesses, is a necessary and positive step towards enlightenment.

Once we have come to terms with our constitution and its pathways to health and disease, and once we have cleared our inherited toxins and miasms and strengthened any weak eliminative channels, we can know that we are ready to preserve and maintain health with all our body's healing powers available to help us.

Only then can we deal effectively with acute diseases, overcoming any onslaughts with our full inherent healing powers supported by natural treatments. The outstanding homeopath, Grauvogel, claims emphatically that 'acute diseases run their course in the track marked out by the bodily constitutions.'

Always, our dominant miasm, like the darkness underneath, waits for weakness, exhaustion, shock and stress to bring us to our lowest ebb, to the point of no resistance, so that it can rise up and pull us down. Whenever a patient says, 'I've never been the same since', you know that incident activated the power of the miasm, the constitutional weakness, so that destructive forces overcame constructive forces and the downhill spiral towards ill health began.

Regeneration not degeneration

The Bible states that we bear the sins of our fathers. We are another link in a long chain, and our parents have created a new being who carries the taints of the past and the hereditary patterns. We are made up of our constitutional inheritance, which we cannot escape. It is most often the cause of our death as the stress of life, old age and the results of poor living habits weaken our resistance to our miasmatic pathways.

However the work of homeopaths and now of iridologists seeks to relieve us from this helpless bondage to our constitution, helping us to rise above them, increase our tissue integrity and overcome our inherent weaknesses. Our purification and regeneration ensures that our children do not inherit our weaknesses. (It is important not to force these ideas on others who are not ready for them.)

Early iridologists recognized that a wide dark scurf rim in an infant indicated a heavy load of toxic inheritance. Usually at the end of the first cycle of seven years the child would attempt to throw off this encumbrance with childhood diseases. However, natural therapeutics can cleanse the system gradually so that childhood diseases are not necessary, and the toxic inheritance is minimized.

Constitutional readings can be taken by iris diagnosis from about six months of age. Homeopathic treatment complemented by strengthening of inherently weak organs and areas by herbal medicine and diet can effectively prepare children for strong and healthy lives.

What weakens constitutions over generations or leads us towards manifesting our constitutional weakness in a chronic disease pattern? Vaccines, drugs, inorganic minerals, alcohol, shock, trauma, extreme emotions, mental obsession, extreme anxiety, depression, stress, deprivation during poverty, famine or war, sedentary living, pollution, chemical poisoning, radiation, poor nutrition.

What strengthens constitutions over generations or leads us to overcome our constitutional weaknesses? Natural living, exercise, good nutrition, fresh air, holistic medicine, correct laws of living, homeopathy, herbal medicine, Bach flower remedies, morality, purity, simplicity, a balanced life, regular purification, attitudes of mind and spirit that enable you to accept life and its ups and downs without extreme reactions.

HISTORY OF CONSTITUTIONAL MEDICINE

Ayurvedic concepts of constitution　According to ancient Ayurveda traditions the basic constitution is determined at conception. When the sperm and the ovum unite, the constitution of the person is determined by the permutations and combinations of bodily ether, air, fire, water and earth from the parents.

Out of the ether, air, fire, water and earth elements, the three humours (*tridosha*) are manifested, being *Kapha* (water and earth), *Pitta* (fire and water) and *Vata* (air and ether). The seven types of constitutions are: vata, pitta, kapha-vata, pitta, pitta-kapha, vata-pitta, kapha, vata-kapha and vata-pitta-kapha, combinations of the main three elements of the tridosha.

The sanskrit word for constitution is *prakruti*, which means 'nature', 'creativity' or 'the first creation'. In the body the first expression of the basic five elements is the constitution.

'The basic constitution of the individual remains unaltered during the lifetime, as it is genetically determined. The combination of elements present at birth remains constant. However, the combination of elements that governs the continuous physio-pathological changes in the body alters in response to changes in the environment.'

(*Ayurveda,* Dr Vasant Lad).

They also recognize that there is a ceaseless interaction between the internal and external environments, which they call the microcosm and the macrocosm. One of their basic principles of healing is that the balance of the internal forces can be adjusted by altering diet and living habits.

The essential aim of Ayurveda is to determine the individual constitution and to treat that constitution.

The Ayurvedic physicians also pay attention to the mental constitutions, called *Gunas*, which correspond to the three humours of the physical body. These gunas are *Sattvas, Rajas* and *Tamas.*

Sattvas people express pure behaviour and consciousness and as a result their physical humours are in balance and they enjoy health as well as exalted states of compassion, love and understanding.

The Rajas people are active and creative, involved in the worldly passions of power, greed and status. They enjoy wealth and the fruits of their labours. Religious attitudes are more superficial and political.

Tamas individuals have selfish and lazy attitudes and may seek destructive or criminal ways of getting what they want. They are so egotistical that they do not consider the feelings of others.

It is clear the Ayurvedic constitutions are similar to the Greek and Islamic concepts which follow. The elements of nature are observed within and without the body and treatment is aimed at balancing any excess or deficiency. It is clear that the ultimate goal is the sattvic state of mind and a balance of the elements and humours in the physical body, and the attainment of both physical and mental health and well being.

In *Ancient Indian Medicine* P. Kutumbiah explains the significance of the examination and diagnosis, and mentions the following points:

1. normal constitution in health
2. abnormal constitution which has developed
3. predominance of an element in the constitution
4. body appearance and type (stature, build, etc.)
5. what things are suitable for the constitution
6. mental disposition
7. power of assimilation
8. power of exercise
9. age

It is clear from the above how important the constitution is in all aspects of Ayurvedic treatment.

Chinese concepts of constitution

The Chinese believe that the basic constitution comes from the parents at conception, and they call it congenital Chi, or Before Heaven Chi. This corresponds to the Genotype constitution, the basic constitution we inherit from our parents. Chi means life force. Heaven means clear, rarified, immaterial. After birth, Before Heaven Chi becomes concentrated in a place called the Dandien in the lower abdomen. Here the Before Heaven Chi combines with the After Heaven Chi, or acquired Chi, which is made up of the essence of the foods, drink and air. This corresponds to the Phenotype constitution which is the result of interaction with the environment. The kidneys are seen as 'the foundation of the native constitution' in the Nei Ching.

The mixing of the Before Heaven and After Heaven Chi creates the Yuan Chi or the fire which is the source of the 'yang' or masculine energy of the body and the Jing or the kidney essence which is the essence of the 'yin' or feminine energy of the body.

It is clear that the balancing of the two types of Chi which is fundamental to the balance of the yin and yang energies is a prime object of the Chinese medicine; whether through acupuncture, herbal medicine, exercise, diet or philosophy. These essential constitutional aspects form the foundation of constitutional health.

Greek concepts of constitution

In ancient Greek writings the humours are blood, phlegm and yellow and black bile. Hippocrates writes that each of the elements preserves in the body the power which it contributes.

> 'Each of the elements must return to its original nature when the body dies; the wet to the wet, the dry to the dry, the hot to the hot and the cold to the cold. All things have a similar generation and a similar dissolution ...'

> 'Health is seen as that state where the constituent substances are in the correct proportion to each other, both in strength and quality, and are well mixed. Pain occurs when one of the substances presents either a deficiency or an excess, or is separated in the body and not mixed with the others.'

When Hippocrates discusses treatment, he says that each of the factors of regimen (bodily habits) must be sought out and changed, having regard to the constitution of the patient, his age and appearance, the season of the year and the nature of the disease.

In Hippocrates' discourse *A Regimen for Health* he describes both the constitutionally moist person and the constitutionally dry person and their appearance and advises diets that balance these excesses.

In his discourse on *Airs, Waters, Places* he also discusses the effects of different climates on the humoral constitutions. Here it is clear he has also observed heredity and the continuation of social and family characteristics. After many fascinating descriptions of the peoples of that time he concludes that 'the constitutions and the habits of the people follow the nature of the land where they live.'

Further reading:
Hippocrates *Writings*, edited by G.E.R. Lloyd. (Penguin)

In the Islamic tradition, there are four humours (blood, phlegm, yellow bile and black bile) and blood relates to the element of fire, phlegm to the element of water, yellow bile to the element of air, black bile to the element of earth.

Islamic concepts of constitution

Nasr states:

'Each humour is related to two natures and two elements and possesses qualities which are at once the same and different from other humours. The humours form the foundation of animal activity and the body of all animals, including man, is comprised of them. In fact each person possesses a unique temperament as do the organs of his body based on the particular combination of the humours comprising his constitution.'

Nasr's comments on the tradition of Galen which was absorbed into the Islamic medicinal tradition include the following:

'The more refined the mixture of humours the greater the perfection and the more complete and perfect the possibility of receiving the soul. Moreover, in each man, health means the harmony of the humours and illness the disruption of the balance of the constitution. Of course, harmony is never perfect in any person, but relative to his own constitution. Health means the re-establishment of the balance of the humours'

But it is clear that they did not view the humours or the mixture of them as the cause of life. They are only the vehicle which makes possible the manifestation of life. The spirit descends upon this mixture of humours, as the subtle body which stands between physical body and the force of life from above. This was how they envisioned the genotype, as a pattern of elements translated into body humours.

They also were aware of the phenotype interaction between the internal climate of humours and the external environment. They keenly observed how different climates influence temperaments and caused people to be different and to suffer from different diseases.

Nasr gives the last word:

'It is for man first, and secondly for his physician, to discover the nature of his temperament, the tendencies within his constitution to move away from the state of harmony, and the means necessary through diet, medicament, exercise or other factors to re-establish the harmony which is synonymous with health.'

Further reading
Islamic Science, Nasr.

Galen's concepts of constitution

The Greek physician Galen organized the humours into temperaments which greatly influenced medical thought. He also began to integrate constitutional elemental humours with psychology.

1. Anyone who has a dominance of the earthy humour is known as a Melancholic, easily recognized by their excesses of eating.
2. Those with a dominant watery humour sleep a lot and are known as Phlegmatic type.
3. The airy dominant type, identified by mental activity and thinking, is identified as the Sanguine.
4. The Choleric firey dominant type drinks excessively.

Paracelsus' concepts of constitution

Paracelsus, a Renaissance alchemist and physician, believed that medicine was a sacred task, a priestly mediation between God and patient, both a duty and a high privilege.

He built a profound and deep philosophy which describes the principles of true medicine. He founds his theories on four main pillars:

1. Philosophy of the earth.
2. Astronomy (the microcosm in relation to the macrocosm) – the philosophy of the heavens.
3. Alchemy – explanation of the elements.
4. Virtue – that which supports the other three pillars.

According to Paracelsus, the constitution of man consists of seven modifications of one primordial essence, which are:

1. The Elementary Body. (The Physical Body)
2. The Archaeus. (Vital force)
3. The Sidereal Body. (The Astral body)
4. Mumia. (The Animal Soul)
5. The Rational Soul. (The Human Soul)
6. The Spiritual Soul.
7. The Fully Realized Man.

Five Ens Doctrine

Paracelsus created a system of five groups which organized the causes of disease. Research has not clarified the origin of the word 'ens', but it seems likely it refers to essences or principles.
The groups are:

1. *Ens Venini* – Poisons which cause disease.
2. *Ens Naturale* – Morbid conditions of the body which cause disease.
3. *Ens Astrale* – Astral or emotional causes of disease.
4. *Ens Spirituale* – Spiritual causes of disease.
5. *Ens Deale* – Diseases caused by breaking the moral laws.

In response to the above Paracelsus also organized five different ways of removing disease.

1. *Naturale* – treatment using the opposites of nature for balancing.
2. *Specificie* – the employment of specific remedies having affinities for specific morbid conditions.
3. *Characterales* – physicians who cure with their will power, by suggestion, inspiration and hypnosis.
4. *Fideles* – those who cure by faith and magic.
5. *Spirituales* – healing through someone who is in possession of the keys of mysteries of life.

He also believed that there are certain physical and personality types whose character was determined at the moment of conception. The set of dominant characteristics was inherited from the parents, a reflection of the hereditary line or character inherited (*Ens Seminales*). This hereditary constitution and not planetary influences was responsible for the expression of character.

The only interference with the operation of the *Ens Seminales* came through the imagination of the parents at the time of conception. This could lead to minor deformities but an imagination distorted by immorality would in the extreme lead to monsters. The extreme personality types included the witch, the deformed, the disabled, the thief and the murderer.

Within his framework also exists an important consideration of the four elements of man and the cosmos (earth, water, fire and air) and the three basic substances (sulphur, mercury and salt).

This is complemented by understanding of psychology, sexuality and psychic realities and how they influence disease.

'Just as a man can see himself reflected exactly in a mirror, so the physician must have exact knowledge of man and recognize him in the mirror of the four elements in which the whole microcosm reveals itself.'

According to Paracelsus there are three kinds of physicians:

1. Those born of nature and given gifts by astrological divination.
2. Those taught by men and trained in the healing arts.
3. Those given by God and directly taught by God.

Further reading
The Life of Paracelsus by Franz Hartman MD (Routledge and Kegan Paul, London)

Goethe's concepts of constitution

All organisms accord in structure to a certain quite limited number of patterns or plans, 'ideas in the mind of God'. Each human is born with his own distinct internal finalism which constitutes his innate character (or 'Daemon'), that which we are in essence. This determines his behaviour and his actions.

MIASMS

Hahnemann's concepts of miasms

Hahnemann, the German physician and founder of homeopathy, believed that chronic infection agents, or miasms, were the cause of chronic disease.

> 'Those afflicted appear in perfect health ... and the disease that was *received by infection or inheritance* seems to have disappeared. But in later years, after adverse events and conditions of life, they are sure to appear anew and develop the more rapidly and assume a more serious character in proportion as the vital force has become disturbed by debilitating passions, worry and care, but especially when disordered by inappropriate medicinal treatment.'

Hahnemann defines a chronic miasm as an infectious principle of chronic action, a chronic infection agent. Chronic diseases are seen as being caused by dynamic infection with a chronic miasm.

Hahnemann lists the avoidable noxious influences which precipitate disease inappropriately named chronic: liquor, dissipation of many kinds, prolonged abstinence from things necessary for life, residing in unhealthy localities (especially marshes), housing in cellars or other confined dwellings, deprivation of exercise and open air, overexcitation of body or mind, constant state of worry.

Because these conditions disappear spontaneously with improved conditions (provided no miasm was activated) they cannot be called chronic diseases.

Psora

Psora is imbalance or irritation which manifests as skin eruptions and disharmony of the body's natural rhythms, and emotionally as tiredness, depression, worry, timidity, anxiety and fear. It is considered the mother or source of all disease.

The skin eruptions are vesicles which are accompanied by intolerable itching and a peculiar odour. Sulphur or Psorimum are the prime homeopathic remedies for the psora state.

Syphilis

The syphilitic miasm is degenerative and destructive, and likewise those who attract this disease have natures that are easily disturbed and which contain cruel and destructive aspects. Mercury, Aurum and Syphilinum are the prime homeopathic remedies. Syphilis begins with the initial chancre sore.

Sycosis (Gonorrhea)

The sycosis miasm is an expression of excess or hyperactivity, the word itself means 'wart' or 'excrescence'. The miasm causes imbalances in digestive, respiratory, cardio-vascular and urinary systems. The nature of the sycotic state is one where an extrovert, ambitious and ostentatious nature indulging in overheated mental and emotional activity leads in extreme cases to mental illness. Thuja and Medorrhinum are the prime homeopathic remedies.

There can be no real cure of this or of other diseases without a strict particular treatment (individualization) of each case of disease.

It is also necessary to differentiate between an acute and a chronic disease where the symptoms are more difficult to ascertain because the condition has been progressing over a period of years.

Homeopathic treatment of chronic diseases commences with the smallest possible dose; however, treatment of the three great miasms while they still effloresce on the skin (as the itch, chancre or figwarts) require and tolerate from the very beginning large doses of their specific remedies of ever higher and higher degrees of potency daily or possibly several times daily.

If the figwarts have existed for some time without treatment, they have need for their perfect cure, of the external application of their specific medicines as well as their internal use at the same time.

Psora

After dividing disease into either acute or chronic disease, the homeopath Kent considers the chronic miasms – psora, syphilis and sycosis (gonorrhea). These become complicated by drug treatment so that it is difficult to treat the pure miasm.

Kent's concepts of miasms

'Psora is the beginning of all physical sickness. Had psora never been established as a miasm, the other two chronic diseases would have been impossible.'

Psora is seen as the primary disorder of the human race – a disordered state of the internal economy of the human race. When man began to will the things that were the outcome of his false thinking then he entered a state which was the perfect correspondence of his interior. The state of the human mind and the state of the human body is a state of susceptibility to disease from willing evils, from thinking that which is false, and making life a continuum of false things. Psora is an outward manifestation of deep cause of disease within man's mind and body. It is the state of mind that is prior, the psoric itch comes as a result of that.

Thus man loses his freedom and his internal order. He moves from a state of balance within the will of God, from the pure state of being, into desire and will. This precipitates original sin or original disease – which are one and the same.

Psora affects everything and causes a general breakdown.

Syphilis

Syphilis is the result of actions of the body resulting from thinking and willing evil, and of physical impure coition.

The symptoms come on strongly in robust constitutions and faintly in weak ones.

Syphilis affects the soft tissues, ulcerations and the bones.

Sycosis (Gonorrhea)
There are two kinds of gonorrhea, chronic and acute, and both are contagious. Suppression of chronic gonorrhea is very serious.

Gonorrhea affects the soft tissues (growths) and the fluids of the body.

The contagion of gonorrhea between man and woman produces many of the troubles which they suffer from in this day and age.

Infants inherit the interior nature of the disease and are extremely sensitive. 'The susceptibility is laid out by this inheritance, as it is with all three miasms.'

Further reading
Organon of Medicine, Hahnemann.
Repertory of Homeopathic Materia Medica J.T. Kent

Miasms and flower essences In the more subtle world of flower essences miasms are seen through the fresh shift of the kaleidoscope as a vibratory pattern which is stored in the etheric, emotional, mental and astral bodies. When the pattern inhabits the molecular level of the physical body, the genetic code, then it is passed on from generation to generation as a potential for disease. Miasms are seen as a crystallized pattern of karmic potential.

These patterns lie dormant, sometimes not emerging for several generations, or for most of a person's life. When the pattern emerges as karmic destiny it has penetrated all the subtle bodies and individual cells until it manifests in the physical body.

The miasm should not be seen as negative, but rather as an absence of the life force which usually arranges harmonious patterns. Not only must blockages be elminated, but positive life force must be allowed to enter so that harmonious energy patterns fill the space left by the cleansing. The void will only attract the miasm.

Miasms and esoteric healing Alice Bailey (author and metaphysical teacher) refers to karmic liabilities and miasms which are useful contributions to the understanding of constitution.

The main points to be considered are:

1. Disease is either traced to the individual etheric body or the planetary etheric body (epidemics, war, etc.)
2. We are becoming more aware of the need to increase the potency or vitality of our etheric and physical bodies.
3. The condition of the etheric body predisposes the subject to disease and protects it from disease or fails to do so.
4. The connection and interrelationship between the etheric and physical bodies comprises the new medicine.

5. The main causes of all disease are either the stimulation or lack of stimulation of any centre in any part of the body. These tendencies create the true planetary diseases: Cancer, Tuberculosis and Syphilis.

6. The etheric body focuses energy from the interior of the body which is qualified by astral or emotional aspects. These things together indicate the state of his karma. Thus physical disease becomes psychological and karmic.

7. These focusing patterns constitute the patient's karmic liabilities or his freedoms.

Seen from the viewpoint of esoteric healing the following is the result of the soul choosing the parents to match the required tendencies:

'The vital body is therefore of such a nature that the man is predisposed to a particular type of infection or of disease; the physical body is of such a nature that its line of least resistance permits the appearance and control of that which the vital body makes possible; the incarnating soul produces, in its creative work and in its vital vehicle, a particular constitution to which the chosen parents contribute a definite tendency. The man is therefore non-resistant to certain types of disease. This is determined by the Karma of the man.'

The process of healing is seen as one of either stimulating activity or withdrawing energy, or balancing energies between centres, to produce a harmonious interaction rather than one which contributes to the disease process.

Further reading
Esoteric Healing, Alice Bailey

Miasms and the vibrational pattern of disease

The psora miasm, being the primary irritation of mental processes turning towards evil, represents the first movement from the sattvic state of balance or harmonious union.

The syphilitic miasm is the degenerative tamas guna (or the Chinese yin), the hypoactivity of the system that leads to inertia, neglect, darkness and death.

The sycotic miasm is the outgoing, creative, rajas guna or yang principle which expresses itself as hyperactivity when out of balance.

We can deduce that Hahnemann's miasms reflect these polarities, the duality of activity and lack of activity, as a part of the dynamic movement of life in this world.

Eliminating the miasms brings us back to the source, towards balance and harmony. It is clear that freedom from miasms must also include mental and spiritual evolution towards purity, and freedom from desire for evil.

Grauvogel's concepts
of miasms

1. Any variation to the plus or minus of the basic elements of oxygen, hydrogen and carbon-nitrogen determines the basic differences in constitutions.
2. The symptoms manifested by the differences provide indications for remedies more accurately than if the symptoms are understood separately from their constitutions.
3. The human body is envisioned as a whole, not as made up of separate concepts.
4. Once the constitution is recognized and remedied, all the rest of the symptoms clear.
5. The constitution counts for more than the symptom. Thus symptoms arise from the constitution. The practitioner must observe the conditions under which a symptom occurs, or is worse or better.
   (a) times of recurrence and disappearance.
   (b) associated (concomitant) circumstances – when is a symptom worse or better.
6. He considered constitutional classifications in terms of the tissues themselves, not as diseases or symptoms as in Hahnemann's teachings.

Following Hahnemann's insistence on the necessity of observing concomitant circumstances, Grauvogel proceeded to a deeper level by asking the question, 'What changes take place in the organism during seasonal, climatic and daily changes?'

As the air we breathe is composed of oxygen, carbon, hydrogen and nitrogen, as is the whole organism and its blood, changes of atmospheric constituents affect the constant whole of the organism.

Phenotypic constitution by homeopathic evaluation – the symptoms reveal the individuality of the patient in relation to the world since their birth. There was no way by observation to observe genotypic constitution in his time, yet iridology now gives this opportunity.

Grauvogel claims that if the organism is not able to adapt itself to varying conditions there is something wrong with the organism.

He also believes that understanding a disease or a cure is utterly impossible unless one knows the history of its development.

He believes that acute diseases run their course in the track marked out by bodily constitutions.

As long as general conditions of a disease are not removed no thought can ever be logically entertained concerning the cure or improvement of its special form.

No form of psychotic disease can be cured without good food.

The human race is divided into two sections – the born *analysers* and the born *synthesizers* (logic and intuition, male and female). Grauvogel claims the homeopath should be born both an analyser and a synthesizer.

The constitution determines which disease is communicated. He observed that men exposed to the same venereal disease will manifest different miasmic diseases.

He based his theories on the fact that the molecule was the unit of living processes, not the cell.

The human body is made up of three quarters oxygen, and hydrogen, carbon and nitrogen account for most of the remainder. Grauvogel's constitutions are arranged according to excess or deficiency of certain elements in the tissues and in the blood.

You can see the similarity to the elements and humours, except that he takes a scientific chemistry perspective, rather than that of recognition and harmony with the elements of nature.

IRIDOLOGY, CONSTITUTION AND MIASMS

Heredity and iridology

Hereditary factors (genotype) make it possible for human beings to produce offspring like themselves. Once in the world, environmental influences (phenotype) contribute towards making people what they are. These two factors are complementary forces which represent our inner and outer worlds and their interaction.

As the science of genetics develops, the term *genotrophic condition* has been coined to mean a condition that is predisposed by heredity and precipitated by nutritional factors.

In iridology there are two approaches to constitution, the genotype, or inherited factors, and the phenotype, the acquired factors. Both determine the actual quality of the blood and lymph, which in turn determine the integrity of the organs and tissues.

The evaluation of a constitution assesses the ability of an individual to withstand diseases, and the pathways of weakness which would precipitate disease.

The genotype inheritance may be modified (within limits) by the phenotype (nutrition, climate, home and social life, etc.) Purification and regeneration accomplished through natural therapies allows the patients to rise above constitutional weaknesses. Correct living habits will then preserve health.

Heredity and iris colour

The colouring of an individual's skin, hair and eyes is collectively referred to as their complexion. All known complexion colours are produced with only a few pigments, the primary pigment being melanin. All the variations between light and dark complexions occur because of the amount, concentration and distribution of melanin throughout the body.

One's complexion is pre-determined by the genetic blueprint of the 'colour genes' and will be modified by environmental factors.

The concentration of melanin in the iris determines the iris colour. The more pigment there is, the darker the iris. Iris colours such as blue, brown and grey are due to the distribution of melanin in the iris and the way it reflects light. Green is the result of the abnormal yellow colour affecting the basic blue iris type. The grey colour is the result of extra melanin deposits in the front of the iris. Dark irides contain the heaviest concentration of pigments, and albino eyes are the result of a lack of melanin pigment. Pink colours occur because of the vascularization of the blood vessels. When an individual has one brown iris and one black iris, genetic factors are involved.

Melanin pigment is transported via the blood, lymph and body fluids. The observation of the varying levels of melanin pigments in the iris which give rise to the three basic eye colours – brown, blue and grey, also gives us an indication of the hereditary characteristics.

Blue iris constitution
The blue iris is the result of thin blood which contains a lower concentration of hereditary pigments. Generally considered a 'lymphatic-rheumatic-tubercular' constitution (Kriege) the blue iris has a predisposition to disturbances of the lymphatic and respiratory systems. The typical blue iris reaction is an overexaggerated defence mechanism.

Grey iris constitution
Another thin blood type containing a lower concentration of hereditary pigments, the grey iris centres more on 'rheumatic-catarrhal' (Kriege) predispositions to disease with septic skin disorders.

Brown iris constitution
The dark colour is the result of a higher concentration of chromatophore pigment cells and a greater thicker concentration of blood and body fluids. The predisposition here is of deficient digestion with liver and gall bladder complications. Kriege refers to this type as a 'gastric-bilious-carcinomatus' constitution.

Fibre structure
Constitutional readings also take into consideration the fibre structure. Generally the iris is graded according to how finely or coarsely woven the iris fibres are.

Theodore Kreige measures the ideal structure as an *ideal iris* which is the fine textured iris without breaks in the structure, crypts or contraction rings. The *first-grade* iris begins to have small crypts, especially around the iris wreath. The *normal* iris reveals a looser texture, a greater prominence of the iris wreath and varying distribution of pigment. The *degenerative* iris is a honeycomb network of open weaving with a distorted iris-wreath.

Dr Bernard Jensen marks his patients' constitutions on a scale from 0–10, 10 being the perfect iris of someone who has a strong constitution. Inherent in this system is the judgement of 'good' iris and 'bad' iris which may leave those listed under 5 as being deficient. Dr Christopher also taught this approach.

Dorothy Hall rescues us from constitutional judgement as she helps us see how every constitution has its strengths and weaknesses, and how the different constitutions and their psychological counterparts are invaluable for the differing needs of different times. Thus the *silk iris,* the so-called 'ideal' iris or the *number 10* iris, is suitable for a pioneer, but not for a confined sedentary worker where sympathy, compassion and flexibility are more highly valued and needed.

Theory of determination of iris markings (Deck)

After the coupling phase of fertilization, the new formation of chromosomes is comprised of dominant and recessive structural and regulatory genes which partly determine the iris structure and partly determine the regulation of metabolism.

Irreversible structural markings are formed in the iris by structural genes. These are genetically stable, and are subject to Mendel's Laws.

Iris constitutions and iris colours (Deck)

An iris constitution is a definite shade of iris colour, the basic colour which is characteristic for a particular constitutional type. This constitutional colour is never reversible because the base leaf and the cryptic leaf of the iris have a genetically stable chromosome.

There are three constitutional types – blue eyes, brown eyes and mixed eyes. Within these types are subtypes based on their predisposition to certain diseases (diathesis).

(1936) The constitution is the product of the creative principle of the soul as a unit of existence: anima + animus = corpus (female + male) = body.

(1956) The constitution is a product of somatic, psychic, manifest or latent characteristics, which are a result of endogenous factors (mostly hereditary) and which decide and regulate the ontogenetic development.

1. Diathesis
Hereditary or acquired susceptibility of the body to one or more diseases. In iridology diathesis is correlated to a physiological disease marking which is conditioned by the constitution. It is not actually the result of a structural gene but the product of a pathological regulatory gene. It is in effect another term for constitution in that it refers to the pathway of disease of a constitutional type as a disorganization of physiological processes.

2. Partial constitution
Partial constitution is genetically localized in an organ and determined by the structural genes of the iris. The organ is insufficent because of its predisposition due to genetic weakness.

3. Genotype inheritance (Deck)
Genetic hereditary disposition accounts for 80 per cent of all defect markings (lacunae, transversals, honeycombs and crypts).

4. Network of genetic influence (Kuhn)

The various metabolic pathways are connected with each other in a network of genetic influence. Each characteristic requires a chain of gene-dependent biochemical reactions, in essence a chain effect of genes.

Deck proves that degenerative diseases, especially cancer, can develop from a diathesis (constitution) via the network of genetic influence.

A pre-cancerous state becomes a cancerous state due to organ weakness disposition after toxins block defence mechanisms. The disease develops at the place of least resistance.

Time should not be wasted by treating symptoms. Through naturopathy therapists should aim for a release from constitutional weakness.

Genotype iris markings (Deck)

1. Transversals

True transversals are inborn and are seen in the infant as genetically determined markings which indicate degeneration. They cannot be broken down, but they can be activated by a focus in a segment which is in an active irritative phase. At that time they exhibit pink or red discolouration or vascularization. Their shape varies – they can look like forks, antlers or roots.

2. Lacunae

The iris tissue is connective tissue which gives information on connective tissue of the various organs and areas of the body. Wherever lacunae appear, genetic inherent weakness predisposes pathways to chronic disease.

3. Honeycombs

Weak connective tissue usually expanding out from the autonomic nerve wreath.

4. Crypts

Dark markings usually at the autonomous nerve wreath and often diamond shaped. They occur in heart, adrenal or major organ areas.

5. Defects

Small dark markings which appear innocuous, but they are often the site where breakdown occurs when constitutional factors are the cause of death.

6. Nerve rings

7. Lymphatic rosary

8. Constitutional types

9. Basic iris colour: blue, brown, mixed

With colleagues in Germany Deck observed that latent cancer will develop when a patient falls into a state of hopelessness. When the patient gives up, the constitutional factor is activated and the progress towards death is quick and inevitable.

Psychology and the constitutional factor (Deck)

All children are born with light blue irides and a gradual change via yellow to brown eyes takes place commencing one or two weeks after birth until the third month.

Constitutions during infancy (Deck)

The child obtains its definitive eye colour at the age of two to three months. The chromatophorous cells of the iris are photodynamic and photosensitive and need two to three months to complete this phase. Deck has observed that iris structural markings as specific constitutional characteristics are complete in the second and third years of life. Like the development of photographs these processes take time to complete. The structural genes take time to form during the development of the child in response to light. Deck calls this process 'phase of generalization'.

Mendel's laws are also valid for iridology. Deck has proven that whole syndromes can be determined solely from the iris by heredity. From infancy early recognition of organ weakness and hereditary syndromes can be made through iris diagnosis.

Heredity and iris constitutions

Where organ weakness or syndromes occur through generations of constitutional inheritance, the iris diagnosis guides the treatment to relieve the symptom by strengthening the organ to function normally again. Thus one works toward achieving a reversal of the constitutional factor.

It is valuable if the iridologist can determine the constitutional factor, the disposition towards disease and hereditary succession through generations. This can be achieved even years in advance of any symptoms. Thus the great value of the iris constitution and its recognition through iridology is a great contribution to preventive medicine.

After years of practice and research Deck recommends these steps towards utilizing iridology for positive eugenics.

1. At age six each child should have an iris diagnosis and an iris photograph.
2. If death of parents or grandparents has occurred from any severe chronic disease, the constitution should be evaluated for inheritance of that predisposition.
3. Regular review examinations should be given to evaluate severe constitutional weakness, especially for cancer.
4. Positive cancer types should consider whether to have children or not.

5. Research should be directed as to how harmful genes can be rendered ineffective or eliminated, especially as geneticists assume the disadvantageous genes can remain effective for up to forty generations.

Aside from the analysis of internal constitution by iridology, other constitutional systems observe the external appearance and its reaction with the environment. Therefore the other systems are based on the phenotype. The iris alone reveals the genotype constitution.

Further reading
Vol I *Principles of Iris Diagnosis* (1965): Vol II *Differentiation of Iris Markings* (1980), Josef Deck

Dr Bach and constitutional medicine

Dr Edward Bach states in his book *Heal Thyself* that 'disease in general is due to some basic error in our constitution ...'

He sees these defects as pride, cruelty, hate, self-love, ignorance, instability and greed, each being adverse to Unity. It is these defects which precipitate the physical symptoms we know as illness.

There is one primary affliction – action against the Divine Law of Love and Unity. It is clear this corresponds to the concept of Psora, that initial wrong thinking and desire which leads man away from Union with the Divine Will and its attendant harmony.

He leads us 'to discover the wrong within ourselves, work to eradicate this fault by developing the virtue which will destroy it, not by fighting wrong, but by bringing in such a flow of its opposing virtue that it will be swept from our natures.'

American iridology constitutional types

American iridology evolved out of the naturopathic tradition. It forms an indispensible part of holistic approaches to treatment, complementing the work of chiropractors, osteopaths, herbalists and nature cure physicians.

The emphasis of iridology in America is focused on cleansing procedures combined with nutritional regeneration. Pioneers such as Dr Jensen worked on understanding the chemistry of man, using organic juices, foods and supplements, while Dr John Christopher's system of purification and regeneration was based on the superior nutrients of herbal formulae which contained the full range of vitamins, minerals, enzymes and tissue salts etc., from which the body selects what it needs. Both approaches complemented purification and regeneration work with exercise, diet and reinstruction in living habits as well as supplementary treatments like enemas, reflexology, massage, cold sheet treatments, water therapy, etc.

Recently, a new approach to iridology has emerged as a part of the development of kinesiology, or muscle testing. Iridology indicates which are the most significant muscles for testing, thus saving a lot of time as it is not practical to have to test every muscle every time. Their version of the iris chart shows the position of the muscles along the ciliary edge of the pupil where it meets the sclera. The individual muscles are mapped and identified.

Many American holistic medical and dental practices often retain the services of an iridologist or recommend iris readings so that preventive medicine, constitutional factors and obstructions to function or healing may be considered as a fundamental part of treatment.

Iridology, like other natural treatments, opens the door to a more humane medicine because it enables us to consider each person as an individual. Every case of arthritis, cancer, multiple sclerosis, etc. is uniquely different both in cause and required treatment. Errors of diagnosis and treatment are minimized, and progress is more efficient because all decisions are based on the patient's own body, not on symptoms or disease indications.

Generally, the American approach to iridology is based on an evaluation of structural strength. A strong structure is considered good, and a weak one, poor. It is clear this developed out of the regard chiropractors, such as Dr Jensen, had for a strong spine and muscles which allowed free and unhindered nerve supply to all the body parts and organs. Treatment was directed to improve the integrity of tissue, both in this life and in future generations.

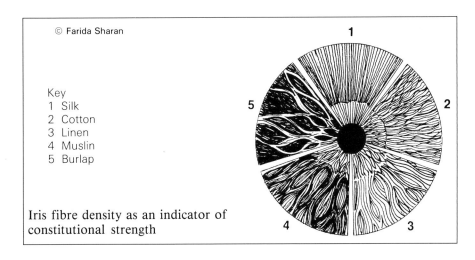

© Farida Sharan

Key
1 Silk
2 Cotton
3 Linen
4 Muslin
5 Burlap

Iris fibre density as an indicator of constitutional strength

Australian iridology constitutional types

Dorothy Hall's psychological approach to the influence of mind over body, both in disease and in iris markings, releases us from constitutional judgement. Her work reveals that each type of structure or constitutional type has both negative and positive aspects. She sees the iris as fabric, describing the finely woven constitution as silk and the loosely woven one as hessian. Both structural tissue integrity and corresponding personality types provide an approach to life as well as a potential pathway to disease. Understanding our constitutional type will provide guidelines for areas of our life which we need to develop, or reveal areas of resistance which need to be overcome.

Her approach to treatment combines herbal medicine, Bach flower remedies and radionic homeopathy (in the same bottle) so that both physical tissue and mental aggravations are treated at the same time.

She strongly emphasizes that structural weakness can result from emotional shock trauma as well as from nutritional, inherited or environmental deficiency. Her latest research shows that marks on specific areas of the iris from pterygium, surgery or accidents actually inhibit the functioning of the corresponding area in the body. This means that the iris is a two way screen. The interior life influences iris markings and iris markings influence the interior functioning of the body.

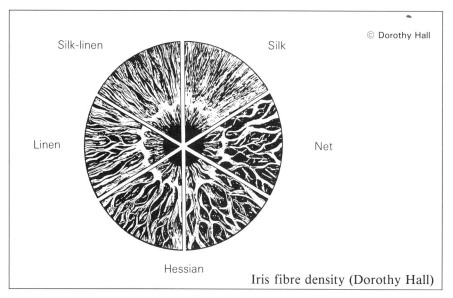

© Dorothy Hall

Silk-linen

Silk

Linen

Net

Hessian

Iris fibre density (Dorothy Hall)

Dorothy Hall's approach to miasms

Syphilis

The syphilitic iris reveals an overlay of white and a white autonomic nerve wreath. There are active, agitated, radiating patterns, corresponding to the hyperactive or highly active personality, which may also give rise to a genius level of intelligence. Usually, however there are strong tendencies to suspicion and jealousy as well as perverse tendencies.

Impatiens, White Chestnut and Sweet Chestnut are useful Bach flower remedies to aid these personalities who live at a high rate of revolution, but the main Bach remedy is Vervain. Use vervain herb as well.

A classic actual syphilitic ancestry displays heavy-lidded, constantly blinking eyes and a loose walk where the foot is slapped down from the ankle. They are often shortsighted and wear thick lenses early in life.

The high activity of intelligence also causes further eye strain combined with adrenal and nervous exhaustion. They can resort to suicide. This type can actualize (the opposite of the Gonorrhoea type) but they suffer from shock and stroke, coming to sudden ends, due to their extreme overactivity.

They are adrenal types, and are found to say things like 'I can't cope', or 'I can't get away', typical reactions bound up in frozen 'flight or fight' adrenal responses.

Syphilitic types should always carry around a bottle of Rescue Remedy to lift them out of adrenal paralysis. Shock is the most dangerous trigger to this type and must never be left untreated.

At some point of treatment the inherited chancre 'sore' may reappear. When that happens the miasm will be cleared. But it must be allowed to complete its cycle and not be suppressed. Use naturopathic, homeopathic and herbal methods to relieve discomfort.

Gonorrhoea (sycosis)

This is the most common miasm today, and lies at the root of many women's urinary and reproductive problems which are difficult to diagnose, including infertility, fluid retention, cysts, discharges and periodic discomforts. The brown Hessian iris with weak connective tissue in the pelvic organ areas is particularly prone to this miasm.

Gonorrhoea can also be the foundation miasm for some allergies, hormone imbalance and inconsistent small symptoms which change quickly. Whenever excessive mucous secretions are combined with irritable gastro-intestinal problems, consider the gonorrhoea miasm.

Rock Rose is given to balance their extreme overexaggeration. Endocrine imbalances may otherwise cause a panic reaction to new experiences. They excuse things, saying 'That's my karma' and so they don't fight or resist. These tendencies are very much a part of the new generation of allergy-prone children who react to everything.

Cerato Bach remedy is used because the gonorrhoea type is easily led astray. They never stay anywhere very long, because they want change and new experiences.

Psora

The miasmic itch is often activated after shocks, wounds or surgery. It is aggravated and surfaces at times of hormonal change such as puberty, pregnancy, lactation and menopause.

Tuberculosis

Tuberculosis miasm is recognized in the iris by dark shadow lacunae in the lung area, sharp-edged structural lacunae in the respiratory zones around 3 and 9 o'clock, lymphatic tophi pearls, which also can go up over the brain area, and segments of the autonomic nerve wreath which droop loosely (like fine threads) over the pupil. Psoric spots can also be mixed in with the tophi. Also look for marks on the thymus gland and psoric spots on the spine or gonads.

The TB miasm is a mixed miasm, part syphilis and part psora. TB types are chunky with an oval shaped head. They have limp hair (which often recedes early). Other signs are an over-developed chest and a high pink spot on the cheekbone, sensitive, sore eyes, lymph swellings which go up and down, especially at the neck and catarrhal discharges. The skin is often smooth and transparent. The fingers are long and tapered. Their energy is low. They are chronically tired people. Night sweats are often a problem.

There is a violent miasmic upsurge at puberty, especially in racially mixed types. Use homeopathic remedies and Walnut, Honeysuckle and Larch Bach flower remedies. We suffer miasms which have been carried forward from our ancestors. Lay the ancestors to rest. Purify for the benefit of the generations to come as well as for freedom from their influence during your own life.

Herpes
Dorothy Hall considers herpes as a new miasm of the venereal contact type. She suggests treatment with a tincture made of one half comfrey and one half thuja.

What triggers miasms?

When the immune system loses its strength the miasmic signature appears. What causes immunity to weaken?

1. Suppressive treatment
2. Toxic buildup from poor elimination
3. Shock
4. Stress and extreme events such as war, floods, famine, etc.
5. Exhaustion
6. Poisoning from foods, pollution and poisons.

Shock
It is important to realize that there are three main stages in the body's response to shock. If a person does not clear the first stage the damage proceeds to the next stage until the miasm is activated.

You often hear during consultation patients repeating the same phrase, 'Since this happened I've never been the same'.

The first stage after shock is *loss of coordination*. The shock sets you off balance, sets you back, sends you off course, and out of alignment. You can even lose your physical balance, fall over or faint. Mentally and emotionally there is mental confusion. This condition can last quite a while before the reaction proceeds to the next phase.

If you study the Rescue Remedy Bach flower formula it will describe all the nervous aspects of this state of mind very fully.

It is very important to get through the first reaction so that you can proceed to the second reaction and *realize the reality of the shock* and its damage so that you can accept and integrate it into your life. At this point the shock must be cleared and physical damage must be repaired so that life can go on. Use Rescue Remedy immediately as well as appropriate homeopathic remedies.

If the first and second reactions are not cleared then *the immune system becomes affected.* The person begins to have infections, acute symptoms, fatigue and just doesn't feel right. Eventually this leads to the third reaction, activation of the miasm. This is a dangerous time. Inherent weaknesses rise to the surface when the immune system is weak. Illnesses become very uncomfortable. Symptoms can no longer be denied. The patient seeks help.

The fourth reaction of *auto-intoxication* is the inevitable result of the breakdown of body functions after the miasm is activated. Not only can the immune system no longer deal with the miasmic disease symptoms, but it is not even able to deal with the daily metabolic requirements.

A person who can handle shock and can release it will never die of terminal cancer and can never produce a malignant tumour!

Dorothy Hall's 'Shock Mix' of Bach flower remedies is made up of Holly, Scleranthus for balance, Oak for standing up strong to work through it, and Crab Apple for getting rid of the experience quickly.

When the shock process is complete it doesn't leave any recording on the iris.

Allergies

Dorothy Hall believes allergies are diseases which are caused when the immune system is working too well. This is the opposite of the miasmic condition where the immune system is deficient. Therefore the allergic person is in a constant state of overprotective reactions and exudations.

British iridology – the commonwealth approach

We are in the fortunate position of being able to look at all the approaches to iridology and to learn from each one. It is important to keep an open mind and to refrain from judgement or criticism. Varying approaches are the result of cultural differences and involvement with different methods of treatment. The iridologist will only observe what comes before him. Because he has not seen something does not mean it does not exist. Thus a homeopath who has never practised purification methods and observed the iris changes which accompany the elimination of toxins may not be aware of this possibility. The Germans who concentrate with great skill on intricate reflexive fibres and lesion markings will understand things that an iridologist who works with systemic purification, regeneration and balancing may not need to be concerned with.

As iridologists we can look at the wide range of approaches with an open mind and respect the possibilities we may not necessarily incorporate in our own particular synthesis. Different cases may suit one approach or another. Practitioners can use a wide range of knowledge for the benefit of the patient.

The British School of Iridology maintains a relationship with all the major iridology centres in the world and each approach is represented in our school. Dr Jensen from America, Dorothy Hall from the Australia, Willy Hauser of West Germany are all honorary patrons of our school. They regularly attend our conferences to offer their advanced knowledge and experience for the benefit of our students. With this firm and wide international foundation students can build their knowledge and practice with the added benefit of a sympathetic communication with others working with iridology.

We have much to learn from each other. Britain is in a key position, having come only recently to the practice and study of iridology. Thus we can respect and integrate present knowledge into a universal system. Because iridology is true for all living beings, representing a truth of the body, we can use it to attain world-wide communication and understanding. The different approaches will heighten and expand our own work. Certain patients manifest iris displays which correspond more accurately to one of the European constitutions, or perhaps to one of Dorothy Hall's or Dr Jensen's constitutional types. When an iridologist has respect for and knowledge of all the approaches he has the complete language at his command.

CONSTITUTIONS – PATHWAYS OF SYSTEMIC WEAKNESS
The chart below shows how the European Constitutions relate to specific body systems. Our foundation level treatments relieve the body of its bondage to constitutional weakness, by clearing obstructions and activating normal and harmonious function of the body systems.

European Constitutions	Systemic Weaknesses
Lymphatic	Lymph System
Neurogenic	Nervous System
Hydrogenoid	Exudative Lymphatic System Reaction
Uric Acid Diathesis	Urinary System
Flower Petal	Muscular/Digestive System
Connective Tissue	Structural/Muscular System
Cholesterol Ring	Circulatory System & Liver and Heart
Biliary	Digestive System
Haematogenic	Digestive, Endocrine and Blood Making
Anxiety Tetanic	Nervous and Digestive Systems.

Disease will occur through the body systems according to the constitution.

Treatment is directed towards eliminating toxins, strengthening weaknesses and balancing harmonious function of all body systems and organs.

European constitutional types

European iridology is based on an approach which considers constitutional types and fine fibre and lesion detail which proves medical diagnosis of degenerative disease. It also gives clear understanding of the individual pathways to disease.

European iridologists consider very little about the psychological or emotional aspects of life as revealed in the iris, except perhaps what can be gleaned from the homeopathic remedy.

Although nature cure, homeopathy and sophisticated methods of herbal medicine and natural medicine are used, the patient is usually dependent on clinical treatment. Superb naturopathic and iridology clinics in West Germany have fine facilities, treatments and results. One MS patient reported that her monthly visit for treatment and medicines kept her almost normal. She was very pleased and happy with the help they were giving her, and was content to attend the clinic monthly for treatments for the rest of her life.

Treatments included ozone inhalation, Kneipp water cure, lymph massage, spinal manipulation, reflexology, blood cleansing (a sophisticated method involving cleansing of a sample of blood before returning it into the body) and removal of toxins by rolling skin puncture and blistering. After a short time blisters formed as toxins were drawn out. A wide range of herbal and homeopathic medicines also accompanied the treatment.

The naturopath Willy Hauser, founder of the Pastor Felke Institute of Iridology (West Germany), commented in his lecture at the British School of Iridology Conference in 1984 that Germans are subject to kidney disease and cerebral insufficiency of circulation due to their living habits. In Germany there are many ice cream parlours, pastry shops, and the people take on excessive amounts of rich dairy products, fats and alcohol; it is clear that there can also be a cultural 'national disease'.

CONSTITUTIONAL TYPES (Deck)

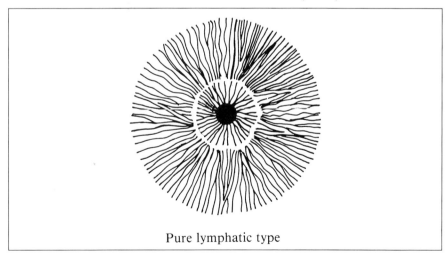

Pure lymphatic type

Constitution	Lymphatic
Type	Pure Lymphatic
Iris colour	Blue
Description	Loose wavy stroma, blue iris, grey iris.
Pathways to disease	White autonomic nerve wreath (ANW), highly

irritable lymph system, exudative reactions – acute eliminations, diseases of the mucus membranes.

Symptoms   Allergies, swollen glands, arthritis, rheumatism, eczema, sinus, coughs, dandruff, flaky dry skin, acne. Water retention, nasal congestion, stiffness, aching muscles, vaginal discharge, sneezing, eye and adenoids irritation.

Recommendations   Mucous-free diet, vigorous exercise, lymphatic herbal formula, balance acid/alkaline, sufficient fluid intake.

Eliminate   Dairy foods, mucus forming foods.

Psychology   This type corresponds most closely to the Rayid stream structural type who learn through sensitive receptivity and experience. They tune in and are 'touched' by everything, as if they were radars. This continual stimulation and reaction makes them restless. Their greatest challenge is to learn stillness and their lesson is to open the channels of giving and receiving.

Because the physical correlation is exudative release it is important for this type to learn discrimination as to what they take into their body in the way of food and drink so that discharge and irritation is minimized. Dorothy Hall refers to this type as the Linen or Average structure that is capable of tuning into others as well as the inner self. This correlates well to the stream structure where both giving and receiving is the issue.

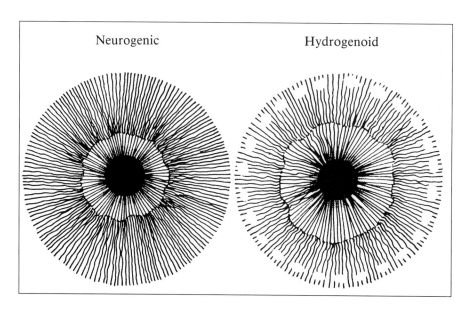

Neurogenic   Hydrogenoid

Constitution	Lymphatic
Type	Neurogenic
Iris colour	Blue
Description	Characterized by elongated fine wavy fibres, like fine silk.
Pathways to disease	Nerve weakness (central and autonomic)
Symptoms	Headaches, vascular spasms, ulcers, skin eruptions, nerve affliction (shingles, multiple sclerosis), migraine headaches, hypersensitivity, calcium deficiency, weak glands (thyroid, adrenal), arthritis.
Recommendations	Relaxation therapy, meditation, massage, nerve formula, calcium formula, adrenal & thyroid formulae, serenitea, lady's slipper before sleep, exercise. Adequate levels of fluid intake.
Eliminate	Stimulants, hyperactive overwork.
Psychology	These fine fibres correlate to Dorothy Hall's Silk type, the pioneer individuals who can push their body to the limit and achieve goals. Socially they lack natural sympathy, understanding and tolerance for others who are not like them. They achieve goals, but ultimately their overdrive results in sudden collapse. They burn themselves out and the adjustment to a life of restricted activity is very difficult. This type needs to learn stillness, to be instead of to do. Releasing energy and tension through activity and exercise is essential to their well-being on every level.

Constitution	Lymphatic
Type	Hydrogenoid (lymphatic rosary)
Iris colour	Blue grey
Description	Concentric white tophi around periphery; when yellow, orange or brown they are toxic.
Pathways to disease	Chronic lymph congestion, lymph afflictions in exudative systems, organs & body areas as indicated by the white 'tophi' markings, water retention.
Symptoms	Allergies, hayfever, rheumatism, acute exudations when tophi are in eliminative areas, swollen glands, oedema.
Recommendations	Drink adequate water, exercise, lymph, blood purifying and circulation formulae. Activate all eliminative channels and support their healthy

action (bowels, kidneys, lungs, skin). Drink fenugreek tea (6-8 cups a day). Skin brushing.

Eliminate   Dairy foods, mucus forming foods, sugar, processed flour.

Psychology   Lymphatic Rosary types hold on to toxins on all levels. They have difficulty processing negativity, releasing and letting go. Lymph should flow in unity, harmony and oneness throughout all the tissues of the body, purifying as it moves passively through the tiny valve hearts towards reunion with the blood before it flows back and through the great heart.

The psychological reflection of the physical system is best expressed by Denny Johnson's Rayid Method wherein he calls the Lymphatic Rosary the 'Ring of Harmony' and describes this type as tranquil, peaceful and loving with high ideals. However they constantly draw people to them who want favours. Because it is hard for them to say no they eventually feel used or bitter. They are always reacting to negativity in the environment. They want perfection. They dream of an ideal heaven on earth. As they respond to beauty and harmony, music, nature and art are excellent therapies. Singing restores balance. When negative, they see the faults of the world too clearly and become depressed.

Constitution   Lymphatic
Type   Uric acid diathesis
Iris colour   Blue iris, occasionally brown

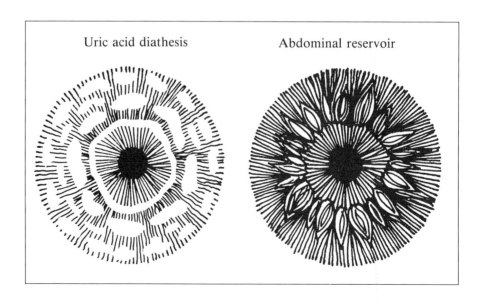

Uric acid diathesis   Abdominal reservoir

Description	Thickened autonomic nerve wreath, lymphatic rosary, whitish catarrh plates.
Pathways to disease	Uric acid retention, hyperacidity, weak kidneys.
Symptoms	Gout, gouty arthritis, rheumatism, kidney stones.
Recommendations	Kidney formula, anti-inflammatory formula, alkaline formula. Fresh vegetable juices (celery, parsley).
Eliminate	Meat, salt, inorganic minerals, dairy foods, processed flour products
Psychology	This type manifests deeper levels of lymphatic toxicity and congestion due to extreme levels of miasmic taints. On the mental and emotional levels, therefore, this person is held in the past. They are shackled to a great weight that resists release and transformation. However, once the resistance is overcome by purification and the fire of will and determination begins to burn away the dross, individuals can work towards being and knowing themselves and experiencing life without the heavy weight of inherited encumbrances. For those that do not attain transformative levels and physical release, the miasmic patterns will keep them imprisoned in limitation.

Constitution	Lymphatic or Haematogenic
Type	Abdominal reservoir (flower petal)
Iris colour	Blue or brown iris
Description	Flower-like lacunae in a regular pattern around autonomic nerve wreath.
Pathways to disease	Connective tissue weakness in the bowel areas. Gastrointestinal weakness. Bowels have an irregular shape. Glandular weakness. Weak nerve supply is caused by the irregular shaped autonomic nerve wreath.
Symptoms	Constipation, poor digestion, fertility problems.
Recommendations	Bowel, nerve, hormone, body building and thyroid formulae. Seaweeds (kelp, dulse) for mineral deficiency. High fibre diet, chew properly, digestea. Exercise.
Eliminate	Clogging foods, rich or heavy foods, and eating late at night.
Psychology	Denny Johnson captures the essence of the Flower type psychology in his Rayid Method, claiming it as one of his

three main structural types. Flower personalities are emotional and spontaneous, responding to life with feeling and visual communication. They learn most easily from auditory instructions. Changeable, social, joyful, flirtatious, they love romantic situations and enjoy creativity. When introverted or quiet, inner dreams, passions and visions fill their minds as they wait for an opportunity to release the energy.

Constitution	Lymphatic or Haematogenic
Type	Connective tissue weakness (Hessian)
Iris colour	Blue, grey, occasionally brown
Description	Very loose widened iris fibres with lacunae & honeycomb structures. Autonomic nerve wreath hard to define or it may be a net structure on the top layer.
Pathways to disease	Skeleton and muscles are inherently weak, therefore recuperative power is slow.
Symptoms	Varicose & spider veins, haemorrhoids, prolapse, hernias, vertebrae misplacement, posture problems, weak disfigured spine, injure easily, weak adrenals, poor circulation, strokes, break easily under stress, complications after operations.
Recommendations	Calcium formula, bone flesh & cartilage formula, adrenal formula, bowel tonic, circulatory formula. Drink licorice tea regularly.

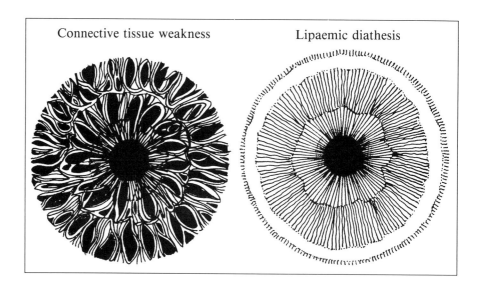

Connective tissue weakness   Lipaemic diathesis

Eliminate	Junk foods, denatured foods, processed foods. Avoid stress and exhausting activities.
Psychology	This is an exaggerated Flower type personality, combining with either the Net or the Hessian type of Dorothy Hall. Whenever the ANW casts a thick raised pattern over the iris structure the individual creates their own version of reality, keeping what is useful and straining out the rest. In this way they make excellent survivors.
	The strength of the Hessian type is social. They are sensitive, adaptable, able to communicate. They reveal their compassion, tolerance and understanding even in difficult or crowded circumstances. Because they are aware of their own weaknesses they understand the weaknesses of others.

Constitution	Lymphatic or Haematogenic
Type	Lipaemic diathesis (sodium, calcium, hypercholesterol ring)
Iris colour	Blue, brown, grey or mixed eyes
Description	White ring around part or all of the periphery (translucent to opaque) of varying thicknesses and widths.
Pathways to disease	High cholesterol buildup in the blood, high sodium or calcium buildup in the joints and tissues, liver dysfunction, cardiovascular degeneration, hypothyroidism, mineral deficiency and imbalances.
Symptoms	Poor circulation, anaemia of extremities, depression, poor memory & concentration, aches & pains, stiffness in muscles & joints, blood pressure imbalances, arthritis and rheumatism, senility.
Recommendations	Balancing mineral deficiency or excess by regular intake of seaweeds, vegetable juice, alkaline formula, circulatory and blood purifying formulae, liver, heart, thyroid formulae, garlic, lecithin, vitamin E, distilled water.
Eliminate	Fats, aspirin, fried foods, inorganic minerals, cholesterol, salt.
Psychology	Just as this physical condition hardens the arteries and slows the flow of life energy, vitality and nutrition throughout the body, the psychological correspondence is best described as inflexible, resistant, unwilling to adapt

and change, set in their ways and so on. The Rayid Method calls this the Ring of Decisiveness and describes this type as a certain, directed individual who easily takes authority. However they can be judgemental and inflexible because their attitudes are set. Unwillingness to change and impatience are the result. Interestingly enough this sign appears more in older people who may be set in their ideas and who no longer wish to adjust, adapt and change to new life impulses. They become like the pillar of salt and harden their body and mind.

Constitution	Lymphatic or Haematogenic
Type	Anxiety gastric
Iris colour	Brown, blue
Description	Radials and stress rings together.
Pathways to disease	Hyperactive neuro-muscular activity, psychosomatic ailments, gastrointestinal disorders, glandular disturbances (thyroid, adrenals, thymus), blood diseases, calcium imbalances.
Symptoms	Anxiety, thyroid deficiency, hysteria, cardiac stress, angina, muscle tension, headaches, epilepsy, tachycordia, colitis, ulcers, intestinal spasms, nervous stomach, constipation.
Recommendations	Multimineral vitamin, nerve rejuvenator, nerve vitalizer, adrenal, nerve tonic, bowel and alkaline formulae. Raw fruit, vegetables and juices.
Eliminate	Fried foods, junk and refined foods.

Psychology   Here we have energy moving powerfully in two directions. The Radii Soleris need release, yet every time they attempt release the containing nerve rings resist. In their negative expression this type wallows in unresolved conflict, wasting energy moving, stopping, and changing, unable to make a decision or resolve a problem. Exhaustion and breakdown are the inevitable result. However, the positive expression of this type is manifested when the person can express both aspects of their personality with creative joy. Development of the will together with inner wisdom and intuition will guide the person to resolve conflicts by looking at both sides and making the best choice, which may be, in some cases, both choices. They can develop very different parts of themselves and give them full expression. This type should take care never to stay in a situation where they cannot resolve a conflict.

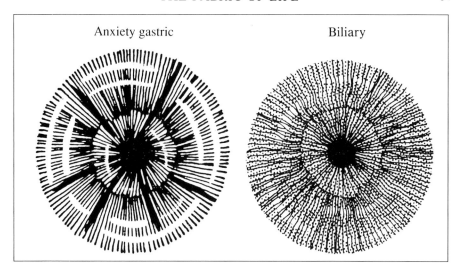

Anxiety gastric   Biliary

Constitution	Biliary mixed
Type	None
Iris colour	Brown overlaid over blue base, blue revealed when there are nerve rings.
Description	Brown markings, blue areas underneath, colour mixture.
Pathways to disease	Gastrointestinal weakness. Pancreatic & liver/gall bladder malfunctions.
Symptoms	Flatulence, constipation.
Recommendations	Vegetable juices (carrot, celery, greens) Bowel tonic, high fibre diet, low protein and low fat diet, plenty of fresh fruits and vegetables.
Eliminate	Fried foods, fats.

Psychology   Because this type contains both the blue and the brown iris colour there is often a confusion of self identification. They are drawn towards both natures and also attracted in turn to both types in relationships. Blending, uniting and combining different aspects of themselves is their work as well as frustration and confusion as to who they really are.

Constitution	Haematogenic
Type	Pure haematogenic
Iris colour	Brown to deep brown iris
Description	Radii Soleris from the pupil or the autonomic nerve wreath combined with some lacunae.
Pathways to disease	Blood making mechanisms weakness,

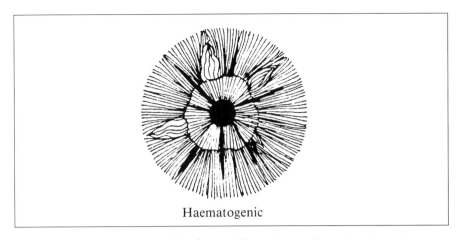

Haematogenic

endocrine malfunctions, digestive disorders, eliminative malfunctions, silent pathology, lack of catalysts (iodine, copper, arsenic, zinc, iron).

Symptoms
Anaemia, blood diseases, digestive pains, constipation, spasmodic aches and pains, auto intoxication.

Recommendations
High fibre diet, regular cleansing diets, bowel, liver/gall bladder, alkaline formula, anaemia, hormone and calcium formulae, hydrochloric acid, liquid chlorophyll. Give trace elements. Stimulate the immune system. Elimination and perspiration must be actively encouraged or silent pathology will develop. Take B12, red clover and red raspberry tea daily.

Eliminate
Processed foods, junk foods, heavy meat intake, tea, coffee, alcohol.

Psychology
Radii Soleris are toxic channels on the physical level distributing wastes instead of eliminating them. Therefore on the mental and emotional levels their presence denotes self destructive attitudes. Their mind goes around and around with obsessive thoughts and desires which they are unable to resolve and release. Once purification prepares the way for positive release of physical toxins, the person can move ahead to resolve psychological negativity. In their positive expression they can release tremendous energy, helping them to achieve goals and express creativity.

Chapter 3

The Symbolic Language of the Interior World

IRIS MAPS

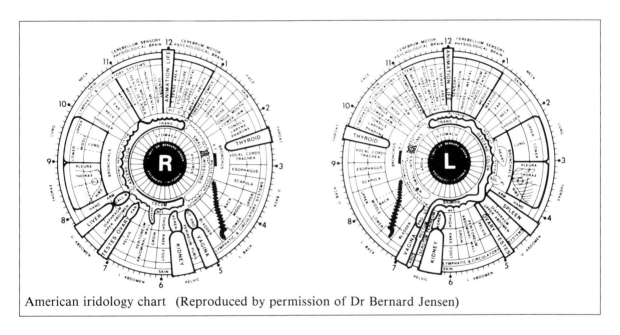

American iridology chart (Reproduced by permission of Dr Bernard Jensen)

IRIS TOPOGRAPHY

The iris mandala is divided in three ways – into radials, circles or sectors. Although there may be small variations in iris charts, the significant information is the same, and all iris charts are drawn up according to the three divisions. (See illustration, page 62.)

Divisions

Radials:
Like a clock or a compass the iris can be divided into seconds, minutes and hours, or degrees along the ciliary edge.

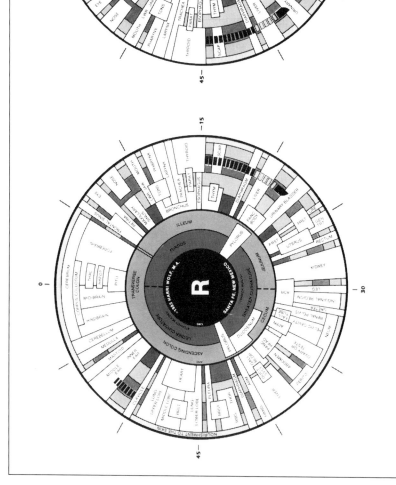

Chart of applied iridology   © Harri Wolf, MA

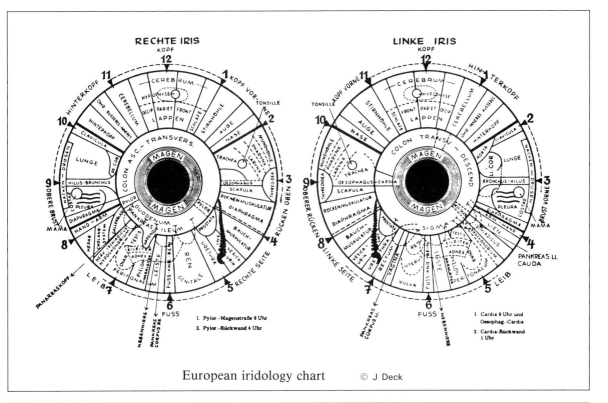

European iridology chart   © J Deck

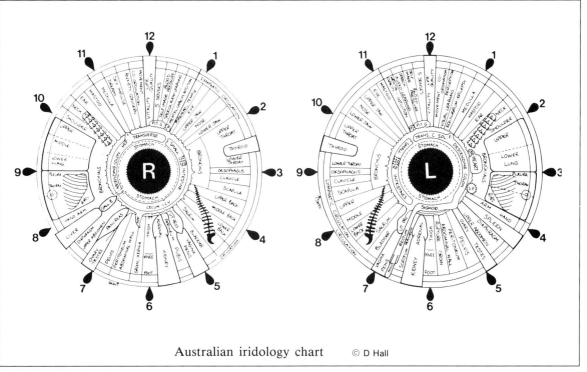

Australian iridology chart   © D Hall

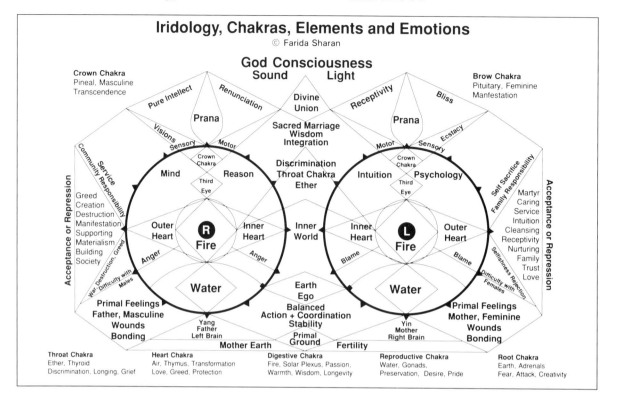

Iridology, Chakras, Elements and Emotions
© Farida Sharan

Circles:

The pupil, stomach ring, ANW, nerve rings and the edge of the iris create circular zones.

Sectors:

Wedges of the iris fan out to encompass main organ, gland or body areas. Sectoral heterochromias often appear in this shape.

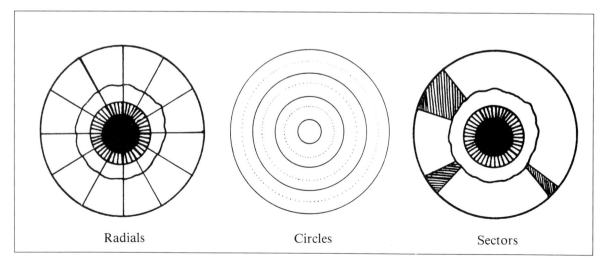

Radials   Circles   Sectors

Iris map terminology

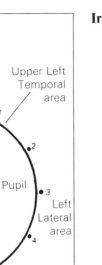

Right
Superior area

Left Superior
area

Upper Right
Temporal
area

Upper Left
Temporal
area

Upper
Nasal
area

12

12

11

1

11

1

Pupillary
Edge

10

2

10

2

Stomach
Ring

Pupil

9

3 9

3

Right
Lateral
area

8

8

Left
Lateral
area

4

4

ANW

7

5

8

7

5

(NOSE)
Medial

6

6

Lower Right
Temporal
area

Lower Left
Temporal
area

Right Inferior
area

Lower
Nasal
area

Left
Inferior area

Iris map terminology

The iris map or photo is flat compared to the living iris which when seen under 4 – 20x magnification reveals significant height and depth. Photos can be misleading because of shadows formed by the flash upon the mountains and valleys of the iris landscape.

Iris depth and height

This is why an iris examination is so important. Iris slides and prints can be misleading. When you look with a torch you can light the iris

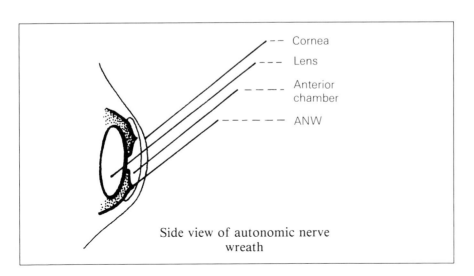

- - - Cornea

- - - Lens

- - - - Anterior
chamber

- - - - - ANW

Side view of autonomic nerve
wreath

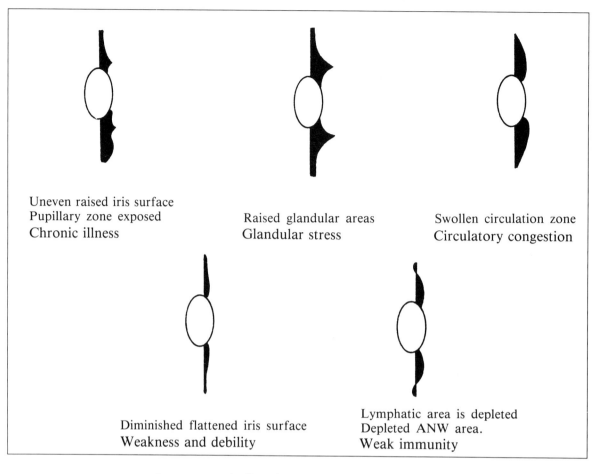

Uneven raised iris surface
Pupillary zone exposed
Chronic illness

Raised glandular areas
Glandular stress

Swollen circulation zone
Circulatory congestion

Diminished flattened iris surface
Weakness and debility

Lymphatic area is depleted
Depleted ANW area.
Weak immunity

from several directions so as to avoid confusing a shadow with a darkened area.

The main areas where shadows are created due to depth and height or where evaluation of depth and height are important are:

1. The relationship of the iris relief to the crystalline lens. Shape and height vary according to the state of health and vitality or the lack of it. Normal levels are smooth and even and disease conditions cause irregularities in height and shape.

2. As shown above the *autonomic nerve wreath* (ANW) can register various heights due to glandular stress, drugs, irritated autonomic nervous system or heart and circulatory problems. It is a significant landmark because its raised ridge circles the pupil.

3. *Nerve rings* are like mountains and valleys. The ring itself, often called a contraction furrow, creates a valley or mountain ridge. Sometimes this ridge is accompanied by a zig-zag pattern of the individual iris fibres. Once the nerve ring deepens the ridge looks like a valley. During healing the nerve rings relax as the nervous system is

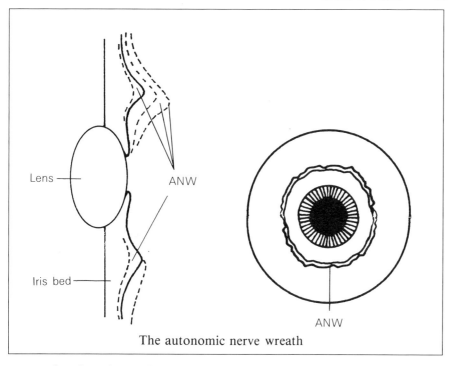

Lens

ANW

Iris bed

ANW

The autonomic nerve wreath

restored and as the pupil size returns to normal. Make sure that shadows from your light source as you observe the iris or take iris photographs do not influence the accuracy of the reading.

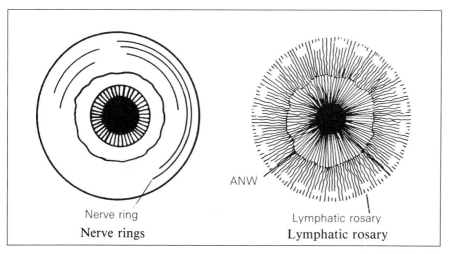

ANW

Nerve ring

Nerve rings

Lymphatic rosary

Lymphatic rosary

4. Lymphatic rosary tophi are raised above the normal iris surface like a film. Although the variation in height and depth here is minimal it needs to be recognized. It may be white or it may be shaded over with yellow, orange, brown or black, according to the level of toxicity.

5. Dark markings which appear as holes in the iris are defects, or crypts, which reveal the deepest darkest layer of the iris. These markings

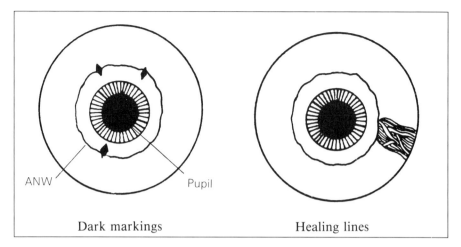

Dark markings   Healing lines

are potential breakdown areas where disease may focus as the body ages or weakens.

6. *Healing lines,* according to Dr Bernard Jensen, appear like darning threads and weave new layers of iris fibres over dark holes, showing the miracle as new tissue replaces old. Although Dr Jensen's theory has credence and many have observed the clearer appearance of these 'healing lines', other iridologists today are questioning this and applying strict research techniques to learn more about these phenomena. Changes in iris colour may account for the fact that the lines were not so visible before. Pupil size also affects the appearance of the iris. This is an exciting area of research where we will learn much more in the next few years.

7. *Pupillary margins* reveal height and depth as they move towards chronic conditions. When healthy the fibres are smooth and even, and when chronic they are ridged and jagged.

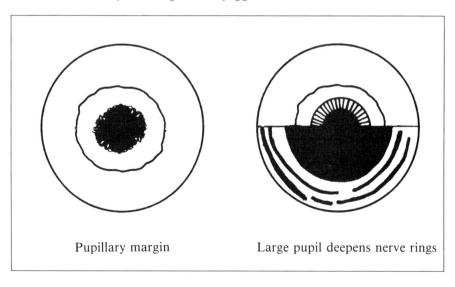

Pupillary margin   Large pupil deepens nerve rings

8.   Large pupils push back the iris, deepening nerve rings and causing more height and depth in the nerve rings.

Small pupils pull the iris fibres towards the pupil, flattening the iris and diminishing the depth of nerve rings.

9.   Radii Soleris are furrows in the iris layers which, in illness, represent destructive, degenerative conditions and attitudes. They appear like cuts, revealing darker layers of the iris. During purification and regenerative treatment they become clearer and cleaner, almost presenting an empty look. In positive manifestation this pattern indicates intense creative energy potential and movement towards expression and realization of ideas in the material world.

10.   Acute white markings are raised above normal fibre levels. Whenever inflammation accompanies iris signs, whether due to the advance of disease or healing, the white layer is superimposed over normal iris levels.

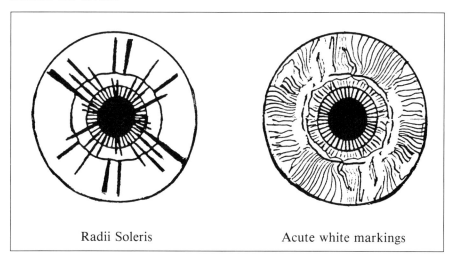

Radii Soleris   Acute white markings

11.   Reflexive fibres are swollen individual iris fibres (actually iris blood vessels) which indicate irritation. They stand out clearly from normal fibres as they are larger, rounder and rise above the normal level of iris fibres. When chronic or irritated they display a pink or red colour and often accompany pain which occurs from sciatica, neuralgia, etc.

12.   Psora are scattered pigments overlaid over a particular iris area. Although psora are above normal iris levels the height and depth factor is minimal. They often reduce, thin and become more transparent during treatment, as the granules of pigment separate, like newsprint under a magnifying glass.

13.   Sodium rings are another iris sign which are minimally raised above normal fibre levels. Like a film which covers the iris, it reduces, thins and becomes more transparent during strong purification treatment, so that you begin to see through it onto the iris.

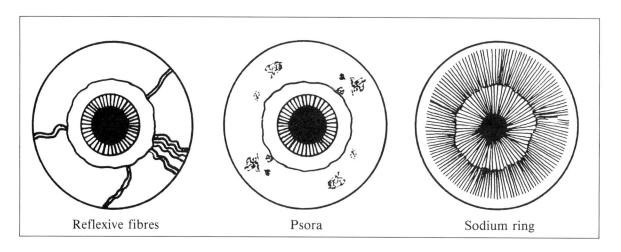

Reflexive fibres   Psora   Sodium ring

Iris colours **Basic eye colours**

There are four main iris colours - blue, grey, brown and mixed. All other iris colours are the result of a mix of abnormal iris colours over the basic iris colour. For instance, yellow over blue creates green eyes or tinges of red over blue create violet eyes. Children of racially mixed marriages have the mixed eye type which looks like a wash of brown through which you can see blue, green or yellow colours emerging. Mixed eyes also reveal these colours in the depths of their nerve rings.

Iris landmark signs

Iridology is as simple or as complex as you make it. The skill is in the selection of significant landmarks. Look at the iris as an overall pattern first. Note the main symbols and then consider important details.

Your eye is immediately drawn to landmarks. They stand out and create the basic pattern. They call out for attention. Separate the significant markings from the background.

Abnormal colours
Anaemia ring
Arcus senilis
Autonomic nerve wreath
Bowel pockets or diverticuli
Crypts
Defect signs
Diamond lacunae in organ areas
Heterochromia (central or
sectoral)
Intrafocal lesion signs
Lesions
Lymphatic rosary or single
tophi
Nerve rings

Psora
Pterygium
Pupillary margin
Pupil shape
Radials
Radii soleris (minoris and
majoris)
Reflexive signs
Sclera markings
Scurf rim
Sodium/calcium/
hypercholesterol ring
Stomach ring
Transversals

Abnormal colours

Abnormal colours are inherited, created by internal metabolism, and manifest as a result of external pollution or by ingestion of chemicals, drugs, preservatives etc. This area can be confusing if you try to determine exactly what the abnormal colour is or where it came from. The complexity of toxic pollution in today's world makes it almost impossible to separate individual metals, drugs or poisons unless case taking reveals direct exposure or intake. It is more important now to progress with eliminative and restorative treatment. Reduction of toxic exposure and intake is also essential, along with strengthening the immune system.

We are the children of parents and grandparents who ingested a higher level of drugs, minerals, dyes, coal tar products, aspirins etc. than ever before in history. Iridologists can recognize these colourations, and guide natural, non-invasive cleansing and regeneration programmes to our children. We are not only working for ourselves when we undergo these treatments, but for future generations.

What I have observed over the years is that whenever psora spots lighten (and they do), the person's behaviour and approach to life changes also. The most stubborn marks, the last to change, indicate a very deep level of the reversal process. First, the spots become diffused, like newspaper print, with spaces in between the colouring. They can also disappear, although this is more rare.

Ten years ago, one of my first patients in England had a reddish brown psora spot over her kidneys. When I first met her she had to pass water constantly, and her feet were so sensitive you could hardly touch them. As time went on, she applied the laws of natural therapeutics very deeply in her life. Herbs and dietary adjustments resulted in a complete disappearance of the mark and restored normal function to the kidneys. Her feet are now so strong she enjoys deep reflexology treatments.

However confusing these colours may appear, they do reveal invaluable information about inherited toxins, nutrition, metabolism, elimination, digestive chemistry, absorption and assimilation of nutrients and the levels of toxins and degeneration in the body.

The main groups of pigmentation are psora, degenerative tissue, heterochromia, heavy metals, poisons, minerals, lymphatic colourations, drugs, chemicals, preservatives, pollution, suppression, inflammation, metabolic pigmentation caused by enzyme activity, nutritive pigmentation caused by water and food, vaccination, liver, gall bladder, pancreas and kidney dysfunction.

The abnormal colours display their pattern over the constitutional pattern. There is no need to be overwhelmed by detail. Each iris manifests its unique combination. Select the main colours, shapes and pattern symbols to determine the individual iris print.

Each person's constitution and inherited tissue and organ weakness will also cause predisposition towards colouration. For example, a person with weak kidneys will manifest yellow colourations in response to toxins while someone else with a liver weakness will manifest brown or rust markings.

Iris colour vocabulary

		Minerals	Vitamins
White (acute)	Pain, shock trauma, inflammation excess mucus, discharges, swelling, heat, overactivity, active elimination, fever, hyper function.	Calcium	A
Yellow-white (Subacute)	Hormone, enzyme and digestive activity increases; eliminative process is more active. Symptoms are fatigue, thirst, low resistance, sensitive to stress, and difficulty in digesting fats.	Chlorine Sulphur	A D
Yellow	Kidney disturbances. Aroteroids are not broken down. The acid mechanism of the digestive system acts as an oxident and converts Vitamin B into a yellow pigment. Toxins collect. Metabolism slows down.	Iron Copper	C
Grey (Hypo-active)	Elimination slows down. Hypoactive metabolism. Symptoms are: low energy, body can't fight back, insufficiency of digestive juices and enzymes, atrophy, poor vitality.	Iron Copper	B Complex C
Browns (red-brown light-brown orange-brown) (chronic)	Abnormal function, toxic accumulation, deficient elimination, low oxygen levels. Symptoms are: exhaustion, slow recovery, weak immunity, diminished activity and creativity, tissue erosion, constipation, diarrhoea. Liver weakness would be indicated in every case.	Complete nutritional spectrum is required. Liver treatment essential.	
Black	Accidents, effects of surgery, degenerated tissue, advanced stages of chronic disease.	Complete nutritional spectrum is required. Treatment for chronic disease.	

Anaemia ring

A full or partial anaemia ring covers the sclera immediately outside the ciliary edge. It is not grey, but a distinct hazy blue. The anaemia ring can

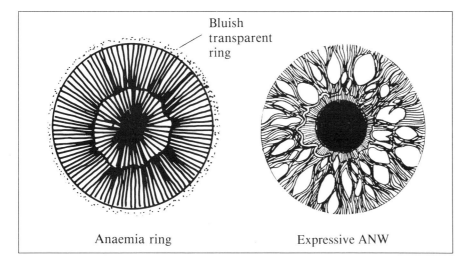

Anaemia ring   Expressive ANW

occur only at the top of the iris, at the bottom on the area near the hands denoting partial or complete anaemia of the extremities. The patient may also have anaemia and not display an anaemia ring.

Autonomic nerve wreath (ANW)

Weak ANW
The large weak connective ANW corresponds to the European Weak Connective Tissue type. Often it is difficult to determine the edges of the ANW in the tangle of fibres. It can also encompass the whole iris.

Flower Petal ANW
This Abdominal Reservoir Constitutional type is created by large lacunae where the connective tissue is weaker. It can be a part of the iris, or the whole iris. Here, the weaker connective tissue is limited to the large and small intestines where it results in poor tone and digestive weakness.

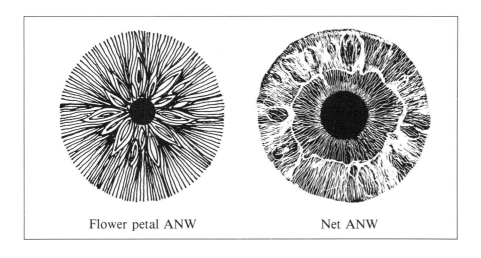

Flower petal ANW   Net ANW

Net ANW

The Net ANW rises much higher than a normal ANW and the fibres which create it are larger and rounder. It is as though the iris is creating another layer of fibres over the primary constitutional fibres. The Net types create their own reality, their own survival and adaption mechanisms, and they filter through the net what they do not wish to confront. Their strength lies in their ability to select and keep only what they choose.

Obscured ANW

White, yellow, orange or brown catarrh, or discolouration from bowel and digestive toxins can obscure the ANW. During purification treatment much of the discolouration will clear away and reveal the ANW. Usually you can pick out parts of it if you look carefully. These clouds are created by toxicity, fermentation, imbalances in digestive and absorption processes, and lymph and blood congestion. Complete cleansing of the digestive tract is indicated.

Partially squared ANW

Squaring of the wreath indicates movement towards chronic and incurable diseases.

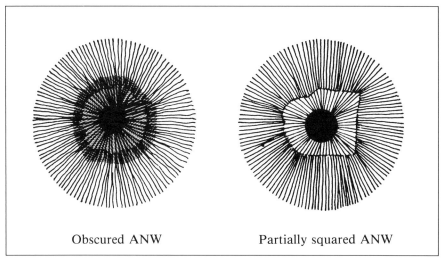

Obscured ANW   Partially squared ANW

Squared ANW

A completely squared wreath is evident in advanced chronic diseases, such as multiple sclerosis. It can manifest in one iris or both.

Stricture in the ANW

A contraction of part of the ANW towards the pupil results in inhibition in the function of the related body area or organ. For instance if it was above the heart, it would mean insufficiency of nourishment to the heart.

Breaks in the ANW

Whether caused by Radii Soleris, crypts, lacunae, weak connective tissue, stress, shock or trauma, breaks in the ANW mean diminished

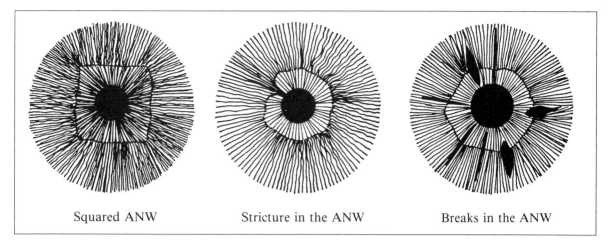

| Squared ANW | Stricture in the ANW | Breaks in the ANW |

nerve supply. They create reflex symptoms in other areas of the body, as well as affecting the function of the immediate area or organ.

Bowel pockets or diverticuli

The shape of the bowel area outlined by the ANW indicates bowel pockets and/or diverticuli when it is ballooned, distended or marked by radials, crypts, or lacunae. The pockets contain toxic faecal matter and are a breeding ground for intestinal infection. Wider systemic consequences occur because the blood and lymph absorb the toxins and distribute them throughout the body. Bowel pockets can occur in crypt or defect areas as well as lacunae and furrows.

Symptoms: Constipation, diarrhoea, fever, pain, flatulence, distended abdomen, gastrointestinal illnesses, malabsorption of nutrient, degeneration of tissues and reflex symptoms in other areas of the body due to toxins being carried by blood and lymph.

Recommended treatment: Bowel Tonic A or B, Intestinal Infection Formula, Castor Oil Pack, Enemas, Colonics. Drink sufficient liquid.

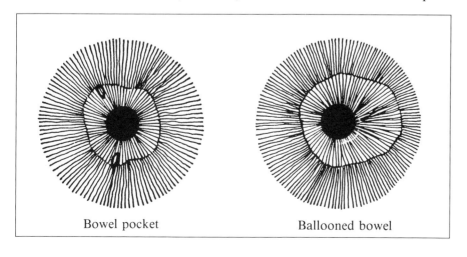

| Bowel pocket | Ballooned bowel |

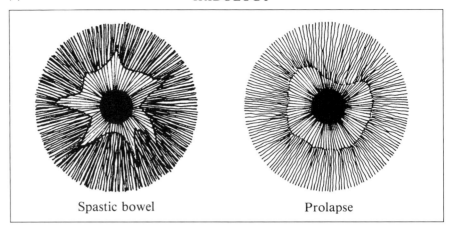

Spastic bowel　　　　　　　　Prolapse

Avoid eating late at night, mucus forming foods, not answering nature's call to relieve the bowels, processed food and purgatives.

Ballooned bowel

Whenever constipation causes enlargement of the bowel, the ANW balloons out. The more toxic this area is, the darker it is. During bowel cleansing treatment the colour lightens. It is important to improve the bowel by increasing nutrients while it is being cleansed of impacted faecal matter.

Spastic bowel

This irregular ANW of almost star-like points and strictures indicates a highly reactive ANW which plays a major role in creating pathways to disease. Instability and changeability are also aspects of this iris pattern. Treatment would be directed towards nourishing and strengthening the nervous system.

It would be important to take a careful reading of the adrenals and to strengthen these important glands as well.

Prolapse

The transverse colon is shown on both irides, across the top of the digestive area. When prolapse occurs the ANW wreath falls below the normal curve. Often the opposite inferior iris area can be pushed out and down as it records the pressure and adaption caused by the prolapse.

Crypts

Crypts are constitutional weaknesses which occur along the ANW at major organ and gland sites. They manifest as disease potential or at any stage from acute to chronic illness. When degenerative they appear as black holes. This shape should always be considered as a serious indication for primary treatment.

Stress, shock, operations, accidents and extreme emotions, particularly of hopelessness or despair, can activate the potential of crypts, and progression towards disease and death can then be quite swift.

Crypts are a magnified version of defect markings. They pierce both

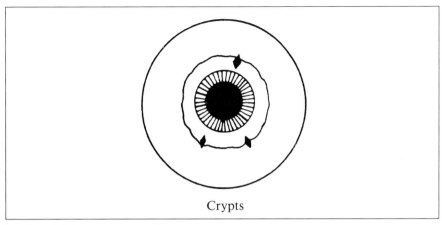

Crypts

levels of iris stroma and usually appear in the ANW area. They are rhomboid and usually small in size. They should not be confused with larger diamond-shape lacunae. The extent of the substance defect is determined by the deepness and darkness within the crypt. During acute irritation the crypt is surrounded by bright fibres, or when more advanced towards chronic conditions, by red vascularized reflexive fibres. Crypts occur along the ANW, either in the stomach zone or the digestive areas. Disease develops as an ulcerative process with a tendency towards perforation. In the pancreas they indicate cysts leading to necrosis. Complete crypts are black holes indicating full loss of tissue which would be surrounded by scar tissue. Incomplete crypts have one or more radial fibres left inside the crypt and the borders of the crypt are thick and bright.

Other iridologists consider these markings to indicate diverticuli, and bowel pockets. Certainly the connective tissue weakness could cause bowel pockets in these areas; however, the markings remain even after intensive colon cleansing, showing that the iris markings indicate a tissue weakness and the manifestation of the condition depends on the life of the patient at any particular time.

Symptoms: ulcers, bowel problems, potential for carcinoma.

Recommended treatment: Treat early in life to prevent the manifestation of this marking (from infancy to 2 years of age especially). Later in life treat the complete digestive system and apply chronic therapeutics whenever advanced symptoms occur. Defect sites can be the weak link that causes death in chronic illness, as proved by Deck in *Differentiation of Iris Markings.* However we must not live in fear of these weaknesses. Our physical death needs a pathway. The body has to break down and the cause of actual death has to occur in some weak part of the body. An understanding of our weaknesses and consciousness, acceptance and compensation will give us quality of life and death. Much can be done to help us rise above these weaknesses and minimize their effects.

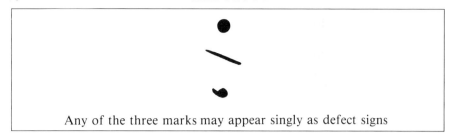

Any of the three marks may appear singly as defect signs

Defect signs

Genetic markings which often appear along an iris fibre are referred to as inherent defects. They are usually very black because the degeneration has reached the lower iris stroma. Although small, their effect can be great if it manifests during times of stress, shock or mental hopelessness.

Symptoms: depend on the site and which organ or area is affected. Defect signs can also accompany cysts and precancerous areas.

Recommended treatment: Full activation of the eliminative system combined with constitutional treatment will diminish their potential. Constitutional treatment during infancy may arrest their development in the iris. When activated only full chronic therapeutics will compensate for their influence. The mental, emotional state is significant and must be considered and included in the treatment.

Heterochromia

Heterochromia (central or sectoral) is a sector or zone of the iris displaying an abnormal or different colour to that of the basic iris. This is the result of the breakdown of normal body functions and constitutional predisposition. It can be inherited or acquired.

Darkness in the centre of the iris as in central heterochromia indicates a concentration or holding towards the centre. Physically this may mean constipation or toxins, and on the mental and emotional levels, the inability to release or to let go. The Rayid method correlates this iris pattern to introversion tendencies.

Collarette heterochromia

The ANW and the absorption zone directly outside the bowel walls can be a completely different colour. Yellow, orange, rust brown, or brown will signify specific organ insufficiency. Purification diets and bowel cleansing will help to eliminate much of the cause of the toxic colour, when combined with treatment of the organs involved (yellow for kidney, orange for pancreas, bright orange for gall bladder, and browns and rusts for the liver). As treatment progresses the area becomes clearer and the murky, cloudy and abnormal colours become less intense.

A yellow ANW suggests fermentive bowels, urinary infections, catarrhal exudations and connective tissue weakness. A yellow spillover from inside the bowel is caused by sulphur imbalance. When it is orange-brown it is caused by pancreas insufficiency.

A grey-yellow colour around the ANW indicates bacterial infection (staph).

Dark lymph tophi around the ANW obscures pelvic abcesses, appendicitis and other degenerative conditions.

A white mucoid ring around the ANW reveals a high level of mucus and catarrh affecting the circulation and absorption zones.

A dark brown colour around the ANW is caused by liver insufficiency and accumulated toxins. This indicates sluggish, insufficient function, and poor absorption and distribution of nutrient. A blue iris can have a dark brown digestive central heterochromia.

If dark brown radiates out over the liver gall bladder sector, the person would suffer from a weak liver and react to fried foods and fats with pain, nausea and vomiting. There are many possibilities for interpretation according to the iris areas involved.

Symptoms: Insufficiency. Weakness. Aggravations. Diminished functions and vitality of the area.

Recommended treatment: Lymph and blood purifiers, bowel tonic, liver/gall bladder formula, cleansing diets and juice fasts. Activate all eliminative channels. Counselling. Avoid: inorganic minerals, drugs, environmental pollution.

Central heterochromia
This manifestation of abnormal colouration covers the entire digestive zone, pupillary margin or ruff, stomach, bowels and the ANW in a different colour from the true iris colour. The central heterochromia is usually yellow, orange, rust or different shades of brown. In a brown iris, it will manifest as a darker, or blacker shade of brown. This is a hereditary and constitutional marking.

Sectoral heterochromia
Extending from the ANW outward, this heterochromia roughly covers a gland, organ or body segment, influencing or inhibiting basic functions in that area.

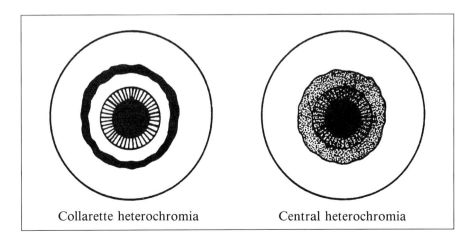

Collarette heterochromia   Central heterochromia

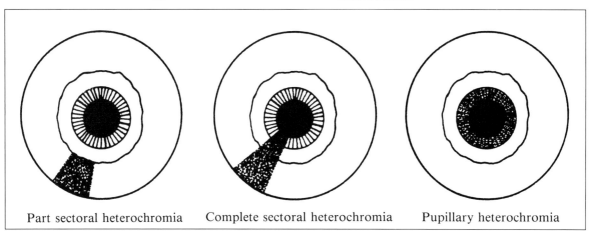

Part sectoral heterochromia   Complete sectoral heterochromia   Pupillary heterochromia

Complete sectoral heterochromia

This pattern extends all the away from the pupillary margin to the ciliary edge of the iris, covering a complete, organ, gland or body area. The effect will be to diminish normal function and increase susceptibility to aggravations and the progression of chronic conditions. It will also influence the psychological life according to the appropriate correspondences of the organ or body area that it covers.

Pupillary or stomach heterochromia

When the central heterochromia is incomplete it may only extend from the pupillary margin to the stomach ring in yellow orange, rust or brown colours. Digestive functions would be impaired by this influence. Note the colour and relate to the appropriate organs.

Heterochromia colours

Yellow central heterochromia is caused by sulphur. Check the iris for kidney and adrenal problems.

Orange-brown central heterochromia is caused by the liver and pancreas.

Orange mucoid heterochromia a thick orange mucus around the bowel is a result of poor liver and bowel function. A very bright orange is more specifically related to gall bladder dysfunction.

Honeycombs

These are differentiated from lacunae by the fact that they are formed by thickened conglomerations of several strands of iris fibres. They indicate organ weakness with deficient metabolism. Both nutrition and elimination are insufficient. They most often occur in lungs or digestive areas. The fibres are similar to the raised net ANW fibres except that they extend outward into the iris.

Symptoms: Insufficiency of absorption and elimination in the area. Symptoms vary according to the acute to chronic progression of disease.

Recommended treatment: This depends on the area affected. Increase circulation, oxygenation and metabolism. Body building, anaemia and circulation formulae are useful.

Honeycomb structure
Thickened fibres form a structural honeycomb. When they are augmented by bright white fibres, psora, nerve rings or radii soleris their insufficiency is even more chronic. This represents functional metabolic problems.

Intrafocal lacunae signs
There are various signs that appear inside a lacuna:

Calcium luteum lines or healing lines
According to Dr Jensen, these are healing lines where the iris fibres are being knitted together like weaving or darning. They occur as the disease moves towards the acute healing stage. You can observe the miracle of new tissue replacing the old. Acute symptoms can appear at this time and it is essential to support with natural treatment, not resort to suppressive drugs.

Many iridologists are questioning this theory as we have more time and better equipment to observe the iris during natural healing treatment. Better iris photography combined with 20X magnifiers helps iridologists to see more clearly what the iris is manifesting. As always, the iris will teach us the truth of the human body as we have the consciousness and the sensitive equipment to record what the irides present to us though the continuum of life. New theories suggest that the fibres were always there, but have been revealed as the colour lightens.

Neuron lattice structure
This sign is a neuron net which indicates nervous disorders due to nutritional imbalances and acidity. These are angular net-like structures, a neuronic network (Schnabel) which indicates nerve depletion and possible neurosis. It is of course most significant which area of the iris manifests this sign.

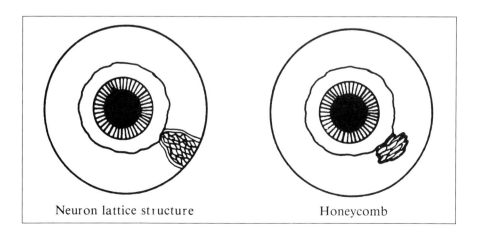

Neuron lattice structure   Honeycomb

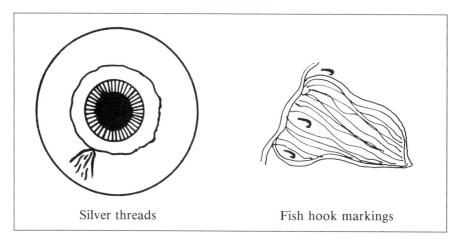

Silver threads   Fish hook markings

Reflexive fibres
Bright white iris stroma reflexive fibres indicate a tendency to spasms and irritations. These actually originate inside the lacunae, and may be fully contained inside or extend outwards into the iris.

Silver threads
These fine, bright threads run in the same direction as iris fibres but they are not reflexive fibres. They indicate a tendency to spastic etiology.

Fish hook markings
These will augment any structural weakness. They usually appear in the stomach or digestive zone.

Lacunae
Lacunae indicate an area where the normal structural strength has broken down. Here the body's strength is not sufficient to maintain normal levels of blood and lymph flow. Therefore, both nutritional flow to the area and eliminative flow out of the area are deficient. Toxins collect easily and weaken the area.

Lacunae can be inherited or caused by extreme stress, overwork or prolonged incorrect living habits. It is possible to cleanse and strengthen these areas so that one can live above one's weaknesses. However, whenever tiredness, stress or improper nutrition occur these weak areas will be the first to signal discomfort or malfunction.

The four stages of disease manifest in these weak areas and their abnormal colours range from acute white, subacute grey, yellowish brown to chronic darker brown or degenerative black. The more chronic the condition, the darker the colour.

As the weak area progresses towards the disease the iris fibres disintegrate and fall away, creating a hole in the eye. According to Dr Jensen, as it progresses towards health, the iris fibres rebuild and weave new fibres called *calcium luteum lines* which build up and eventually fill in the space. The healing crisis occurs when positive regenerative force dominates destructive force. Toxins are eliminated so that the healing can be accomplished. This theory of the healing lines is being questioned

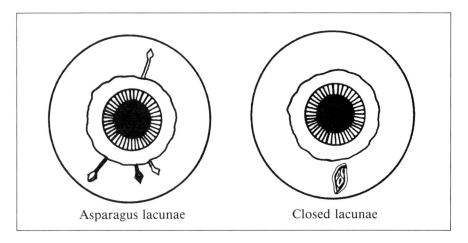

Asparagus lacunae   Closed lacunae

by researchers; as more sophisticated measuring techniques are developed we will have clearer, more scientific proof of whether and how this phenomenon occurs.

Lacunae begin to appear in irides in the silk linen type and proliferate in the hessian and net type (Hall). The types liable to excessive lacunae are the flower petal, chrysanthemum, polyglandular, combined lesion, abdominal reservoir, pancreas triad and cardio-renal syndrome types (Deck).

Lacunae are genetic structural markings which reveal the quality of the connective tissue. Usually found in significant body areas, organs and glands, the potential for organ insufficiency manifests as old age progresses or during stress, fatigue or acute conditions. The degree of toxicity in the body determines to a large extent how further deterioration of the lacunae progresses. The lacunae are formed of raised iris stroma.

Asparagus lacuna When found in reproductive glands it most often appears in the prostate or ovary areas. In the brain area it denotes obsessions. It is considered a precancerous sign.

Closed lacunae indicate severe disturbances of function because they represent the inability of lymph and circulation to distribute nutrition or to eliminate toxins within the area.

Diamond lacunae represent chronic conditions and carry the same weight as crypts in that they appear at major sites, such as heart, adrenal, gall bladder or pancreas. When they are degenerative they are quite black, but when they exist as potential they are close to the iris surface and similar to the normal iris colour. This shape represents a completed disease process whether it is inherited or not.

Divided lacunae
These lacunae extend outwards in segments showing the weak connective tissue.

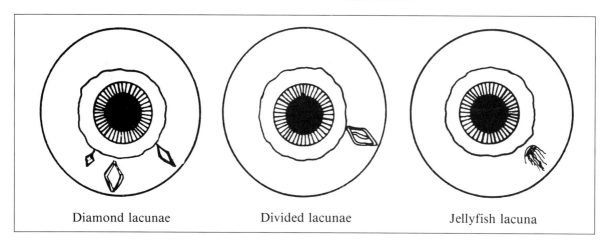

| Diamond lacunae | Divided lacunae | Jellyfish lacuna |

Jellyfish lacunae
When an open lacuna contains raised reflexive fibres it resembles a jellyfish. This lacuna indicates irritation and acute sensitive conditions.

Leaf lacunae
Interior veining causes a progression of the divided lacunae, a further development of weakness and insufficiency. This lacuna is most commonly found in the chest areas in the lung or heart zones in the iris.

Lance lacunae
This lacuna is considered to indicate the first sign of the degenerative process which results in an asparagus lacuna. Once the toxic deposit is collected at the end of the lance, it develops into the asparagus lacuna, which is more serious precancerous sign.

Liver stakes
These appear in the liver zone as an indication of inherited weakness. The base of the triangle is on the outside of the iris and its peak points towards the pupil. It is most often a dark colour.

Medussa
The kidney and lung iris zones are usually the sites of medussa lacunae. These wide, thick fibres represent a high potential for sudden failure of the organ. This sign is often accompanied by bright, white perifocal fibres which indicate irritation. Observe carefully any other iris organs or zones that the medussa covers.

Open lacunae
Open lacunae are the iris sites for active, acute disease processes which may progress towards degenerative conditions. However, they are easier to treat because they are open, and the lymphatic and circulatory fluids have access to the area both for bringing nourishment and releasing toxins.

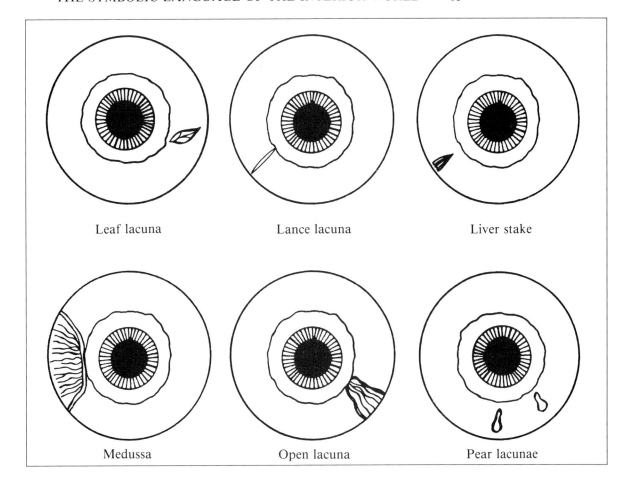

Leaf lacuna   Lance lacuna   Liver stake

Medussa   Open lacuna   Pear lacunae

Pear lacunae

This lacuna indicates another preliminary sign of progression towards the asparagus lacunae. Consider this sign as precancerous and treat accordingly. Work towards increasing circulation and nutrient into the area and eliminate toxins.

Shingle lacunae

The German school of iris diagnosis considers this sign a strong weakness. However, a healthy life style, elimination, and positive mental and emotional expression enables one to minimize the effects of these signs. In advanced cases it is difficult to turn the tide of degenerative processes, but if a patient immerses themself in purification and regenerative treatment with a strong will to attain health, much improvement can be accomplished.

Step lacunae

Another weakness considered to suggest predisposition to cancer. This is not a fatalistic reading but a genetic tendency. Conscious awareness can lead a patient from the position of a victim towards victory as they

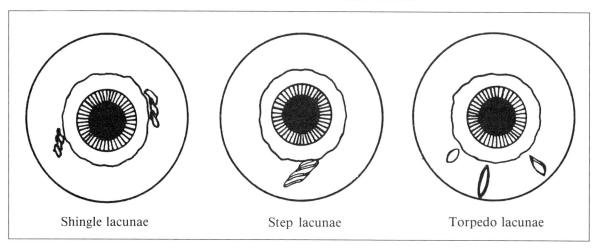

| Shingle lacunae | Step lacunae | Torpedo lacunae |

overcome weaknesses, and avoid degenerative potential.

Torpedo lacunae

The size, colour and depth of torpedo lacunae reveal information about hereditary weakness and predisposition towards tumours. Larger than a pear lacuna this sign is also considered precancerous.

Symptoms: depend on the area of the body, the influences of constitution, the condition of the tissue around the area, the other signs influencing it and the level of toxicity or inflammation. General weakness and insufficiency accompany any degeneration of this site. Mental attitudes and emotional states also influence symptoms.

Recommended treatment: Cleanse the area by stimulation of blood and lymph flow so that accumulated toxins are eliminated. Concentrate on the gastro-intestinal tract and make sure that all sources of infection and toxicity are removed, including bowel pockets and diverticuli. Relieve nerve stress and rebuild tissue with appropriate nutrition and herbal foods. Cleanse, balance and rebuild the whole body so that any stress or

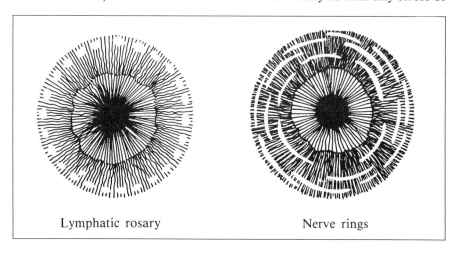

| Lymphatic rosary | Nerve rings |

malfunction affecting this area will be eliminated.

Lymphatic rosary or individual tophi

A lymphatic rosary is a string of wisps or 'tophi' (like clouds or beads) in the lymph zone. Although they are usually white they can become yellow to brown if the toxins in the body increase to high levels. Tophi can also appear individually or in group body areas or organs to augment other metabolic stress or toxic disease manifestations.

Symptoms: Swollen glands, exudations, catarrh, allergies. (See the section on the Lymphatic Constitutions in Chapter 2).

Recommended treatment: Lymphatic formulae, allergy formula, circulation formula, alkaline formula. Drink at least six glasses of liquid daily. Exercise. Activate all eliminative channels to reduce the burden on the lymphatic system. Avoid: all dairy products and the other mucus forming foods.

Nerve rings (or sensitivity rings)

Nerve rings are contractions in iris tissue indicating nerve stress and muscular tension. Where they stop and start is significant as they point to sources of irritation. They can be light colours if they are in the hyperactive stage or if they are on a mixed eye where the nerve rings reveal the underlying blue colour, and darker if they reflect a toxic hypoactivity. The number of rings can indicate the level of stress, especially if the nerve rings are in the hyperactive stage, as four acute stage nerve rings could accompany nervous breakdown levels of stress.

Nerve rings can also be different in colour, height and depth. The type and number of nerve rings can be different in left and right irides. This reflects the influence of the right and left or masculine and feminine aspects in our life. They can also occur only on one side of an iris, reflecting the interior of the body when medial and the exterior of the body when lateral. The Rayid Method contributes excellent research on right and left brain dynamics, as related to right and left iris markings. Refer to the Nervous System, Chapter 5.

Energy held in the body creates nerve rings. Conscious realization of the source of tension together with release on physical, mental and emotional levels will relieve the situation.

Certain constitutional types are based on strong nerve ring pathways. Whatever the symptoms, these types require treatment of the nervous system in order to overcome illness.

Pupil size plays an important part in the number and depth of nerve rings. Large pupils produce deeper nerve rings and small pupils straighten out the iris fibres and reduce nerve rings. Consider the reading of nerve rings in relation to the pupil size.

Symptoms: Running on nerves, exhaustion, nervous breakdown, pain, anxiety, stress, tension, muscular spasms and contractions, effects of toxins, injuries, irritations, etc. spreading out and influencing tissues.

Recommended treatment: aromatherapy baths, Bach flower remedies, counselling. Reduce overwork, worry, stress. Avoid stimulants. Take massage and exercise. Herbal formulae: nerve tonic, adrenal, nerve vitalizer, nerve rejuvenator. Drink serenitea herbal tea.

Perifocal markings around lacunae

A variety of perifocal markings appear around lacunae, honeycombs and crypts. Their presence warns of added complications and insufficiency, and degeneration.

1. Pigmentation augments structural weakness. Peppercorn pigments indicate malignancy. Their presence increases concern to accomplish relief through eliminative and regenerative treatment.

2. Bright reflexive markings, whether transverse or radial, indicate adhesions, a further complication to the focus.

3. Defects are tiny black genetic marks which appear adjacent to or near major structural markings. They indicate predisposition to cancer. They most often occur in the stomach and digestive area.

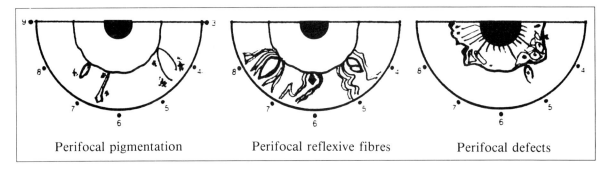

Perifocal pigmentation   Perifocal reflexive fibres   Perifocal defects

Pigmentation, psora, drug spots Psora or drug spots are irregular markings of pigment (often granulated) which indicate the accumulation of chemicals or by-products of faulty metabolism. These markings when inherited are considered miasms or inherited taints from ancestral disease. We are still learning about these markings as their interpretation and effect can vary greatly from person to person. They are almost haphazardly scattered on various parts of the iris. If they have settled on an organ this indicates weakness, insufficiency and an inhibition of function. Psychological traits may stem from these marks. Hahnemann, the founder and father of homeopathy, used the Greek work 'psora' meaning 'itch', or skin diseases marked by severe itching. Lindlahr describes the psora theory as having its origin by 'age-long persistent suppression of itchy, parastic skin eruptions and of gonorrheal and syphilitic diseases which have encumbered 'civilized' humanity with three well-defined hereditary taints or miasms.' These were named by Hahnemann as psora (or itch), gonorrhea (or sycosis) and syphilis. Lindlahr further claimed that the greater part of chronic diseases had their origin in these hereditary miasms and that many acute diseases are

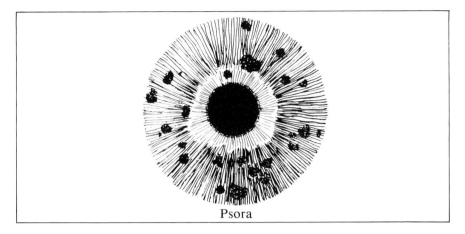

Psora

merely external manifestations of these internal latent, chronic taints.

The iris signs which indicate these hereditary miasms are:

1. Psora spots.
2. Darkening of the iris colour.
3. Darkening and thickening of the scurf rim.

Lindlahr believed that the darkness and width of the scurf rim in a child is an indication of the level of the psoric taints they have inherited. Childhood diseases are an attempt to throw off these inherited miasmic taints. Unfortunately, suppressive treatment drives these conditions deeper and lays the foundation of chronic disease. The use of correct diet as well as working with the body's eliminative functions from an early age would ensure good health and prevention of further and deeper taints. The psora spots, not usually seen in the new-born, appear later in life.

Early iridologists thought they could observe first the spots appear in the iris after suppressive treatment, and then more serious illnesses appear at a later date. As symptoms recurring after cleansing treatment brought about the disappearance of the spots, they recognized the long-term harmful influence of inorganic drugs and medicines. They also observed and catalogued the markings and effect of commonly used substances such as coal tar products, mercury, sulphur, quinine, iodine etc.

Dr Kritzer's work on zymoid spots is invaluable. The medical meaning of zymoid is 'any poison derived from a decaying tissue'. In the iris these deposits show as black or muddy brown spots on the superficial layer on the surface of the iris, often looking like a speck of dirt or dust. They may be congenital, hereditary or acquired. They may be found anywhere in the iris, as they occur in any part or area of lowered vitality. He maintains these spots occur wherever there are 'depositions of toxins resulting from putrid tissues such as boils, carbuncles, fistulae, abcesses, cysts, necrosis – all forms of dead tissue, also vaccines and serums'. It is also the case that 'Zymoid spots may often indicate effects of suppressed measles, scarlet fever, smallpox, various skin diseases and often suppression of pediculosis (lice infestation)'. Dr Kritzer feels that the terms 'itch' spots or 'psora' spots are misleading. After informing us that Peczeley was the first to discover and interpret these spots as suppressed scabies, he tells how he discovered that they also indicate other suppressed external conditions and local hereditary encumbrances. Further, he claims that these conditions lead to the development of malignancy and cancer. Zymoid deposits are eliminated through boils and carbuncles.

Dr Kritzer also defines vaccination spots as black or muddy brown, similar to zymoid, and often surrounded by white circles. He then makes the point that 'immunity against disease must come from within, from a revitalized organism in which the individual cells are strong enough to resist and expel all foreign substances and to resist invasion of pathogenic bacteria'. Instead of eliminating toxic material which is the breeding ground for disease, vaccinations and serums add to the load of foreign substances already weakening and irritating the system.

Dr Jensen differentiates between the inherited 'psora' spots and acquired drug spots in the following way. He believes that the psora spots are on the surface of the iris stroma and drug spots are in the stroma itself. The psora spots are confirmed by iris analysis of parents and child, showing that they were inherited. Modern research has not indicated that there is any relationship between drug intake and the appearance of psora spots on the iris, except in a few isolated cases.

Although some modern iridologists seem to want to dispense with the theory of drug accumulation and put it all down to enzyme deposits and organ cell damage, the fact is that early iridologists were able to see irides change colour dramatically after the intake of certain drugs. In the 19th century Liljequist saw his own irides turn green from quinine and develop red spots after the intake of iron. They are the results of inorganic substances settling in tissues and abnormal chemical and enzyme processes.

Another point to consider is that the drug, mineral, chemical or poison is affecting the whole system. While it may show up more strongly in one part of the eye or another, it is also collecting in the other weak parts of the body and influencing all body functions.

Both inherent weaknesses and the effects of toxic drug and chemical deposits are passed on to the next generation. This is significant in that this combined weakness makes it impossible for that part of the body to throw off toxins, therefore it attracts more and more accumulation. The iris area becomes darker and the predisposition to disease is stronger.

Dr Jensen observes that 'miasms' occur in dark murky eyes, indicating catarrhal settlements which are in a state of chronic stasis. One or more miasms may be present and the more there are, the slower the patient will respond to treatment. He also makes the point that there is an emotional/mental disturbance for each physical miasmic taint and that chemically imbalanced bodies produced imbalanced minds and irrational behaviour, often leading to insanity and criminal behaviour.

Dorothy Hall's psychological interpretation of the psora as

'inefficiency producers' or 'blocks' on the personality, helps us to understand the mental and emotional aspects of psora.

A completely fresh intepretation of concentrated colour-markings in the iris of the eye is presented in the *Rayid Method of Iris Analysis* by Denny Johnson in America. He calls these markings 'jewels' and says that they correlate to the forces in nature that concentrate, crystallize and organize matter. He believes their presence indicates a thinking, intellectual person who possesses many talents of analysis and verbal dialogue, and who learns by observing, as they enjoy visual stimulation. Self acceptance and change are most difficult for the jewel iris type within the Rayid Method.

Denny Johnson also observes that the psora spots or jewels are not manifest at birth. They begin to appear in the iris anywhere from three to eight years of age. It is now believed that the theory that psora spots appear after vaccinations and drug use is inaccurate. First, everyone that has vaccinations and drugs does not manifest psora spots. Second, they appear at this time whether the person has had vaccinations and drugs or not. Therefore they are a constitutional factor, the result of metabolic processes. It is most interesting how our knowledge increases as we observe the iris in continuum, over lifetimes, and from different viewpoints.

In his book, *Applied Iridology and Herbology,* Dr Donald Bamer refers to 'microscopic examination during cadaveral research which indicates these (spots) to be deposits of various enzymes such as LDH, SGOT and others that are associated with organ cell damage'. In other words, certain pigmentation is released by various organs and/or systems as a chemical reaction to improper and weak function.

Dr Bamer lists four major pigmentations:

1.	Dark Brown	Hepatotrophic	Liver
2.	Reddish Brown	Porphyrin	Hemalytic/Blood destruction condition
3.	Orange	Pancreatic	Pancreas
4.	Yellow	Nephrotic	Kidneys

He also renames the 'psoric' spots as 'Pigmented Nervi' and mineral deposits are called 'Pathological Polychromia'.

Dr Bamer's psora colour variations

Brown to black spots involving second and third iris layers indicates serious metabolic disturbances, possible organ degeneration or pre-cancerous conditions.

Rusty-red to red-brown spots indicate iron deposits from red blood corpuscle destruction.

Light yellow to black-brown spots on the iris surface suggest liver, pancreas or kidney imbalances.

Josef Deck's colour variations

Brown –pancreatic insufficiency and disturbance of liver function.

Ochre –Hepatic/spleen imbalances.

Yellow – Kidney/urinary malfunctions.

Gold – Vitamin A breakdown problems.

Frequency of psora exists whenever the pancreas is insufficient or when it manifests cysts and necroses. Usually the condition is a result of the breakdown of both pancreas and liver functions.

Theodor Kriege places the emphasis of the pigment deposits on their chemical process, not on the initial causes, which would be either the intake of various inorganic substances, or inherited psoric taints. The presence of these substances set the processes in motion by weakening the body and bringing about chemical and enzymatic imbalances.

Kriege does not discuss the hereditary miasmic taints, but divides pigmentation into either exogenous (intake of minerals and metals from outside) or endogenous (developing or originating within the organism). Even if we do not always understand why these marks occur it is clear that the pigment signs indicate irritation and weakness and the presence of toxic buildup. They do respond to cleansing programmes and in many cases become very faint or disappear altogether. However, in all cases, their effect on the whole person becomes lessened by natural therapeutic treatment.

Denny Johnson's Rayid Method of Personality Analysis through the iris of the eye calls the psora 'jewels in the rough'. They represent the raw material, the potential, the resistance which encourages transformation.

It is clear that psora and drug spots give us the opportunity to transform poison into medicine. By striving to eliminate their toxic influence on the physical level we attain personal evolution. On the psychological level transformation of the jewels in the rough to diamonds, the polishing of resistance and inhibition to consciousness talents and achievements would be a positive expression of this type.

Symptoms: Depend on the area of the body and all the other factors of constitution and tissue indications. Symptoms may be active or may only exist as potential. They may influence basic attitudes towards life.

Recommended treatment: Bowel tonic. Blood purifying formula. Lymphatic formula. Chronic purifier formula. Heavy metal formula, kidney formula and epsom salts baths. Cleansing diets and juice fasts. Distilled water. Avoid: inorganic minerals, synthetic drugs.

Pterygiums Yellowish thickened cells of opaque gelatinous tissue on the sclera are indicative of congestion and possible liver weakness. They are usually placed laterally rather than towards the nose. If the pterygium covers part of the iris, its effects are related to the corresponding part of the body.

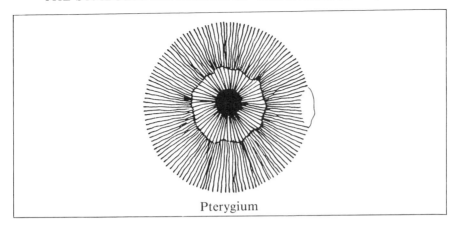

Pterygium

Whenever liver damage is suspected check for other indications such as:

1. Pupil flattening in liver area.
2. Sclera sign near the liver area.
3. Radii soleris, psora mark, lacunae or reflexive signs in the liver area.
4. Nerve rings breaking at the liver zone.
5. Lymphatic congestion.
6. Bowel pockets (ballooned or spastic).

Whether accomplished by natural therapeutics or by operation, diminishment or removal of the pterygium may restore lost function to the related body area.

Symptoms: Diminishment of function of related area.

Recommended treatment: Full eliminative and systemic treatment to make the body work efficiently will allow natural processes to diminish the pterygium.

Pupil flattening
Flattening of the pupil shape indicates strong disturbances in the adjacent iris areas. The more severe the disturbance the flatter the side of the pupil.

Pupil shapes

Superior

Inferior

Church peak

Superior angled pupils are related to central nervous system (CNS) brain function and accompany mental illness, depression, paranoia, mania, psychosis, fatigue and melancholia.

Inferior angled pupils relate to the leg and foot area indicating muscle weakness and flat feet. Pelvic organs are also affected. Headaches and poor elimination may also occur.

Superior double nasal/temporal (church peak) pupils This rare condition would accompany strong mental imbalances and psychotic disturbances.

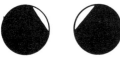

Superior nasal

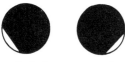

Inferior temporal

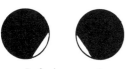

Inferior nasal

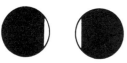

Medial

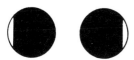

Lateral

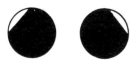

Superior temporal

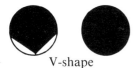

V-shape

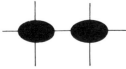

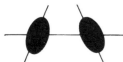

Superior angled nasal pupils relate to liver and digestive insufficiency with related eye problems. The left eye relates more to hormonal imbalance and the right eye to liver congestion. The cervical spine is affected. The upper abdomen will be disturbed causing bloating and stomach pains.

Inferior angled temporal pupils correspond to shoulder and arm weakness with impaired movement. The right iris may relate to liver and gall bladder insufficiency. The left iris affect the arms, solar plexus, diaphragm and possibly the spleen and liver. Digestive functions would be impaired.

Inferior angled nasal pupils accompany such conditions as reproductive and urinary weakness. The lumbar/sacral spinal areas are affected. Sexual weakness, impotence or infertility may result.

Medial angled pupil sides augment spinal disorders with accompanying heart weakness and breathing difficulties. Thoracic vertebrae are also affected. There may be nervous stomach symptoms.

Lateral angled pupil sides relate to respiratory weakness and breathing disorders. This may be caused by inhalation of environmental toxins. Cardiac and circulation problems may also accompany this sign as well as nervous weakness. Weakness of the thoracic vertebrae will contribute to the above conditions.

Superior angled temporal pupils relate to psychic deafness and tumours. The manifestations of the inability to register normal sound may range from genius to madness. The person cannot relate psychological truth to the words. Sexual imbalances may also complicate the illness. As this area relates to the cervicals, neck and shoulder pains may also occur.

Inferior double nasal/temporal (V-shape) pupils A severe condition indicative of syphilitic ancestry. The condition may only improve under miasmic, homeopathic treatment, and the most strict naturopathic regimen.

Pupil ovals

Vertical oval

This occurs when a seriously ill person is near death. If it is in both eyes it is even more serious. It can indicate sudden apoplexy or cerebral haemorrhage resulting in coma, paralysis and death.

Horizontal oval

An oval pattern accompanies severe depression and suicidal tendencies. Cerebral pressures may initiate this development. It may also suggest a predisposition to asthma or respiratory distress accompanied by glandular disturbances.

A-shaped ovals

This configuration indicates muscular weakness, paralysis and painful spasms. Pressure affects the limbs and pains may extend downward from the buttocks. Thyroid and parathyroid glands may register disturbances.

V-shaped ovals
This configuration indicates a disposition to cerebral apoplexy, haemorrhage or paralysis accompanied by muscle spasms. The person will also suffer from mental/emotional neurosis, anxiety and grief.

Right oblique ovals
A right imbalance may result in right-sided paralysis and urogenital disturbance. Legs may suffer weakness.

Left oblique ovals
Left-sided paralysis may occur with this sign as well as sexual disturbances. Legs may suffer weakness.

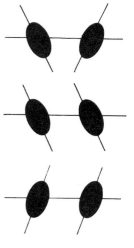

Pupil ovals

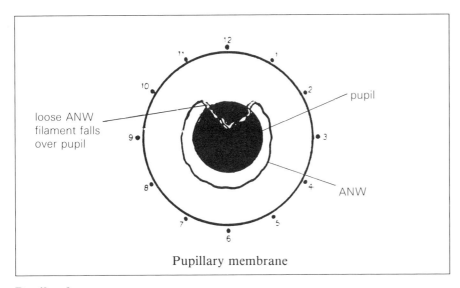

Pupillary membrane

(labels in figure: loose ANW filament falls over pupil; pupil; ANW)

Pupil colours
A film of colour, either greenish or grey, often covers the pupil. In early stages this may appear only as a slight cast, but it is important to know how it will develop. The green cast indicates a tendency to glaucoma and the grey cast a tendency to cataract, in possible combination with diabetes and arteriosclerosis.

Pupil threads or remnants
Although this looks as though the ANW wreath is falling over the pupil, it is actually the remains of the foetal pupillary membrane, when it bursts during the last few weeks of pregnancy. It can also look like granule deposits over an area of the pupil. Dorothy Hall believes this relates to the TB miasm and would enquire whether a patient had parents or grandparents who had had TB.

Dilated pupils (mydriasis)
This accompanies exhaustion, epilepsy, anaemia, TB, drug addiction and

Pupil variations

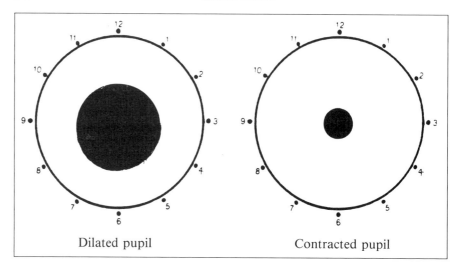

Dilated pupil   Contracted pupil

mental illness. Sympathetic dominance occurs when the parasympathetic nervous system (PSNS) is weak.

Contracted pupils (miosis)
Weakness of the sympathetic nervous system (SNS) results in
parasympathetic dominance. Tension and too much control of the will
cause this tight pupil. There is little interaction or response to others and
the environment.

Fluctuating pupils
Weak adrenals combined with a sympathetic nature causes a sensitive,
responsive nervous system which succumbs easily to shock, stress or
trauma. These people often have difficulty saying no, and they can
become drained and depleted when they continually consider the needs
of others and deny themselves. They feel the needs of others more than
their own because their sympathetic nervous system is overresponsive.

One dilated/one contracted pupil (anisocoria)
This imbalance registers severe diseases which have affected the nervous
system to an extreme degree: diptheria, meningitis, syphilis, insanity.

Pupil placement

Medial position pupils
Digestive, respiratory or cardiac weakness.

Nasal superior position pupils
Liver and spleen insufficiency

Superior position pupils
Intestinal weakness. Tendency to ulcers or tuberculosis.

Inferior position pupils
Pelvic weakness. Possible kidney, bladder, reproductive or
haemorrhoid problems.

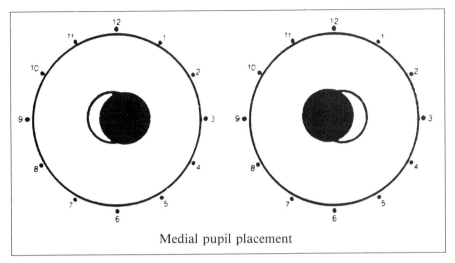

Medial pupil placement

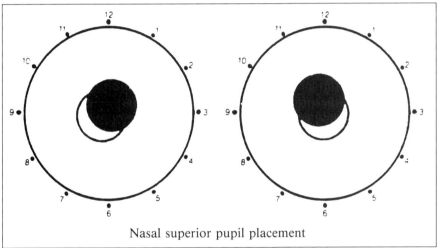

Nasal superior pupil placement

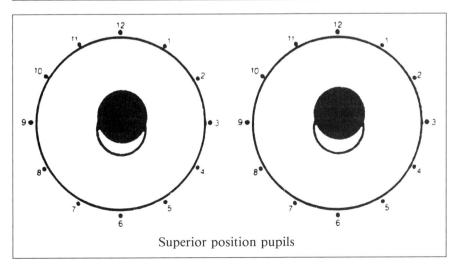

Superior position pupils

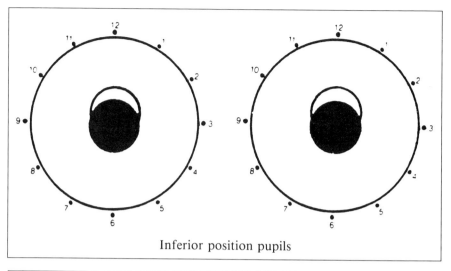

Inferior position pupils

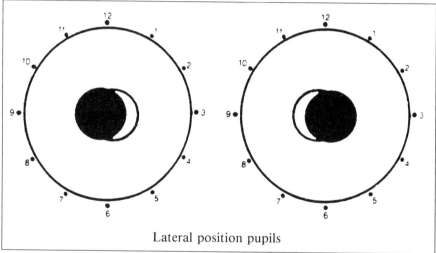

Lateral position pupils

Lateral position pupils
Gastrointestinal weakness. Cardiac problems.

Pupillary margin
The edge of the pupil reflects both the condition of the stomach wall and the CNS. In health it has an even smooth appearance, a thin line of a medium brown colour. The more degenerated the condition the more jagged, dark and uneven the pupillary margin.

Symptoms: Lack of hydrochloric acid (HCl), digestive atrophy, degeneration of the CNS.

Recommended treatment: Full chronic treatment, juice diets, HCl replacement, nerve tonics.

For more details refer to Chapter 5 (CNS).

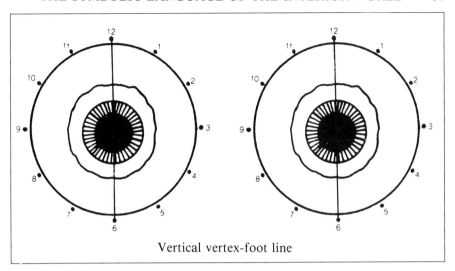

Vertical vertex-foot line

The radials divide the iris first in halves, then in quarters, then in **Radials** eighths, into sixteenths, and so on.

Vertical vertex-foot line
This is also called the equilibrium line or will line. This line divides the iris in half vertically, into lateral and medial sections. The line can be white or dark and both sides of the iris can also be different. For instance, one side can be darker than the other, or have nerve rings while the other does not. This line can also indicate disturbances of equilibrium and balance.

Horizontal throat-neck line
Also called the disharmony line or the hyperthyroidism line. Because this line divides the body at the throat, it represents disharmony between

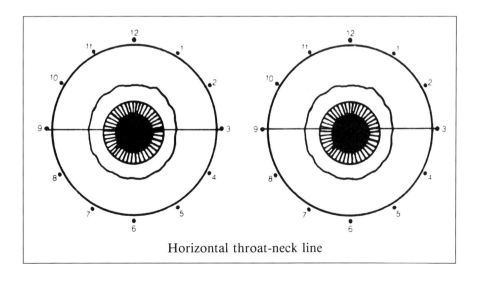

Horizontal throat-neck line

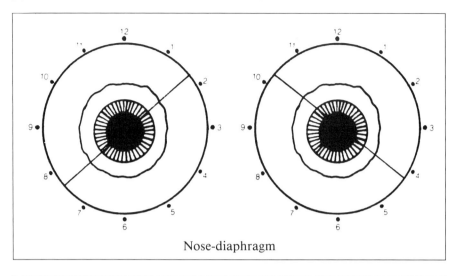

Nose-diaphragm

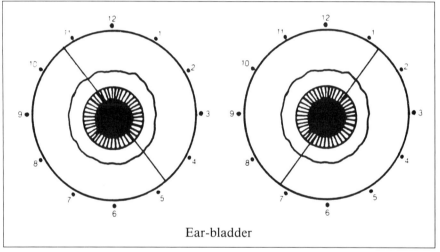

Ear-bladder

the head and the rest of the body. Whenever this line occurs, check out the thyroid, heart and lung for disturbances, as they lie near the line.

Nose-diaphragm line, or the pain line

This runs through the liver in the right eye and the spleen in the left eye, dividing the chest from the abdomen. When acute it represents organ pain in either the liver or the spleen. The digestive belt which runs across the body from the liver to spleen is associated with strong and angry emotions.

Whether one vents one's spleen or raises one's bile, hot tempers are associated with flaring nostrils. Yogic exercises to calm one's temper involve alternate nostril breathing. The spleen transforms prana and distributes it throughout the body chakras, and the nostrils breathe in air which circulates oxygen via the lungs and blood throughout the body. The diaphragm also produces sneezes, hiccups, vomiting, etc,

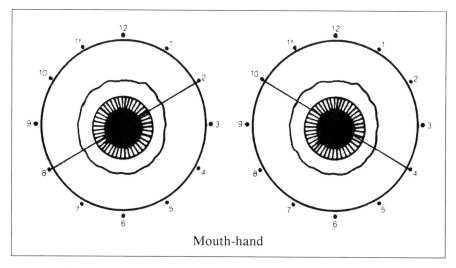

Mouth-hand

once again showing the relationships of these two areas.

The ear-bladder line

Also called the hereditary transmission line or the infection line. This line reveals the connection with inherited encumbrances. If a child has inherited chronic bladder disease, the line will manifest in the right iris, and if the infection is associated with venereal disease the line will appear in the left iris. This is also related to the line which runs from the anxiety sector of the brain to the adrenal/kidney area. Bedwetting will cause anxiety which will cause reflex adrenal stimulus with resultant hyperactivity.

The mouth-hand line

Also known as the nutrition line. The hand that feeds the mouth is guided either by wisdom or emotions. When a radial occurs it signifies that this normal function is out of balance. The person suffers from compulsive eating and nutritional defects and cannot or will not change these eating habits. The will cannot overcome the compulsive feeding. Once again, negative or repressed emotions affect living habits, as the jaw tenses under strong emotions, and the need to relieve the pressure with chewing, eating and drinking, shows the relationship with the adjacent liver. If we chew completely, instead of eating quickly, this tension is relieved in a normal way.

The forehead-ovary/testes line

Also known as the brain-ovary line. The 'mental ability' area of the brain deals with higher thought. It is here that an individual's choice or destiny between the development of maternity, family and a sex life or a mental, spiritual life where controls such as family planning, chastity or continence are practised. While it is possible to have a harmonious balance between the two, many times the balance shifts completely and a radial will manifest in a woman completely given over to child bearing and rearing without any time or opportunity to develop the mental aspects of her being.

She will suffer from headache, travel-sickness, giddiness, bedwetting, short stubby fingernails and small breast nipples. The strain of child bearing takes its toll. The concentration of energy required to produce and rear offspring registers in the iris as an imbalance. In fact, either ovarian deficiency or fertility affects the forebrain, which also houses the sex instincts for preservation of the species.

Ovarian cysts often result from conflict between two potentials of a woman's life: either a strong drive for creative mental or spiritual fulfilment or motherhood and a normal family life. It is significant whether the iris marking is on the left eye or the right eye or both. Periods come from alternate right and left ovaries. Therefore, alternately or occasionally, a woman will have a painful period. It is important to observe and determine which ovary causes the difficult period and if the iris signs confirm this.

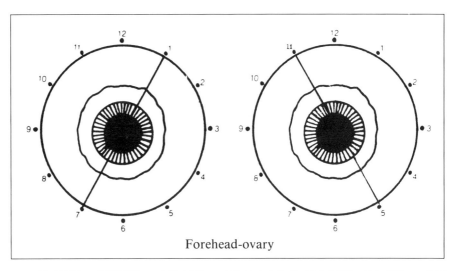

Forehead-ovary

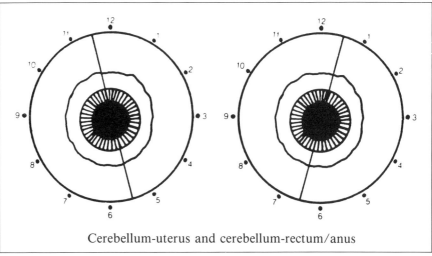

Cerebellum-uterus and cerebellum-rectum/anus

These same principles apply to the male. Does he choose to express his energy in sexual ways, or does he transmute this power into creativity, study or spirituality? Sexual excesses manifest themselves as dark or white signs. As many of these toxic signs originate in the bowel, these conditions can be relieved by cleansing and regenerative programmes.

The cerebellum-uterus line and the cerebellum-rectum/anus line

The right iris radial manifests a relationship between the sex impulse brain flair and the uterus, prostate area. The left iris manifests a relationship between the equilibrium brain flair and the rectum/anus area. The right mental area when activated or underfunctioning results in fantasies, dreams and lack of reality about one's normal sexuality and produces a hysterical noisy patient who suffers from headaches. Extreme fear of sexuality and hysteria can manifest as obsessional mental disorders, or influence a person's life so that normal love and sexuality are denied them. The left mental area, associated with equilibrium and balance, is related to the rectum/anus, producing a patient inclined to hypochondria and guilt. The rectal centre is the chakra associated with the earth element and the emotion of fear and attachment. The self obsessional hypochondriac is demanding love and attention. This focus on oneself denies the necessity to deal with the world and other people. Their world becomes small and morbid.

The axilla-loin line

Also known as the endurance line, it manifests when sensitive people cannot endure much. The practitioner must offer considerable support and not ask too much of the patient. The axilla and loin areas are two of the three main glandular terminal areas of the lymphatic system. They also form the squares of the torso, the pelvic foundation and the shoulders. Both areas are tender and delicate. Legs and arms extend into the world from the underarms, shoulders and the groin areas. With weakness here, movement from legs and arms is limited.

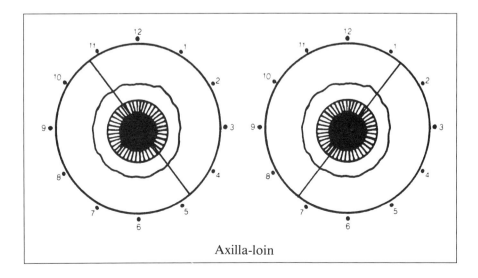

Axilla-loin

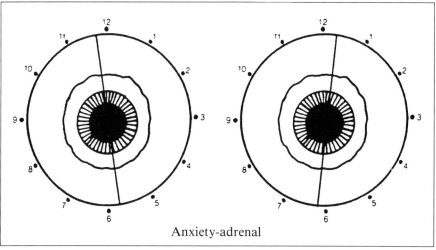

Anxiety-adrenal

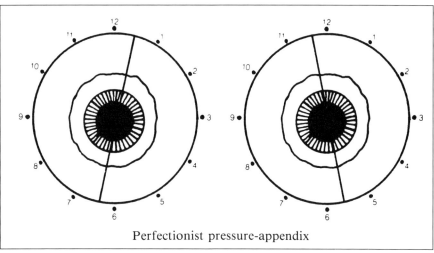

Perfectionist pressure-appendix

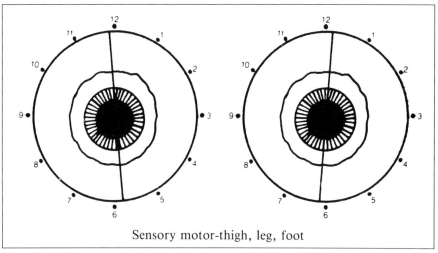

Sensory motor-thigh, leg, foot

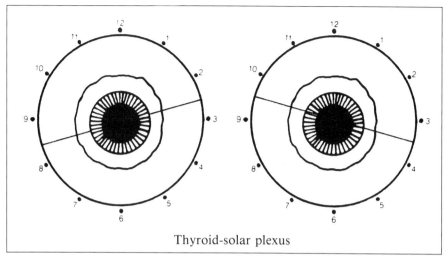

Thyroid-solar plexus

Anxiety-adrenal line

This radial marks the cause that sparks off the overstimulation of the adrenal response and eventually leads to exhaustion and hypofunction. Constant worry, fear or stress does not give the adrenal system a chance to rest, and the SNS becomes unbalanced in its relationship with the PNS.

Perfectionist pressure-appendix line

It is a well known fact that acute appendicitis often coincides with times of pressure or stress, such as exams, speeches or interviews. If pressure and striving for success is accompanied by extreme fear and anxiety the body breaks down.

Sensory motor-thigh, leg, foot line

The radials manifest the relationship between the brain areas coordinating the sensory input and the motor response which determines locomotion.

Thyroid-solar plexus line

Also known as the throat abdomen line. The solar plexus is a nerve plexus in the abdomen which reflects the emotional life in physical tension. Here, if emotions are repressed, the diaphragm hardens like a valve to prevent expression of feelings too strong or fearful to be dealt with on the conscious level. In natural expression they rise through the heart centre to the throat where they are expressed by the voice, in the throat area. The thyroid governs the speed of metabolism, thus affecting all the body functions below that area. If the flow of energy is not two-way, pressures build up, and imbalances, illness and disease result.

Radii Soleris or radial furrows

Radii Soleris fan out like spokes of a wheel. They represent auto intoxication on the physical level, and self destructive attitudes on the

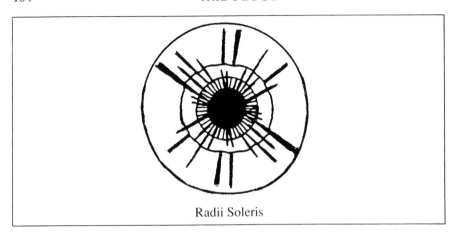

Radii Soleris

mental and emotional level. They are actually troughs for toxic poisons. Instead of eliminating what is impure, whether physical or mental, it is recirculated. Discrimination has been neglected. The power to let go of negativity has been lost.

Radii Minoris come from the pupillary edge and do not break through the ANW.

Radii Majoris come from the pupillary edge and break through the ANW or start at the ANW and radiate out into the iris.

Symptoms: Parasites, circulation of toxins, negative habit patterns, auto intoxication.

Recommended treatment: Bowel tonic, blood and lymphatic formulae. Bach flower remedies.

Reflexive fibres   High magnification (10–20x) reveals that individual iris fibres pulse and breathe with life and the ebb and flow of blood. The bio-microscope reveals the intricate living reality of this minute, but highly complex area of our body. The iris takes on a dimension that one cannot appreciate from viewing at only 4x magnification.

These iris fibres are actually formed by layers of blood vessels coated

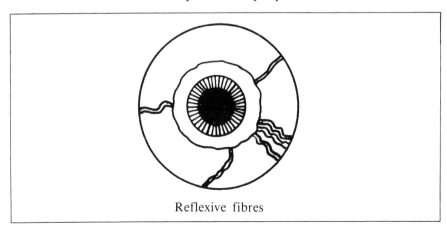

Reflexive fibres

by connective tissue. When certain individual fibres become swollen so that they stand out clearly this is the result of the acute irritations. The fibre may stand out by itself or it may appear in groups. When chronic the reflexive fibres become vascularized which causes a pink or red colour. While this sign may accompany great distress it is still reversible.

An Exudative Arc is when a group of reflexive fibres weave together towards the ciliary edge of the iris. This indicates a larger area of painful irritation.

Symptoms: These signs are accompanied by pain, inflammation, irritation, cysts, exudations, etc.

Recommended treatment: Systemic treatment accompanied by activation of all the eliminative channels.

Aberrant and Transversal Reflexive Fibres are covered in this chapter under Transversals.

SCLEROLOGY

Sclerology is the study of the marks on the sclera, the white of the eye surrounding the iris. The sclera is the tough fibrous outer coat which is in front of the eye with the cornea. The sclera both maintains the shape of the eyeball and protects it.

Like the iris, the sclera tissues have a close connection with the brain. In fact, the sclera tissues are continuous with the dura matter of the brain via the fibrous sheath of the optic nerve. The sclera develops in the fifth week of embryo development from the outer layer of loose tissue surrounding the developing eye.

A clear white sclera is a reflection of health and balance in the body and the life of the individual. Blood pressure and the integral relationship of the eye extending from the brain explains the patterns that appear. Reflex back pressure in the vascular system produces the sclera markings which indicate and point to problems in the body.

There are three main sclera colours:

Red sclera markings: These are caused by arterial active congestion and inflammation. Red markings mean excessive body heat, congestion of local blood vessels and excessive intake of starch, sugar and fats.

White and yellow sclera markings (pterygium): White and yellow congestions on the sclera (sometimes they cover over part of the iris as well) indicate high cholesterol levels, excessive bile in liver disease, blood loaded with impurities, tendencies to diabetes and jaundice, imbalances in digestive chemistry, and inability to digest and assimilate fats.

Blue sclera markings: This colour occurs when there is passive venous congestion due to circulatory weakness, and poor blood flow to and from the head.

Sclera markings fade, lessen and even disappear during the natural treatment based on iridology readings. As the body organs, systems and eliminative channels begin to function properly, the blood is purified and circulation is equalized, pressure and congestion which caused the markings disperses.

Sclera markings augment iridology diagnosis. Often when there are strong chronic or acute markings in the iris, a sclera vessel occurs nearby. In many cases there is either a sclera marking pointing directly to the area or one that follows the curve of the edge of the iris. A practitioner can confirm or extend the diagnosis by checking the sclera chart.

In Germany, sclera markings are combined with iridology during diagnosis. Recent research there has focused on the early detection of cysts and tumours. Unfortunately translations of this work are not yet available in English.

As with iridology, sclerology does not attempt to name disorders. It reports on tissue disturbances, drawing our attention to malfunctions that may exist in organs, glands or areas of the body and in the function of the various systems.

Right eye sclera markings display problems on the left side of the brain and vice versa. Because the sclera is partly covered by eyelids, it is necessary that the patient look in each of the four directions (up, down, left and right) so that all the sclera becomes visible to the practitioner.

SCLERA SIGNS

Arterial system

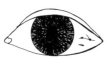

Lake sclera vessels

Lake sclera vessels
Overflowing sclera vessels indicate narrowed arteries. This may be part of arteriosclerosis. Look to the constitution and treat the entire circulatory system, including the heart. The liver may also need support.

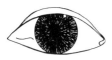

Engorged vessels

Engorged vessels
This strong sign indicates a local dilation of the walls of an artery, due to weakening through injury, infection, hereditary or degenerative conditions. Liver and heart will also be involved and will require herbal treatment. Weak blood vessels may create other problems.

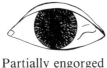

Partially engorged vessels

Partially engorged vessels
This sign usually curves more than the fully engorged sign. This indicates localised thrombosis and arteriosclerosis. Look at the pancreas and consider blood sugar levels and possible diabetes. This is a chronic sign requiring full systemic treatment.

Parallel ciliary vessels
This can mean either arterial or venous congestion in the adjacent iris area. It often appears by the liver/gall bladder or heart/spleen areas. If it is in the hand areas it suggests cerebral congestion. Treat the constitution and the eliminative system and add specific medicine for the area where it appears.

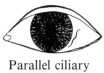

Parallel ciliary
vessels

Venous system

Curved sclera marking
This curving snake-like pattern indicates venous weakness which manifests as varicose veins and haemorrhoids. When it is even more curved and swollen in the iris it suggests hypertension. Calc. Fluor. and Silica tissue salts will assist this condition.

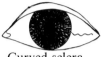

Curved sclera
markings

Parallel sclera marking
When veins are congested this sclera sign will occur. Usually congestion is more severe in the legs, rectum, anus and throat areas. The sclera sign may be near these areas.

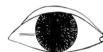

Parallel sclera
marking

Pearl chains
This sclera sign indicates a tendency to spontaneous bleeding. The main chain may also be accompanied by red spots.

Other sclera signs

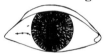

Pearl chains

Cholesterol deposits/pterygium
White or yellow congestions on the surface of the sclera indicate high cholesterol, liver malfunction, digestive disorders and toxic blood.

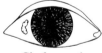

Cholesterol
deposits

Pointers
These sclera pointers draw our attention to a specific organ, usually the liver or the spleen. This sign accompanies chronic conditions and the organ would require primary treatment. Treatment of the constitution and eliminative channels will relieve the workload of the primary organ.

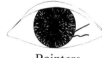

Pointers

Vessel network
Whenever the ciliary iris edge meets the sclera with a network of small red sclera vessels, allergies are present. The stronger the network, the more pronounced the allergies, though the allergies may be latent only. The mucous membranes will be affected, as well as the skin. When it manifests in the head area it is called the migraine net.

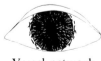

Vessel network

Curls
Corkscrew curls are indications that the blood pressure is abnormal. Take tests and observe symptoms to determine whether it is high or low.

Curls

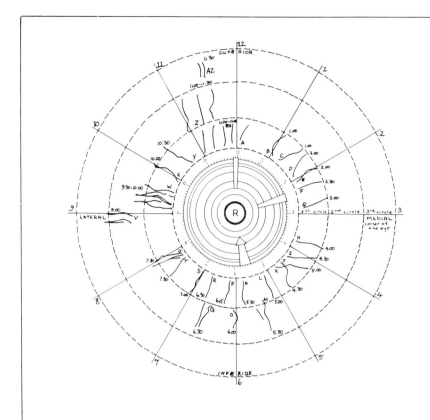

RIGHT EYE | FIRST CIRCLE | SECOND CIRCLE | THIRD CIRCLE

A 12:00	Nervous disorder
B 1:00	Right eye (upper line)
C 1:15	Tonsils, throat (lower line)
D 2:00	Nose (upper line)
E 2:00	Thyroid (lower line)
F 2:30	Trachea
G 3:00	Oesophagus
H 4:00	Upper back
I 4:30	Middle back (upper line)
J 4:30	Sciatic nerve, problem in right leg
K 5:00	Lower back (upper line)
L 5:00	Prostate or vagina (lower line)
N 5:30-6	Kidney adrenal
P 6-6:15	Uterus
R 6:30	Pancreas
S 7:00	Ovaries, testes
T 7:30	Liver or gall bladder (lower line)
U 7:30	Thorax congestion (upper 2)
W 9:30-10	Lung congestion
X 10:00	Right ear or mastoid
Y 10:30	Right ear or neck
Z 11-11:30	
AZ 11:30	
BZ 11:00-12:00	Nervous disorders (5 lines)

SECOND CIRCLE:

M Small intestine

O Transverse colon
Q Ascending colon

V Right shoulder 9:00

THIRD CIRCLE:

Z Sinusitis (3 lines)

AZ Brain concussion or injury

Sclera map © Farida Sharan

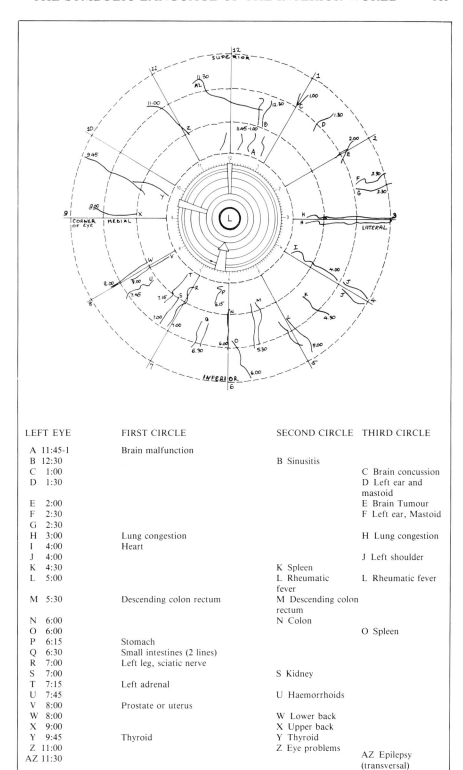

LEFT EYE	FIRST CIRCLE	SECOND CIRCLE	THIRD CIRCLE
A 11:45-1	Brain malfunction		
B 12:30		B Sinusitis	
C 1:00			C Brain concussion
D 1:30			D Left ear and mastoid
E 2:00			E Brain Tumour
F 2:30			F Left ear, Mastoid
G 2:30			
H 3:00	Lung congestion		H Lung congestion
I 4:00	Heart		
J 4:00			J Left shoulder
K 4:30		K Spleen	
L 5:00		L Rheumatic fever	L Rheumatic fever
M 5:30	Descending colon rectum	M Descending colon rectum	
N 6:00		N Colon	
O 6:00			O Spleen
P 6:15	Stomach		
Q 6:30	Small intestines (2 lines)		
R 7:00	Left leg, sciatic nerve		
S 7:00		S Kidney	
T 7:15	Left adrenal		
U 7:45		U Haemorrhoids	
V 8:00	Prostate or uterus		
W 8:00		W Lower back	
X 9:00		X Upper back	
Y 9:45	Thyroid	Y Thyroid	
Z 11:00		Z Eye problems	
AZ 11:30			AZ Epilepsy (transversal)

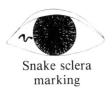

Snake sclera
marking

Snakes

A snake sclera marking is indicative of high blood pressure. Check the heart, liver and circulatory zones for confirmation.

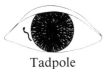

Tadpole

Tadpoles

A thinner, more loosely curved snake with a small head, suggests predisposition to anaemia. Do other tests and look for an anaemia ring when you see this sign.

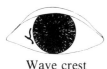

Wave crest

Wave crest

The unique wave crest sclera marking may appear after accidents which caused injury to the head, and may guide the practitioner to diagnose concussion.

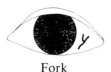

Fork

Fork

The sign, reminiscent of the fork transversal, indicates rheumatism when it is present in the sclera.

Sclera melanin

Brown sclera markings occur around the iris in African, Caribbean and East Indian irides. Dorothy Hall's theory indicates a possible constitutional factor, a leprosy miasm, a valuable indication for treatment with radionics and homeopathy. The sclera does become clearer during purification regimen, but usually the melanin remains.

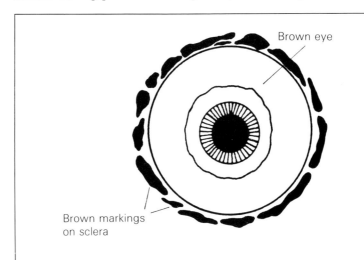

Markings on the sclera, the white of the eye surrounding the iris

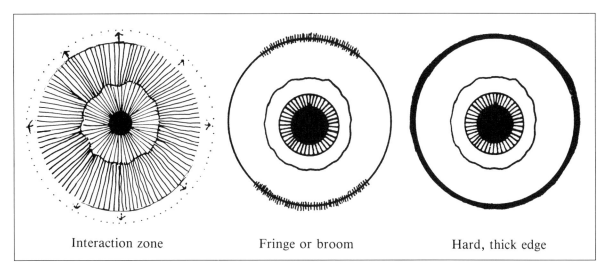

| Interaction zone | Fringe or broom | Hard, thick edge |

Sclera-ciliary interaction zone

The zone where the sclera meets the ciliary edge offers many clues to both physical conditions and the personality. The interaction of the person with the outside world is revealed where the ciliary edge meets the sclera reflecting the person's non-physical auric envelope. There are various types of interaction zones.

Fringe or broom – open interaction with circumstances and people, showing vulnerability, psychic sensitivity and the need for protection. On the physical level it correlates to skin, capillary and lymphatic functions.

Defined – a defended ego, yet still there are reasonable levels of interaction and reciprocity with the world. A sharp clear edge indicates normal relationships and normal body functions.

Hard thick – insensitive, overprotects self, reduced interaction and reciprocity with others and the environment. Strong will, fear and tension accompany the armouring. A thick edge may also go inward (increasing the scurf rim) and indicating accumulated toxins as this person finds it difficult to let go as well as to receive. Their tension inhibits movement inwards and outwards.

Soft indistinct – represents easy interaction with the world and a relaxed reciprocity in relationships. On the physical level this indistinct grey haze over the edge of the iris relates to circulatory insufficiency or lack of power. Often the haze may be at the top and bottom of the iris, or only at the top or bottom.

Migraine neuron net – the sclera sign is composed of an intricate web of red capillary markings that interweave between the ciliary edge of the

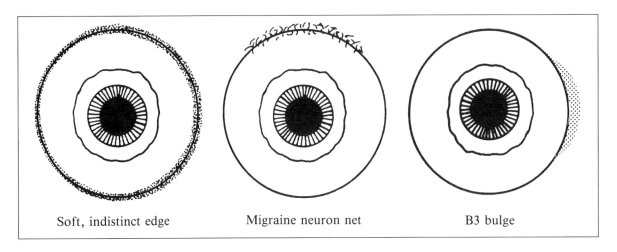

Soft, indistinct edge   Migraine neuron net   B3 bulge

iris and the sclera, causing a webbed, hazy reddish edge to the iris. This indicates sensitivity and irritation in relationship with the world, as well as pain and irritability. It can also manifest as allergy symptoms.

B3 bulge - (between 2 and 4 pm and 8 and 10 pm). A grey transparent curve extends outward on both sides of the iris, usually lateral, but sometimes, both lateral and medial, which changes the shape of the iris. Dorothy Hall claims that it is the result of B3 deficiency, and certainly I have seen this sign reduce when B3 is added to the treatment programme, when accompanied by constitutional and eliminative treatment. It often appears when patients have digestive troubles.

The sodium ring
The sodium ring starts in the circulatory zone, often moving out and covering the skin zone. It appears to be a part of the sclera, following or covering the cornea and overlying the tissues of the iris without being a part of the iris fibre itself. The ring can be narrow or it can spread over as much as half the iris and the heavier it gets the more of an opaque white it becomes. The sodium ring can be different shades of white and may be opaque, translucent or transparent. The thicker and wider it is, the more chronic the condition.

The anaemia ring
Here the transparent sclera draws up over the skin area in the iris and you can see the iris underneath it. The more area is covered by the anaemia ring, the more serious is the condition. Often the anaemia is concentrated in the head and in the feet, and is then called anaemia of the extremities.

In either case, the blood is not reaching the skin and extremities due to excess blood in the internal organs, poor circulation, nutritional deficiencies, lack of exercise and incorrect living and bathing habits. The anaemia ring is a distinct blue colour. The Rayid Method names it

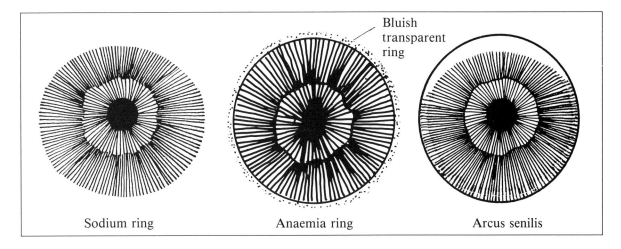

| Sodium ring | Anaemia ring | Arcus senilis |

the Ring of Purpose because individuals with this ring have a strong sense of purpose.

The arcus senilis
The sclera is pulled down over the upper part of the iris. The colouring can be white, yellow, brownish or transparent, depending on whether other materials are settled there, the presence of an accompanying sodium ring, lymphatic toxins or scurf rim.

Insufficiency of circulation in the extremities
Grey fog covers the interaction zone at the ciliary edge of the iris when poor circulation, combined with thyroid, liver/gall bladder, heart or lymphatic weakness creates capillary, skin and lymphatic congestion. This may occur only at the top of the iris, only at the bottom or may manifest on both top and bottom at the same time.

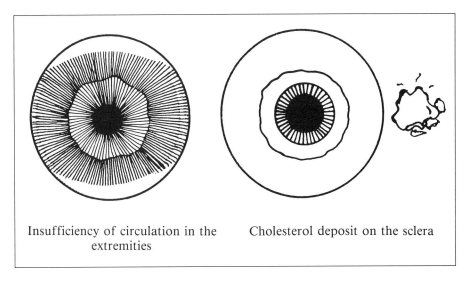

Insufficiency of circulation in the extremities   Cholesterol deposit on the sclera

Cholesterol deposits on the sclera

Lumps of white and yellow-white appear on the sclera, when heart, liver and circulatory problems occur. The Lipaemic Diathesis constitutional type has a predisposition to their manifestation.

Scurf rim

The scurf rim appears at birth indicating the toxic inheritance from the parents' blood stream. It usually diminishes if the child is raised without suppressive treatment, but it can increase if every attempt at elimination (childhood diseases especially) is met with drugs.

People who live in cold climates usually have larger scurf rims. Contributing factors are: synthetic clothing and bedclothing, skin never exposed to fresh air, insufficient bathing and skin scrubbing, overuse of anti perspirants, lack of exercise, overheated rooms and diminished natural perspiration.

Symptoms: Poor skin elimination. Skin rashes, eczema, psoriasis, pimples etc. Insufficient lymphatic function. Poor circulation. Poor adjustment to hot and cold temperature changes.

Recommended treatment: saunas, Turkish baths, skin scrubbing. Drink six to eight cups of fenugreek tea daily. Blood purifying and lymphatic formulae. Increase the function of all the eliminative channels.

Sodium/calcium/hypercholesterol ring

Iridologists have different ideas about the sodium ring, which is called by several different names – sodium ring, calcium ring, cholesterol ring, circulatory ring, hypercholesterol ring, lypaemic diathesis constitutional type or the arteriosclerosis ring.

The ring may be inherited or it may develop due to incorrect living habits or the intake of excess sodium in salt, food, water, soil or medicines. It may also be caused by excess cholesterol deposits or calcium out of solution.

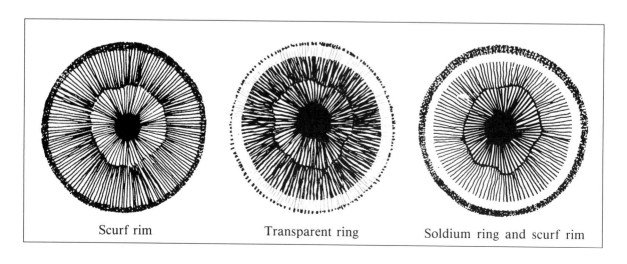

| Scurf rim | Transparent ring | Soldium ring and scurf rim |

The lypaemic diathesis constitutional type occurs in either blue or brown eyes. Troubles with fat metabolism and hardening of the arteries precipitate the overlay of white over the ciliary edge of the iris. This condition invariably points to diabetes, liver involvement and possible heart weakness.

The ring may extend in a full circle around the iris, or it may concentrate in a specific area, sometimes only on one eye, but usually on both eyes. Wherever you find this marking there is diminished circulation and venous congestion, causing inhibition of function. When the brain area is affected, mental processes become confused and the person usually suffers from poor memory, fatigue and inability to concentrate.

The plaquing of the vascular system is caused when the body tries to find a place to store the buildup of inorganic sodium. When the condition is chronic it usually indicates arteriosclerosis. These rings are found in the irides of persons who habitually use sodium and other inorganic salts in large quantities, but they also occur from other causes. It is significant to note that these salts are neither assimilated nor eliminated. They act as a foreign agent in the body, becoming a contributing factor in producing disease.

The ring may entirely surround the iris or cover only a part depending on the quantities of inorganics, salts, fats, etc. used, the powers of the various eliminative organs of the person and the part of the circulatory system that has the least resistance.

The sodium ring is found in the circulatory zone within the iris, with a noticeable margin between it and the extreme ciliary border. It may be present in advanced dropsy. The arcus senilis is a whitish blue outer covering which seems to raise the sclero-corneal coat causing it to overlap the iris. The anaemia ring is recognized and differentiated from the above two signs by its bluish colour which is seen at the point between the ciliary border, the outer edge of the iris and the sclero-corneal coats.

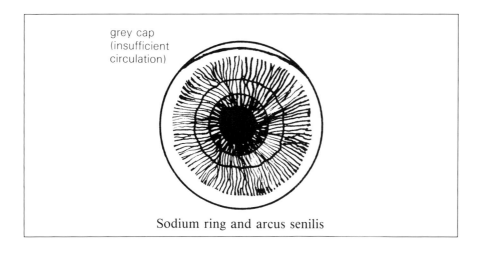

grey cap
(insufficient
circulation)

Sodium ring and arcus senilis

Another main cause of the arcus senilis is reduced blood flow to the brain cells. This process apparently begins as partial blockage in the arteries of the head and neck. Further accumulations of triglycerides, inorganic sodium and other deposits collect and form a blockage of the arteries which diminishes circulatory force to the brain area.

The sodium ring may lead to recognition of any of the following causal factors:

1. Sodium salicylate used to treat rheumatism.
2. Sodium bicarbonate used to treat stomach acidity.
3. Large quantities of baking soda consumed in baked goods.
4. Excessive use of common table salt.
5. Saline cathartics.
6. Use of mercurial salts, especially when combined with potassium iodide.
7. Artificial sweeteners, antacids, aspirins etc.
8. Diminished liver function, excess of fried foods.
9. Heart insufficiency.
10. Parathyroid malfunction.

Symptoms: Patients who manifest the Sodium Ring and/or Arcus Senilis often complain of stiffness, aches and pains on waking in the morning, high blood pressure, lack of suppleness and mobility. When the sign occurs in brain areas they despair of loss of memory, confusion, mental fogginess, difficulty in thinking and lack of concentration. They may also swing from one extreme to another.

When this sign manifests check out the following:

1. Liver.
2. Heart.
3. Circulation.
4. High blood pressure.
5. Brain anaemia.
6. Pancreas (diabetes).
7. Parathyroids.

Recommended treatment: The elimination of these inorganic salts can be accomplished by the following regimens over a sustained period of time. Relief of symptoms occur before visible change of the ring.

1. Elimination of salt for dietary or medicinal purposes.
2. Increased consumption of organic fresh fruits and vegetables.
3. Body massage and general hygiene, including improved skin elimination.
4. Spinal manipulation to tone up organs of elimination.
5. Restore liver and heart function.
6. Activate all eliminative channels.
7. Strengthen circulatory and lymphatic activity.
8. Use only distilled water, the empty water which draws out inorganic minerals.

9. Blood- and lymph-purifying herbs, heart, thyroid and liver formulae.
10. Epsom salts baths, saunas, skin scrubbing.
11. Fresh juices.
12. Exercise.

Stomach ring or halo

The halo surrounding the pupil in the first zone of the iris gives a reading of stomach hypo/hyperactivity and acid balance. This halo is found in some of the lymphatic blue or grey irises. It may also appear in brown eyes. These colours indicate the following conditions:

1. Brilliant white – hyperactive stomach with excess HCl.
2. White – normal reading for lymphatic constitution.
3. Grey – first stages of hypoactivity with insufficient HCl.
4. Dark grey – hypoactive stomach with lack of HCl.

Symptoms: The hyperactive stomach will experience pain, flatulence and stomach swellings as the food moves through too quickly. The hypoactive stomach will have a slow digestive process, fermentation, feelings of heavy stomach and difficulty with digestion of proteins. Chronic conditions of hypoactivity can lead to degeneration.

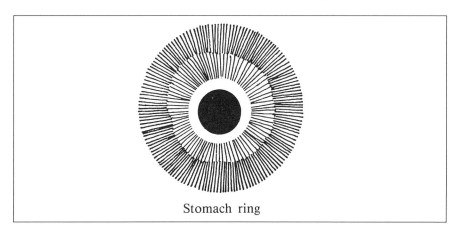

Stomach ring

Recommended treatment: Stomach acid/alkaline balancing formula. Digestive tea to help balance the acid/alkaline levels. Slippery elm and wild yam root herbs. Can be cleansed by purifying diet and juice. Natural chlorophyll drinks or wheatgrass. Avoid: acid foods and bad food combinations. Foods should be combined properly by eating proteins first and not mixing fruits and vegetables together in the same meal. Do not eat late at night and avoid taking snacks.

Transversals

Transversals are reflexive fibres that cross over normal fibres. The ends of the transversals do not pass into the normal radial fibres. These transverse fibres are hereditary and irreversible vascular disease markings. Although they usually occur in the lower half of the iris, they may also be found in the head areas. As discussed under reflexive fibres, the fibres become swollen, then vascularized during active irritation. At this time they can display various shades of pink or red. The most common transversals are in the liver, heart/spleen or reproductive areas. Some transversals begin at the ANW and move outwards. Others run across the normal fibres closer to the ciliary edge. Whenever other organ signs accompany the transversal, consideration should be that it is a primary focus for treatment.

When swollen or vascularized they accompany irritated conditions in organs, glands and tissues.

Symptoms: change of organ position, cysts, varicose veins, adhesions, pain, acute irritation, hernia, organ weakness and insufficiency, venous congestion, phlebitis, dizziness, insomnia, tumours, abdominal plethora, pain in joints, degeneration of joint cartilage and collagen fibres, and connective tissue weakness.

Recommended treatment: This depends on the organ, gland or body area affected. Proceed as usual with constitutional and eliminative treatment, with emphasis on purifying the blood and lymph and equalizing and activating the circulation. It is important to relieve tension and congestion around focus areas, whether by poultices, enemas, osteopathy or chiropractic, deep tissue massage or purifying diets and juice fasts. Water therapy can be very useful to reduce congestion and pain.

Straight transversals
When transversals appear as straightened lines they are usually white and active, indicating functional disturbances.

Curved transversals
The more wavy or curved the transversal, the more serious is its indication. It has also been called the phlebitis transversal.

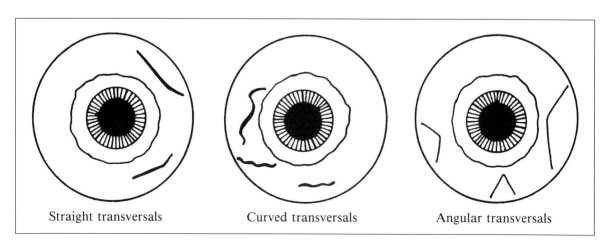

Straight transversals   Curved transversals   Angular transversals

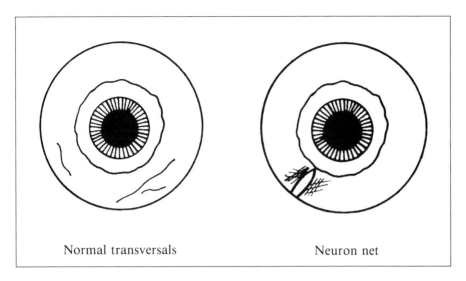

Normal transversals   Neuron net

Angular transversals
These are usually associated with joint pain, especially the hip or knee. These irritated fibres would be accompanied by other signs indicating the degeneration of connective tissue, cartilage, collagen and bone.

Neuron nets
When this net pattern appears outside lacunae it is due to the crossover patterns of small transversals. This weaving of the fibres increases vulnerability to stress, extremes of hot and cold, pollution, exhaustion, the effects of drugs, etc. This pattern often accompanies nervous conditions such as neuralgia.

Normal transversals
Connective tissue weakness is indicated by transversals, with tendencies to adhesions, cysts, hernias, as well as weakness and insufficiency of the organ or body areas. The normal transversal is a genotypic sign which

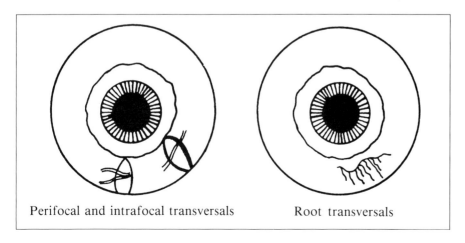

Perifocal and intrafocal transversals   Root transversals

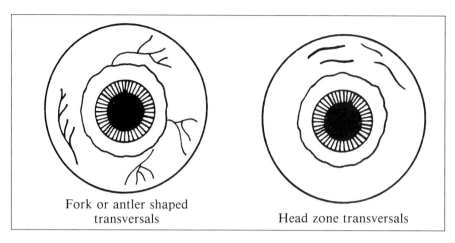

Fork or antler shaped transversals

Head zone transversals

has not yet become aggravated by living or developed its phenotypic potential into the swollen or vascularized condition.

Perifocal and intrafocal transversals
These transversals indicate irritation and congestion around (perifocal) and/or inside (intrafocal) a lacuna. The transversal may cross over the lacunae, but if it originates inside the lacunae it is called an intrafocal transversal.

Root transversals
Congestion and obstruction to function occur in areas or organs marked by the root transversal. This is a complicated and intricate network and the symptom pattern may be erratic.

Fork or antler shaped transversals can accompany cysts, tumours and constitutional deformities. The more prongs in the fork, the more serious the condition.

Ciliary fork – when the fork opens towards the ciliary edge this indicates congestion. In the head areas this might mean dizziness, pressure or insomnia. In organ areas the excess blood and pressure could lead to a variety of symptoms. Assess individually.

Pupillary fork – when the fork opens towards the ANW it indicates a condition of abdominal congestion.

Head zone transversals can manifest symptoms such as headaches and encephalitis when in the acute irritation phase. These occur from TB miasms. The potential may exist for some time without being activated.

Vascularized transversals
As the irritation progresses the transversal becomes more swollen until it reaches the vascularized state. The phenotypic potential has been activated. First the fibre becomes whiter and brighter. Then a pink or red colour appears from the blood vessels in the iris. This, however, is

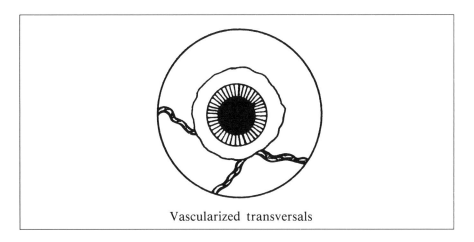

Vascularized transversals

still reversible and the red colour fades as the condition improves during treatment.

Vascularization of a transversal occurs when there is pain in the corresponding body area. It may appear at the focus of serious disease or in a reflex area. Look clearly at the total iris picture.

Significant vascularized transversals often appear in the liver, heart and spleen areas. They swell up and stand out clearly above the normal fibre levels.

Chapter 4

Clearing Space — The Eliminative Channels

THE ELIMINATIVE SYSTEM

Pathways to health or disease The first step to visualizing our transparent body is to gain a clear understanding of the eliminative channels: the bowels, kidneys, lungs, skin and lymph. Unless wastes are allowed free and unhindered passage out of our body, toxins accumulate and obstruct natural functions. The stage is set for the degenerative processes which are the beginnings of disease.

Our body inhales air, absorbs moisture and takes in nutrients from the world. After discrimination, digestion and assimilation, wastes must be eliminated. A rhythmic balance between intake and elimination is

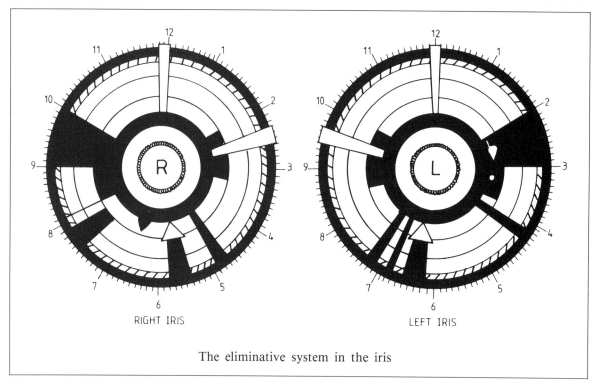

RIGHT IRIS

LEFT IRIS

The eliminative system in the iris

essential for well-being. If there is more intake than outflow, wastes are retained in the body causing fermentation and the spread of toxins throughout the system. Toxicity, degeneration and imbalances of bodily processes result. If there is more outflow than intake, the person soon becomes weak and depleted.

Because it is difficult for a person to gain an understanding of their own eliminative channels, the iridologist acts as a teacher. During the analysis the iridologist can see the condition of each eliminative channel, whether it is working adequately, or whether other channels are compensating. Almost every person lives their life with two or more eliminative channels functioning at low levels. This effectively diminishes vitality and accelerates the ageing process.

The eliminative channels are a reflection of forces within our bodies which are working to preserve health and to protect us. We need to understand and work with these forces and recognize how important they are to our well-being. We also need to understand that these physiological forces are reflections of our emotional, mental and spiritual attitudes. When the physical processes are allowed to work freely, the individual experiences a release on other levels as well. The eliminative forces are powerful friends that work for us at every moment. If we remove any obstructions to their function and then consciously strive to maintain their regular performance, they will keep our bodies clean and clear.

The pathway to the transparent body is a sensitizing, softening process which awakens us to our vulnerable and tender self, the loving child within.The clearer and cleaner our bodies are, the softer and more responsive we are to our inner spirit, the spirits of the brothers and sisters around us, to nature and how we live in the world. Purification has always been a sacred part of religious or spiritual initiations and ceremonies. Once we learn about our own uniquely personal body, and once we bring our body to balanced active function we shall know what we need to do to keep ourselves well. Our body will then serve us, so that we can turn our attention to living a full and productive life.

Before we consider a treatment of the eliminative channels we must clarify our belief system and establish a practical philosophy. Hering's Law of Cure helps us to understand that healing forces come from within and move outward. One of the first manifestations of this healing force would be the clearing of all obstructions to elimination and the opening of their pathways.

Our body is designed to work efficiently, so if we cleanse, support, activate and strengthen these natural functions we will be helping the body to do its work. Orthodox medicine has worked for centuries with the concept that nature is negative, that it is to be feared. Nature causes disease and therefore treatments must be active, even violent, in an attempt to put nature in its place. We prefer to see nature as both positive and negative. How we work with her or against her is the determining factor. Birth, maturity and death are all around us. It is a fact of life that all that is born must die. The body carries the seeds of death as well as tremendously powerful forces seeking to preserve and maintain life. The lesson to be learned is that nature does have laws, and if we break them either through ignorance or rebellion the results are the same. What goes against nature reaps its reactions. We make the choice to nurture positivity by taking responsibility for ourselves and by choosing to respect nature's laws.

Acceptance of Positivity and Negativity

Iridology is a diagnostic tool which helps us look at our positive and negative aspects and to come to terms with them. If we fear the negative realities and try to hide from them we still have to face them sooner or later. Although truth and acceptance of both positive and negative realities connects one with life on deeper levels of being before you realize the potential of death as an every day companion, the reward of this acceptance is consciousness. The negative realities are not condemned to the prison of a shadow self and we are not denied the creative energy that is their counterpart. Negative realities, once accepted, can be raised to consciousness, and transmuted by energies freed from repression and resistance. When we accept nature in its entirety, in both its constructive and destructive principles, we can learn its laws. Only when we know the laws can we strive to uphold them.

Death is inevitable. It comes to us all. How we prepare for it is our choice. Regardless of whatever we do, think, or feel, it comes to us. Death is happening around us every moment of our lives. Cells are born and die. Seasons come and go. Plant life surges upward towards the sun, then withers away. Yet seeds are sown, and roots hold life within for another season. Whenever bodies hold life, death is inevitable. The form will be dissolved and the life spirit freed. Iridology gives us perception and the understanding to accept and work with our positive and negative inheritance. We need no longer fear and hide away from our destructive principle. With consciousness our weaknesses can come into the light of day, and serve as warning signals to let us know we have gone too far.

Elimination and the force of movement from within outward as a part of the healing process also happens in other ways.The release of repressed or unconscious toxicity exists on many levels, and once the main force of crystallization begins to break up, the momentum includes the dispersal of mental and emotional negativity. Tears often accompany these clearing processes and it is interesting to note that they often burn your cheeks, making them red because they contain acid salts.

Women's periods can become an alternative for regular eliminative channels. Many women suffer physical and emotional disturbances, especially from the time of ovulation to the onset of the period. Although this has been tidily named pre-menstrual syndrome, there is more to it than meets the eye. We find that the iris reveals either the accumulation of pelvic toxins or inflammation together with the obstruction of one or more eliminative channels. The menstrual cycle, influenced by endocrine vibrations, attempts to clear pelvic toxins and their effect on the potential womb of life by turning the period into an eliminative channel. These energies reach peak levels during menopause when the surfacing of the unfulfilled aspects of our life, our shadow self, makes a bold and powerful attempt for recognition. If the mature woman can accept and eventually welcome all that she projects or represses as a part of her potentially destructive or creative power, then her energy is relieved from the insidious duty of invisible degeneration. Menopause becomes an opportunity for the self-birth of her complete full psyche. From this balanced, grounded, viewpoint she can offer her creative, nurturing and administrative abilities in the service of mankind as she develops her inner spiritual life.

The sum total of our toxic and degenerative realities are completely interwoven with our unconscious repressions and resistances. Iridology releases us by offering enlightened impartial opportunities for evolution, reassuring us that release from ignorance is not something to be feared but is a positive way of dealing with the realities of this world. By letting go of negativity, we make space to receive positive healing.

Elimination is also activated through secretions and discharges from body openings, such as the eyes, ears, nose, vagina, penis, breast nipples and mouth, when the regular eliminative channels are not functioning properly. Treatment of such exudations must include the return to function of each of the five main eliminative channels. Stopping the exudation and acute activity of any body openings without clearing the main pathways will only result in further suppression until the eliminative energies gather strength once more to attempt release. Repeated suppressions eventually cause a loss of power with the result that the eliminative channels are no longer able to generate the energy to eliminate morbid accumulations.

Taking into consideration all of the above thoughts and principles let us consider a basic approach to treatment. The first consideration is to relieve any obstructions to elimination and the second to support any weak organ and system. With that as the foundation we can then offer tonics to strengthen and stimulate the energy which will be required to overcome inertia and exhaustion. During this transitional period counselling and instruction will give the opportunity to adjust mental and emotional patterns, and to learn new living habits to support the emerging health pattern. The healing crisis (or preferably the healing achievement) is reached when positivity overcomes negativity, and establishes a new pattern of movement towards health and healing.

The healing achievement and the eliminative channels

Many natural medicine practitioners have written about the healing crisis as a potentially dreadful experience, to be sought after and then endured once it has manifested. What we have experienced is that healing crisis aggravations are diminished by the active, continuous flow of eliminations on a daily basis. Occasional disturbances or exudative manifestations are mild and can be adjusted and alleviated by supportive natural treatment. Rashes, diarrhoea, colds, headaches or tiredness are some of symptoms that come up during treatment. Iridology helps us approach treatment so that aggravations are minimal, except in cases of severe chronic disease. The acute stage of uncomfortable symptoms can be minimized by practical treatments such as mustard baths, enemas, juice fasts, aromatherapy baths, herbal teas, poultices, castor oil packs, hydrotherapy, etc.

The healing process is one of softening, opening up and letting go. It manifests when the vital force increases and body fluids and pressures are equalized, thus facilitating the communication of function on all levels. Areas of stress, congestion or depletion are relieved and balanced. Health is a dynamic process of being in the present and allowing life to flow in and out at all levels. There is neither obsession with the past nor with the future. We let go to make space for what is coming next.

In the healing process we let go of negative, toxic, destructive and unassimilated residues on all levels and make way for positive, cleansing and regenerative forces. Treatment provides and releases the level of positivity needed to overthrow the accumulated resistant negativity. This timing is different for everyone. Each person's cycle of healing is unique. Degenerative disease treatment like the Gerson Therapy applies highly intense levels of positive intake to overthrow excessive levels of degeneration. The balance of cell growth must be greater than cell destruction.

Whenever you are involved in a healing and purifying course of treatment it is helpful to ask yourself the following questions and evaluate the answers. Consider the physical, emotional, mental and spiritual aspects of the problem.

What am I taking into myself that is good for me? What am I taking into myself that is not good for me?

What is the balance between what I am taking in and what I am eliminating?

What am I eliminating that is good and what am I eliminating that is not?

What am I holding on to that is good and what am I holding on to that is not?

How am I stopping the elimination of what is good for me?

What can I do to let go of what is harmful to me?

How can I increase my acceptance of what is good for me?

The above questions will help you to take a clear look at what is happening in your life. Once we can see what we have to do, it is only a matter of time until we achieve it. Conscious recognition and acceptance is the first step.

THE ELIMINATIVE CHANNELS

If we imagine the thin crust of earth which sustains life on the edge of our planet, we become aware of the life under the earth's surface, which sustains the growth of plant life which makes it possible for us to live on this planet.

The bowels

Let us, for a moment, imagine the billions of worms, tunnelling and burrowing their way through the earth. This great network in constant motion beneath our feet makes the soil rich and loose. They nourish the soil that nourishes every living thing on this planet.

After expanding your consciousness to include the global activity of these billions of worms and offering thanks for all they contribute to the life we enjoy, turn your attention to your gastro-intestinal tract and imagine the tube that goes through your body as if it were a great worm, passing nutrient through our system. This is our great connection with those humble tireless servants of the earth.

Although doctors, surgeons, anatomists and pathologists see the insides of man's bodies, they never relate the toxic accumulation in the bowels to the cause of disease in any practical way. It is essential to face the reality of body cleanliness in all its aspects and to comprehend the relationship between toxicity and disease. Even the personality changes when the bowels are clean. Irritability, impatience and other difficult behaviour problems are greatly relieved when the bowels are functioning properly. It remains only for each individual to experience the reality of these words in their own bodies.

One hears the most amazing rationalizations for constipation, and very rarely anyone stops to imagine what it might be like inside the body where fermenting putrefactive matter is allowed to stay in a warm temperature. Yet chronically ill people will say things like 'Every other day is normal for me' or 'I go regularly twice a week, and have for years'. Abnormal function is accepted as normal and other symptoms such as flatulence, foul odour, distended stomachs, diverticulitis and colitis are rarely associated with constipation. Many people rely on daily laxatives, pessaries and enemas, thus further weakening the bowel. Even regular eating of bulk foods such as bran will not necessarily clear impacted faeces.

One of the great values of iridology is that it shows us the relationship of bowel toxicity to disease. Bowel pockets, radials, defects and weak connective tissue all contribute to health problems. The fabric of malfunction must be unwoven if we are to enjoy good health. For centuries medicine applied the most violent and drastic purges and laxatives with serious side effects. However, we now utilize safe, gentle and balanced treatment to restore proper function, cleanse toxicity, relax bowel spasms, tone the muscles, heal the colon walls and adjust the micro-environment so that fermentation, parasites and flatulence are discomforts of the past.

Iridology shows how bowel toxins affect the entire body due to the distribution of the toxins via the blood and lymphatic circulation as well as through reflex nerve irritation. There can be no cure if the bowel is flooding toxins into the body on a regular basis. The bowels must function regularly at least twice a day, and preferably three. Although most people eat three or more times a day you will rarely find a person who moves their bowels three times a day. High levels of health and vitality depend on a pure blood stream, colon cleanliness and regularity of function. Also, if the bowel walls are covered in a toxic mucous lining, only a limited amount of nutrient reaches the blood stream. Therefore, people feel hungry and eat excessively in an attempt to alleviate that hunger, opting for instant stimulants, like sugar and coffee, as their fading vitality needs larger and more active boosts. When the bowels are clean and functioning properly a simple diet of vital wholefoods will provide excellent levels of energy needed without strong stimulants.

The bowels in the iris

The bowel signs are centred in the first major zone. Look for bowel pockets, defects, radii soleris, prolapse, and changes of the basic colour and shape of the bowel area. The relationship of the bowel shape to the ANW is very close, as the nervous and digestive systems work intricately together. The bowel is either the key to a healthy body and a clean blood stream, or to toxicity and disease. Cleansing and regeneration of the bowel is an essential requirement for healing. If it is not functioning properly as an eliminative channel, it will be a major contribution to any disease pattern.

Treatment indications

One of the best ways to get to know your bowels is to lie on the floor with your knees up and gently knead your abdomen. Start at the bottom right side of your groin where the ileocaecal valve opens from the small intestine into the ascending colon. Feel if it soft, hard, lumpy or tense. Press as deep as possible, without causing discomfort, and then work your way up the ascending colon to the hepatic flexure, under the bottom of the right rib cage and then across the transverse colon under the diaphragm. When you reach the spleenic flexure gently knead your way down, noting all the tender, hard, or lumpy areas. As treatment progresses you will find these areas soften and release. Eventually your abdomen will be relaxed and clear from obstructions.

It is helpful to know where your bowel pockets are. Iridology gives clear indications and reflexology can corroborate its findings, revealing the tender, tense, reflex congestions on the feet which relate to the same areas on the iridology iris chart. If it is possible to have a series of Reflexology foot massages when you are working on restoring your bowels they will hasten the healing process.

The two pillars to bowel rejuvenation are the bowel formulae and the castor oil pack. Other treatments and additional techniques mentioned below are helpful and applicable to individual requirements.

Bowel Tonic 'A' - (see Appendix I) Because these formulae need to be adjusted according to response they are best kept separate from other herbs. The average dose is two capsules immediately before eating. There are sensitive individuals who may only need one capsule per day and others who need up to 30 or even 45 per day for a short period of time before their impacted faeces are released. Some individuals also seem to fluctuate between diarrhoea and constipation so that the dose needs to be adjusted every day. Individual reactions need to be worked with until the system stabilizes. Eventually the person becomes more aware of how they are affecting their bowels with food, mental attitudes, and emotional anxieties.

It is important to understand that the formulae are more than a laxative. They stimulate peristalsis, relax tension, heal, tone, offer superior nutrient, adjust the microenvironment, balance constipation and diarrhoea, and equalize circulation. The various herbs in the formulae combine together for total bowel cleansing and rejuvenation. The ultimate goal is not dependence, but complete healing so that the formulae are no longer required. Because this formula contains golden seal it should not be taken indefinitely. Give it a break at three months, or alternate with formula 'B'.

Psyllium seed Psyllium seeds form a bulk which moves through the colon like a broom, sweeping away faeces as they press into bowel pockets. Take one or two teaspoons psyllium seeds or husks depending on body weight, one to three times a day or as needed.

Bowel Tonic 'B' - (see Appendix) This herbal combination was created because there was a need for a formula which would work as well as the other bowel tonic, and yet would not rely on continued use of golden seal, which is contra-indicated during pregnancy and should not be taken over long periods of time. Happily, this formula, which has been well tested, achieves the positive results of Bowel Tonic A without continued use of golden seal. Dosage is adjusted according to response, and it combines well with or can be alternated with Bowel Tonic A. Bowel Tonic B is excellent for combined treatment of bowel and liver.

Diet to improve bowel function It is important that diet be corrected so that each person has a regular intake of fresh fruits and vegetables, grains, nuts and seeds. These contain adequate fibre as well as the vitality and nutrient necessary for healthy living. The addition of two tablespoons of olive oil a day will also be beneficial. Adequate liquid intake is important, otherwise the faeces will be dry and constipating. Two glasses of hot liquid herb tea or lemon water taken on rising will help to stimulate bowel activity. It is best not to drink with meals, so that digestive juices are not diluted. Proper chewing habits mix the saliva with food so that the first processes of digestion set the stage for the correct progression of food through the gastrointestinal tract.

Treatments

Heed nature's call. When the urge comes do not postpone moving your bowels. Travelling, work or study environments as well as unsocial attitudes towards bowel needs during school years causes poor habits. We have to break these habits and reactivate normal functions. It is good to take exercise after meals and especially important not to go to bed on a full stomach. Chronic cases will be assisted by alternate hot and cold sitz baths, which will stimulate peristalsis and encourage the flow of energy and circulation.

Another effective treatment is the cold abdominal pack. This wet cloth pack activates and relieves digestive organs by increasing circulation. Moisten a light cotton cloth (100 per cent natural fibres only), wring it out in cold water, then wrap around the abdomen twice from groin to chest. Then wrap or tie a 100 per cent wool cloth twice around to cover. Leave in place about an hour and a half every evening. This seemingly simple naturopathic pack is more powerful in its effect than you can imagine. It is also very helpful to sluggish kidneys. These methods prove themselves. When you find what works for you, you will have aids you can use to keep yourself well. The advantage of trying these methods is that you will learn how to adjust imbalances before they become chronic.

Diarrhoea

Most forms of diarrhoea are caused by a mucous coating which has built up all along the colon walls. Because this has become solid, the colon walls are not able to absorb moisture, so the faeces are thin and watery and move through quickly. Other forms of diarrhoea are caused when the bowels are activated by infection or irritation. Even though diarrhoea is evident is it important to give regular small doses of the bowel tonic so that cleansing processes can continue. Usually the castor oil pack is too strong for a chronic diarrhoea case. As the diarrhoea improves, increase the dose of the bowel tonic, and try the castor oil pack when bowel function is more normal.

The following suggestions need to be tried until the right one matches the right person.

1. Meals of stewed apples with very high doses of cinnamon, alternated with baked potatoes, are an excellent means to slow down the force of diarrhoea.
2. Make a quart of mullein decoction and sip regularly until relief is obtained. Drink one half cup after every bowel motion.
3. Make a tea of slippery elm, comfrey, mullein, red raspberry, witch hazel or ginger and take regularly throughout the day.
4. Periwinkle tea, drunk twice a day, is an effective astringent.
5. Take a capsule of bayberry powder every one half hour until relief is obtained, along with two capsules of iceland moss taken every hour.
6. A rectal infusion of witch hazel tea will act as an astringent, helping

to stop the eliminative force that has gone out of balance.
7. The biochemic tissue salt Ferr. Phos. may also be taken three times a day.
8. Whenever there is a feeling of draining downward, homeopathic Sepia may be indicated.

The eliminative forces are a very real energy. They are activated daily after rising and usually expend their force about noon time. The yogic term 'apana' describes this downward energy, which must be kept in balance or the body becomes depleted, the assimilation of nutrient is impaired and the person suffers discomfort and debility. Diarrhoea must be cured before healing can proceed.

Recommended reading
Tissue Cleansing Through Bowel Management, Bernard Jensen; *Colon Health,* Norman Walker; *The Colon Health Handbook,* Robert Gray; *Herbs of Grace,* Farida Sharan.

The lymphatic system

The best way to visualize the lymphatic system is to imagine all the cells of your body floating in a sea of pale clear liquid. Whatever is life giving is accepted, but toxins or foreign invaders are attacked and eliminated. The cleansing processes of this boundless sea of lymph continue day and night. Stimulated by physical movement, breathing and intestinal pulsations, the lymph fluid pulses towards the centre of the body along tiny pearl-like strands, each one a miniature heart, eventually passing through larger channels into the lymph glands. Once purified it is returned to the venous river that flows back into the heart. Eventually it finds its way into the tissues again when it is lost from the capillaries.

As the lymph system is a mysterious, mostly unknown aspect of anatomy and physiology, it is important to understand and visualize it because it is our main line of defence against infection, viruses and the invasion of microbes. When we know how it works for our benefit, we can also learn to support and care for it so that it may serve us well.

First and foremost the lymphatic system functions as a **drainage system** for body tissues, flushing all the by-products and wastes of metabolism. When this function is impaired, the collection of toxins marks the beginning of disease.

As a **defence system**, the warning devices are the appendix, the tonsils, the peyer's patches in the small intestines and the adenoids.

Although lymphatic fluids move through all the tissues of the body except the central nervous system, they collect in the lymph nodes in the groin, the underarm and the neck where the lymph is purified. Here the lymph nodes manufacture antibodies to fight infection and filter the lymph fluids to remove impurities, toxins and old blood cells. The lymphatic system is constantly at work to reduce excess catarrh, mucus secretions and waste. It acts as a collector and purifier of spent blood flow and assists and supports the kidneys in retrieving and eliminating toxins. The endrocrine member of the lymphatic system, the thymus, secretes 'T' lymphocytes which stimulate organs to secrete a substance which attacks the proteins of tumour cells and foreign cells.

Wherever blockages of the lymphatic flow occur, whether due to mechanical reasons, injuries, damages due to severe high fevers, acid/alkaline imbalances, inherited weakness or incorrect living habits, lymph stasis must be overcome so that it can contribute its valuable purification and protective function.

The lymph system in the iris
The lymph system is seen clearly in the lymphatic zone of the iris next to the skin zone in the ciliary edge. This zone shows imbalances in a variety of ways: as a lymphatic rosary, as individual lymphatic tophi in organs or other areas and as grey, yellow, orange, brown or black abnormal colours indicating the level of encumbrance and malfunction. Nerve rings which run through the lymph zone indicate that muscular tension is inhibiting the flow of lymph. The sodium, calcium or hypercholesterol ring can cover over the lymph zone with transparent to opaque white colouration. Also, whenever catarrh and mucus collect in the circulatory zone next to the ANW this is an indication of impaired lymphatic function. Check the iris areas for groin, underarm (axilla), neck, breast, adenoids in the nose, tonsils in the neck, appendix in the caecum area, and peyer's patches in the small intestines. The area for the thymus is found in both eyes near the sternum. These are all important parts of the lymphatic system and should be assessed if immunity is weak or the person is suffering from lymphatic disorders.

Note the colours of the lymphatic markings, remembering that white indicates an active exudative state, grey means underactive, yellow definitely sluggish, and brownish markings a clearly toxic condition of chronic malfunction.

Treatments
With the treatment of any eliminative channel, the important first step is to realize that iridology clearly shows you which of the channels needs support. For example, if both the kidneys and the lymphatic system are weak, it is proven that each adjusts more quickly when both are treated together. As each of the eliminative channels is brought into clarity of function and harmonious attunement with the others, the body will be kept clean and clear on a daily basis and toxins will not be allowed to accumulate.

The lymphatic formula activates the leucocytes, purifies the blood and lymph, and stimulates and equalizes circulation of both blood and lymph. The lobelia acts as a catalyst and a thinking herb, drawing the herbal formulae to areas of congestion so that balanced communication is restored. Other useful formulae listed in the Appendix are the chronic formula, antibiotics naturally formula and the infection formula.

Diet to assist the lymphatic system Diet recommendations make potent and powerful additions to any treatment focused on cleansing and activating lymphatic fluids. The mucus-free diet and the juice fasts will relieve the lymph system, as will the purifying diet (see Appendix V). Dairy foods must be eliminated from the diet of the lymphatic constitutional types who suffer from chronic or reactive lymphatic exudations.

It is also important to be aware that you are taking in enough fluids on a daily basis and that regular exercise moves the lymph around the body.

Massage and exercise stimulate the movement of lymph. While any massage is effective, skin rolling, lymph massage and reflexology (especially around the toes and ankles) are particularly useful. The addition of aromatherapy oils offer direct absorption into the lymph system, and results can be very quick if the circulation is active. This is especially important for bedridden patients who cannot exercise.

Any local swellings of lymph glands can be relieved by the application of herbal poultices, particularly the swollen glands formula, made up of two thirds mullein and one third lobelia. Support this external treatment by the use of internal lymphatic herbs listed above.

Kidneys

Balance and discrimination are the fundamental energies of the kidneys. They work to maintain the acid/alkaline balance of the blood and to eliminate waste. They also seek to harmonize the influences of the right and left sides of the body, in response to right and left brain, and the masculine/feminine principles.

On the subtle levels these organs represent decision-making, the weighing, sifting and discriminating processes that constitute preparation for choice. We are the sum of our choices. Just as the kidneys decide from moment to moment what will be eliminated and what will be retained, so our minds constantly lead us to choose one thing or another.

The astrological sign Libra perfectly depicts this weighing, adjusting, balancing process, so sensitive, so easily shifted by the addition of anything new. Justice is depicted blind, while the scales adjust the weight of innocence as opposed to guilt. The kidneys work ceaselessly, quietly, seeking always to maintain equilibrium, so that the essential body processes can go on unhindered. What a task they face with all that we do every day!

Acupuncturists connect kidney energy to the emotion of fear. When fear is excessive it is common that a person loses control of their bladder. The kidneys are said to contain the substance which is the source of life and development from conception, maturation through to old age. The kidneys are called the 'root of life' because they hold the underlying material for each organ's existence and the balance of yin/yang.

The kidneys work to filter and purify the blood, removing up to 500 grains of waste matter every 24 hours. If their functions are not complete you will feel depressed, tired, restless at night and perhaps suffer lower back pains. Also, whenever urine is scanty, too frequent or you feel thirsty all the time, or never want to drink, kidney function must be considered. If there is excessive urination there is too much sodium, and if there is fluid retention there is not enough sodium. Balanced nutrition is essential to proper function. Also, both left and right kidneys need to be brought into balance.

Kidneys in the iris
Kidney iris areas very often show large lesions called **medussas** and **radials.** They also appear as white inflammatory, or sub-acute with grey shading. Inherent weakness or kidney lesions need to be carefully assessed and constitutional weaknesses evaluated. Look for lymphatic tophi in the kidney area. Congestion of lymph or insufficient blood circulation to the kidneys will cause problems. Also evaluate the condition of both left and right kidneys. Often one is compensating for another, thus overworking while the weak kidney is hypoactive. See whether nerve rings point to the kidneys and note also where they start. Psora spots on the kidneys will indicate diminished function and radii soleris or bowel pockets in the kidney zone will reveal toxic accumulation and negativity. Observe whether the radial in the brain's inherent mental or anxiety zone is also showing a marking. Radials, lacunae, bowel pockets and radii soleris, which weaken the kidney, may also affect the adrenal glands. If so, treat the adrenal glands as well.

Treatments
It is essential to work towards restoring kidney function from the onset of treatment. If they look chronic or constitutionally weak use the kidney formula. If a major formula is not needed, support the function with waterbalance tea. When the functions of the other eliminative channels are restored, the kidneys will be relieved. Diuretic herbs remove wastes from the blood, maintain the action of the kidneys when impaired, lessen irritation of the genito-urinary tract, dilute urine, relieve the distress of uric acid by their flushing action, soothe and heal inflammation and alter morbid conditions with antiseptic action. They also increase the flow of urine by stimulating kidney cells and improving blood and lymph circulation to the kidneys.

The kidney formula is a balancing, strengthening and nourishing herbal treatment. It is important that it be taken between meals, on an empty stomach, with a cup of water, so that the herbs are taken directly to the kidneys.

Herbal infusions of these herbs, singly or in combination, will also benefit the kidneys: uva ursi, buchu leaves, parsley root or leaves, clivers and couchgrass.

Strong decoctions of any of the above herbs used as foot and hand baths will also influence the kidneys by direct assimilation into the blood stream. Herbal treatment of the skin and lungs which are closely associated to the kidneys and water balance will assist kidney treatment. As it is important that the kidneys receive adequate blood supply and nourishment whenever the heart and circulation are weak, they will also need to be treated.

Liquid taken in drinks and foods must provide sufficient fluid for the kidneys to do their work. If there is not enough fluid, it will be drawn from elsewhere, thus depleting other organs. The bowels, for instance, could become dry, causing constipation, or the lymph may become thick and congested. Both lung and skin respiration would also suffer from insufficient liquid.

Other helpful therapies include acupuncture, reflexology, lower back massage and ginger poultices over the kidneys. Osteopathy and chiropractic would relieve structural imbalance and help restore nerve function to the kidneys. The cold abdominal pack described in the section on the bowels is a valuable naturopathic treatment as it increases the circulation of the blood to the kidneys.

Lungs

From the moment of birth two muscles begin working and they never stop until we die. These two muscles are the diaphragm which causes the lungs to expand and contract, and the heart whose beat measures out our life span. We can only hold our breath for a short time and then we must breathe or die. The incoming waves of air must reach the cells of our body to support basic life processes and the outgoing breath is essential to our eliminative processes. This rhythmic interchange, the drawing in and release of the breath of life, provides the oxygen and the pranic energies which vitalize the body processes.

The lungs also draw in vapour and circulate through the body until it is eliminated through the pores of the skin as perspiration or as vapour released during exhalation.

As your body responds to purification and regeneration treatments, it becomes lighter, clearer and cleaner. As obstructions are released and tensions relax, breathing becomes deeper. The body loosens and allows the ceremony of breath to take place without resistance. The more sensitive and attuned you become the more you merge into a state of oneness with the spirits of the air and the more ecstasy you experience with every breath. Sight, sound and fragrance also enhance the experience. So much is happening at every moment if we only have the time and inclination to open ourselves and participate in the full experience.

Time slows down until each breath becomes an infinity; you feel that you can live on breath, that it would be enough. States of uplifted consciousness are so beautiful. One wishes they could last forever. The more fully you breathe, the more sensitive you become. The very air is filled with spinning light radiations which vibrate throughout your body. Everything melts into one field of dancing energy. You become a transparent being, aware of the sea of prana which flows within and without.

Imagine every animal, bird, insect, every living thing breathing in and out every second of every day. Over and over we learn the lesson that consciousness is everything. We can breathe for years, never noticing or rejoicing and then one day in a meadow, on a mountain top, in a yoga class, or making love, the universe opens up and we become aware of the radiant energy that flows through and between all living beings and everything in the world they live in. Even though we return to rush through our lives, the memory is there. It has left an imprint, and in quiet moments when we return, the path is clearer and quicker each time.

In acupuncture the lungs, called 'the tender organs', are associated with grief and sadness. Physically, they provide the descending inhalation and the propensity for disseminating the air throughout the body.

Practices like meditation, pranayama, yoga or tai chi awaken us to the sacred qualities of breath and fill us with gentle loving awareness for the process that is taking place every moment of our life. Whenever consciousness expands and we re-experience the beauty of breath taken in full awareness, give deep appreciation for this gift of life and the blessings of vitality, energy and power that it floods throughout your being.

Lung signs in the iris

A variety of iris markings reveal information about the condition of the lungs. Inherent weakness shows up as open or closed lesions combined with colours from white to black. Observe whether a bowel pocket or radii soleris magnify the condition by sending toxins to the area. Reflexive fibres (whether swollen or pink) reveals increased levels of irritation. Observe the condition of the absorption ring, the shape of the ANW, the lymphatic rosary. Are there nerve rings, psora or dark spots? How wide is the scurf rim in the lung areas? Medulla markings must always be considered because of its function as the respiratory brain. Observe the differences between the left and the right iris. Often the iris bulges out at 3 o'clock on the left iris, 9 o'clock in the right iris, extending a thin grey shadow over the sclera. Dorothy Hall seems confident that this is related to vitamin B3 insufficiency. The decrease of the shadow has been observed during eliminative and systemic purification and regeneration. Over the years lung cancer patients have either displayed black spots in the lung area or no visible sign. It is clear that observation of many cases would be needed to draw general conclusions. Each case should be considered individually.

Treatment

Often the lung area does not need specific treatment until it becomes active. All the herbal formulae benefit the lungs as circulation, lymph, nervous and digestive functions are improved. However any active condition needs support, with an emphasis on minimizing the aggravation and assisting the process of elimination without allowing infection. Any active or severely chronic lung case, however, should use respiratory herbs along with systemic and eliminative herbs.

The respiratory formula is excellent. However, it is necessary to complement its action by adding the asthma formula which loosens and expels thick mucus, and the antibiotics naturally formula which activates the immune system. These herbs, in combination with the individual eliminative and systemic formulae, work wonders with the strongest cases of asthma and respiratory difficulties. A mixture of two thirds slippery elm and one third lobelia in a poultice will relax the chest and relieve the pain and congestion. Likewise six to twelve drops of lobelia tincture or antispasmodic tincture in comfrey tea releases brachial tension and relieves spasms. Elecampane is a specific herb for the TB bacillus. Even if patients are using drugs, the use becomes less urgent as the herbs detoxify and increase natural elimination. The drug dose can be diminished and often eliminated. It is also important to feed the medulla (the chest brain) with sulphur foods, such as lecithin, amino acids, onions and garlic.

Because posture and muscular conditions are so intimately connected with how we breathe, it is important to receive balancing and restorative treatment with some of the following therapies: osteopathy, chiropractic and Alexander technique. Acupuncture works on restoring balance and allowing the 'tender organ' to free itself from its burden of grief so that the lungs augment our life energy, not inhibit it. Techniques like rolfing free the muscle restrictions and allow more space to breathe. Rebirthing helps to release emotional breathing patterns constricting us from our earliest memories. Any therapy which deepens and expands breathing, including gentle aerobics, rebounding, dance or jogging opens us to receive more life, vitality and prana. Yoga, tai chi and chi kung are excellent exercise methods to restore breathing power.

Sore throats can be effectively treated by making this delicious syrup. Mix the following ingredients in proportions to suit your taste. Although some of the ingredients have a strong flavour, their blending neutralizes the therapeutic essences into a pleasant and soothing drink. Make a big pot and sip it throughout the day.

Ingredients: apple cider vinegar, pressed garlic, honey, lemon, grated ginger, cayenne pepper. Simmer in water and serve warm. Gargle, then swallow.

Thyme tea, which is highly antiseptic, is also an effective aid for sore throats. Drink several cups a day.

Skin

If we see the body as transparent, we can no longer perceive the skin as being only a container for our body. We can visualize our body's inner world of pulsing, muscular churnings, vibrant fluids, digestive chemistry, and cellular metabolism. You might have seen the film which was made about the male and female reproductive processes from a tiny camera placed inside the body. This miraculous filming of the colourful, spectacularly beautiful body processes was a visionary experience which is hard to forget. We can use these visualizations to give us understanding and respect for the body in which we live.

In your mind start an imaginary journey. Become a drop of blood which has been sent out from your beating heart, ready to begin a long journey around the body. Using an anatomy and physiology book for reference, imagine the journey in all its complex manifestations, travelling through organs, being dispersed outside a capillary and eventually finding its way back through the lymphatic system. It takes only a few moments, yet offers a wealth of understanding as it reveals the living interactions that often go ignored in more traditional forms of learning anatomy and physiology. The body is exquisite living poetry.

Once the inner world comes alive, visually surround it with skin that is filled with a multitude of openings, which allow sun, air, warmth, moisture, and energy to be absorbed into the vibrant, pulsing, inner world. Then imagine radiating eliminations pouring out in the form of gases, moisture, heat and energy.

How soft and gentle this absorbing and diffusing process is determines to a large extent how we relate to the world. Attitudes of fear, tension and rigidity limit our interaction with the environment and our fellow human beings. When we are transparent the inner and outer worlds become as one. We neither protect ourselves from the outer world nor resist interaction.

These skills of visualization may also be applied to stimulate the healing process. If we have become identified with a disease and its pain or symptoms, we often feed that process with fear as we surround the area with negative thoughts and tensions. If we can mentally surround the area with loving thoughts, covering any darkness or disease with light and energy, the forces of healing will be manifested by the increased levels of blood, lymph and pranic energy.

Our body does not stop at the skin. Immediately around the skin is a world composed of a variety of subtle energies, micro-environments, radiations, and a heat envelope. Here, bacteria and other micro-organisms, both protective and potentially destructive, thrive. Bathing and elimination habits affect the health or disease patterns of this heat envelope.

The molecular aura, which extends a few inches out from the body, contains keratin (skin) particles, tiny salt crystals, ammonia and other organic materials and gases. These fields, which seem to be interwoven with each other, also contain electromagnetic energy composed of infra-red radiations or heat. Variations in the heat patterns reveal valuable information about the state of the various areas or organs of the body. A field of pure electric potentials reflects changes within physical and psychological makeup, giving indication of both present realities and potential problems. Professor Harold Burr discovered relationships within this field to the electromagnetic variations in the sun, magnetic storms, sun spots, and solar and lunar variations. Changes in electrical potential also occur during ovulation.

The etheric or health aura also extends outwards from the body, enclosing each of us in an egglike shape of energy, colour and light. Although not all of us are able to see this aura, we can feel its presence in various ways. The aura acts as a blueprint for our bioelectronic energy system and our physical body. It contains the chakras, the nadis, the pranas and the acupuncture meridians. These patterns form a subtle communication system that distributes energy throughout the physical body, in close connection with the endocrine glands. The etheric body can vary a great deal in colour, shape and structure, depending on food, emotions, mental and spiritual attitudes, practices and karmic destiny. When the vitality is weak, inherited miasms held in the vibratory patterns of the etheric body are able to penetrate the physical body.

We have a close connection with this field which encapsulates our body. When we open ourselves to it we receive the energy it dispenses. Practices like tai chi, meditation, yoga and other forms of mental, physical and spiritual discipline form harmonic relationships with this body field. Martial arts masters reach such levels of perception that they can literally see through the back of their heads and are able to sense an opponent's strike before it happens.

Emotional and mental energies also constitute the realities of the energy fields around our physical body. We do not end at the outside of our skin. To know ourselves we can expand our vision inward and outward until we can visualize our total reality. We are a microcosm within the macrocosm.

The iris reveals a great deal of information about this body envelope. It can show the hard, sharp defined edge of someone who surrounds themself with metaphorical armour, or the soft, receptive attitude of someone who accepts interaction and relationships in a welcoming way. Often, those who carry the dark, thick, scurf rim find it hard to be in the present. Because they are carrying a heavy load it burdens all that they do.

As we learn to soften and open ourselves, our body develops more subtle strengths and attitudes to protect us in this complicated and difficult world.We do not have to harden our body edge like armour so that we cut ourselves off. When we do that we also cut off our ability to love, to feel and to give. Natural bodily functions related to receiving and releasing through the skin are also inhibited by tension, fear and resistance.

Like the lungs, the skin performs a dual role of respiration and elimination. If either of these functions is diminished the whole body suffers the consequences. If our skin was sealed off, or painted for a short period of time, we would die, yet today, most people wear synthetic fibres and sleep in synthetic bedclothes. Chemical and synthetic creams, lotions, makeup and deodorants are also in common use. Bathing habits do not always include skin scrubbing to remove dead skin. One only needs to experience a skin scrub, taken in conjunction with a Turkish bath, to realize the joy of a truly clean skin. The fresh glowing feeling lasts for days.

The skin has millions of pores from which a constant stream of gases and toxins flow. Moisture is secreted to adjust the body temperature. If the pores are blocked, toxins collect under the skin, and then are reabsorbed back into the blood lymph. The skin is often called the third kidney and any diminishment of skin function burdens the kidneys. Also, when the kidneys are weak, active skin elimination will relieve them.

In Germany, nature cure centres offer Kneipp Water Cure treatments which usually include a 'continuous shower'. For over two hours the patient lies in a tiled room, turning every five minutes or so from back to front, or side to side, so that a light, warm shower reaches all parts of the body. This causes the capillaries to release sluggish toxins. The feeling of well-being and relaxation is remarkable. Patients sleep deeply in total relaxation and wake completely rested. The benefits last nearly a week. Imagine how valuable this treatment would be to bedridden patients whose basic body functions have slowed down due to lack of exercise.

The skin on the feet is also very important. The constant wearing of shoes creates callouses and corns. When we appreciate the wisdom of reflexology or the Metamorphic Technique we learn how any area of the foot which does not have soft, fully functioning skin will both affect the reflex areas and tell us about the condition of that area of the body. A healthy foot is clear of callouses and corns. Daily pumice scrubs (and chiropody when required) are essential for good health.

We can learn so much from our skin. Sensitive healers, osteopaths, massage therapists, acupuncturists and doctors all read messages from variations in temperature, moisture, colour and hair differentiation. Homeopaths, oriental doctors and practitioners diagnose from the facial colours and lines. Studies have been made for centuries based on the lines in the hands. The skin often rebels with rashes and pimples when it is eliminating toxins. Severe skin diseases are a reflection of complex and chronic functional imbalances. Skin markings and discolourations caused by the liver, warts, even freckles, become lighter, and in many cases disappear during purification regimens. Menopausal skin discolourations fade when the woman's body becomes clean and active under treatment. The condition of the skin reflects the condition of the organs and systems.

The skin in the iris
The skin zone is on the ciliary edge of the iris. When it is sluggish, inactive or has collected toxins it shows up in varying shades of grey, brown and black. The darker and thicker the zone is, the more toxic and inactive the skin. When this zone manifests small dark spots, the condition is even more serious. Scurf rims in infants register the degree of inherited toxins. During life they deepen as a result of incorrect dietary and living habits. Childhood diseases are the body's attempt to throw off inherited toxins, and often the scurf rim is left after the illness. Change of climate can make considerable differences to scurf rims. Cold northern climates, where people wear more clothes and are able to expose their skin to air only for short seasons, increase the scurf rim. The opposite is true of warm climates.

Treatment

Choose a quiet time when you can be free for an hour to enjoy rest and rejuvenation. Set the stage for yourself with love. Light candles and incense, bring in music or a book, and if you are the meditative type, let yourself float away and forget the world.

Pour a hot bath, as hot as you can take it. If you suffer from heart problems or high blood pressure, adjust the temperature to suit your personal situation. While the water is running, give your skin a thorough dry brushing. Brush in circular motions, always moving from the periphery of the body towards the centre and the heart.

Epsom salts/cider vinegar bath Add a cup of the commercial variety of Epsom salts, (not the fine expensive internal brand) and a cup of apple cider vinegar. This bath is both eliminative and relaxing and leaves the skin feeling smooth. Mix a tablespoon of vegetable oil in the cup of Epsom Salts and then rub it all over your skin while you stand in the bath. This removes old skin, leaving it smooth and soft. Let the salts fall into the water. This bath is essential when you are on intensive purification programmes. Soak at least 30 minutes. Use cold cloths on your head and neck to help keep you cool. Add hot water as needed to maintain the bath temperature. Complete the treatment with a cold shower, for at least three minutes. Whenever you are in eliminative baths it is helpful to drink stimulating teas which encourage free perspiration from the skin. While yarrow is the strongest, sage, catnip, pleurisy root, peppermint and spearmint will also be effective.

Herbal baths There are various forms of herbal baths:

1. Lobelia – very relaxing, gives an excellent night's sleep
2. Catnip – relaxing and soothing, excellent for children
3. Chamomile – gently relaxing, uplifts the spirit
4. Capsicum, ginger, mustard bath – stimulating, warming; equalizes circulation to overcome chills, colds and flus.

If you have had a very hot bath it is necessary to cool the skin, close the pores and balance hot with cold. You can either pour cold water into the bath while the hot is running out, take a cold or cool shower or splash yourself all over with cold water and walk around naked for at least 5 minutes. If you wish to produce copious perspiration to eliminate the onset of a chill, colds, fevers or flu, go directly from the hot bath to a very warm bed with quilts and hot water bottles. This will encourage profuse perspiration.

If you use oils and lotions, make sure you do not put on your body anything that you would not eat. The body absorbs everything that is put on the skin and has to assimilate or eliminate through its body systems. Almond oil mixed with coconut oil, jojoba oil, and avocado oil makes a beautiful body lotion, especially when you add aromatic aromatherapy oils. Take particular care to pumice any old skin or callouses from your feet, then rub the feet thoroughly with natural oils.

After a bathing experience like the above, it is an excellent and natural time to do exercises, yoga, foot reflexology, deep breathing and meditation.

Saunas, Turkish baths, health clubs There are more of these establishments available now due to a revived interest in health and self care. Saunas and steams are effective for eliminating toxins, stimulating the circulation and relieving tense muscles. Scrub your skin while taking the sauna or steam and make sure you take cold showers or plunges to balance the heat expansion which draws blood to the periphery of the body. The cold sends the blood back to the interior of the body and alkalinizes the blood, making your head feel awake and clear.

Skin elimination When the body throws off toxins through the skin, rashes, lice, pimples, eczema and psoriasis may occur. These are unhealthy conditions which are the result of toxic blood and a body whose eliminative channels are not working properly. Sulphur is also eliminated through the skin. When these conditions are a part of the healing process they will not last very long, usually up to three days. They should never be suppressed.

Herbal infusions and formulae To complement sensible natural living habits and to revitalize skin function, drink diaphoretic teas to stimulate elimination. Excellent teas taken individually, or combined, are sage, yarrow, thyme, catnip, sassafras, sarsaparilla, boneset and pleurisy root. Fenugreek is a herb which activates deep cleansing through the skin. Simmer the seeds very gently for 15 minutes or pour boiling water over fenugreek powder and stir. This herb is also a rare vegetarian source of vitamin D.

   Nourishment is an essential aspect of healthy supple skin. The following formulae will provide the wide range of nutrient to preserve and maintain youthful skin when combined with eliminative and systemic treatment and correct living and eating habits. Both blood circulation formulae will carry the skin or body building formulae throughout the body tissues. The liver/gall bladder formula and the blood purifying formula will help to ensure that toxins are not eliminated in the skin. Whenever there are boils use burdock, two to eight capsules three or four times a day, as well as the systemic treatment.

Itching can be relieved with chickweed ointment, chickweed baths or Balm of Gilead ointment. It is very important not to use suppressive treatment. Treat the cause of the condition from within.

Chapter 5

Restoring Harmony

The purpose of interpretation is to select the outstanding, significant markings. The next step is to determine the relationship and the effect that the significant markings have on each other, and at this stage it is important to understand the interaction of physiological processes.

Thus each body system is seen in relation to every other system and affecting and being affected by every other system. The living ecological processes of the interior world are in constant movement, change and interaction. If one system is hyperactive it may drain resources from other systems; if it is underactive another system may have to work harder to compensate. The permutations are infinite. Every case of arthritis, or any other disease, is different. This is why treatment based

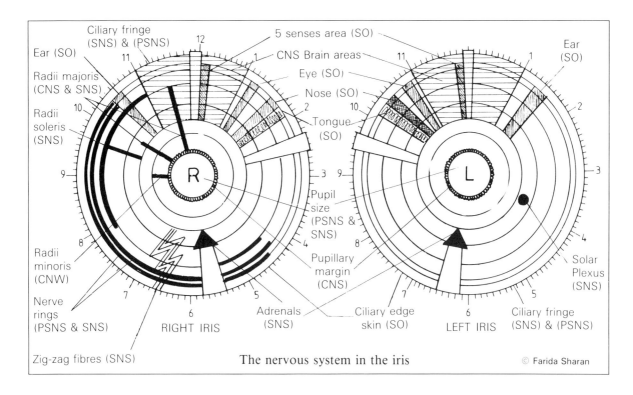

The nervous system in the iris

© Farida Sharan

on individual iridology analysis is so successful.

The aim of treatment is to restore harmonious function so that every part of the whole is doing its work and is in open communication with every other part. Treatment does not have to fight disease. If treatment restores harmonious function disease will not be tolerated. Disease cannot exist in a properly functioning body.

THE NERVOUS SYSTEM

The nervous system – holistic relationships

The nervous system operates from the centre outwards and from the periphery to the centre, connecting every part of the body with every other part.

The structural system provides the framework for the nerves to pass through to every part of the body, and holds the central nervous system in the brain and spinal cord. Any pressure of the skeletal bones on nerves will inhibit the flow of messages, and cause pain.

The nerves pass through the muscular system and provide the sensory means of touch sensation all over and through the skin. Damage to any part of the body tissue will also be damage to some of the millions of nerve pathways, and so the seemingly infinite complex messages will be transmitted to the brain to be acted upon. Muscular response to motor impulses also creates movement.

The circulatory system including the heart is closely governed by the nervous system both from sympathetic/parasympathetic balance and the medulla.

The endocrine glandular system responds to brain messages in the higher centres such as the pituitary and the pineal, and then to the messages these glands pass down. This is a response system to the discriminating brain function of the input of environmental information, both inner and outer.

The adrenals are closely connected with the sympathetic nervous system, reacting, like the solar plexus, to mental and emotional stresses. As the adrenals secrete hormones which excite the body to fight or flee, continued stress will exhaust the body.

The reproductive system, closely allied with the glandular system, is guided in a similar manner by high brain messages and hormones secreted in response to those messages.

The solar plexus unites the digestive and nervous systems. Study how the sympathetic and parasympathetic activate and relax the digestive system in alternation. We have all felt how 'nerves' affect how we eat, chew, digest and eliminate our food.

In the urinary system we can see how the sympathetic and parasympathetic contract and dilate the bladder. The adrenals of the endocrine system sit on top of the kidneys, showing the close relationship.

The respiratory system is closely attuned to the nervous system via the medulla, the 'respiratory brain', which governs respiration, heart and vasomotor function.

The lymphatic system is everywhere in the body except in the central nervous system. Congestion of obstructed lymph may press on nerves and cause pain. Messages via the nervous system will stimulate local healing by the lymphatic system. The lymph system supports the function of the nervous system by cleansing and nourishing tissues and protecting the body from infection.

The nervous system – our communication network

If the nervous system is depleted, exhausted or out of balance, the communications system is not working properly and the whole being suffers, physically, mentally and emotionally.

Because iridology gives such accurate, in-depth readings of the condition of the various parts of the nervous system, practitioners who use iridology achieve good results. If the nervous system is deficient, no matter how effective treatment may be for any other symptom, results can only be marginal and temporary. Health is the result of open and responsive communication from each part to every other part. No part can be neglected or overactive if harmony is to reign.

Consider the nervous system in its various aspects:

1. The peripheral nervous system (PNS) and the sense organs (SO) relay information to the central nervous system (CNS).
2. The central nervous system (CNS) discriminates and acts on all impulses which reach its central computer.
3. The autonomic nervous system (ANS) responds to both inner and outer stimuli, from the inner and outer worlds. It seeks to balance the activity and response of the sympathetic nervous system (SNS) to outer activity, with the rest, maintenance and preservation of the internal environment activated by the parasympathetic nervous system (PSNS).

It is easy to see that failure of one or more parts of the nervous system creates immediate imbalances with far-reaching effects. It also becomes clear that certain personalities and their approaches to life are actually built around imbalances of the nervous system.

Constitutional types

The nervous system in the iris

The Lymphatic blue irides reveal nervous weakness in the Neurogenic Type, the Anxiety Type or the Zig-zag Fibre Type. Haematogenic brown irides reveal nervous weakness in the Anxiety Tetanic Type.

Supplementary signs and colours

Whenever supplementary markings or colours point to or augment the above nervous system indications, they are a significant factor in the interpretation.

For example:

1. *Radii soleris:* Whenever Radii Majoris break through the autonomic nerve wreath (ANW) the function of the ANW is impaired. If the Radii penetrate the brain area, sense organs or the adrenals the nervous system will be directly affected in that area. Radii from the pupillary margin reflect degeneration of the CNS. Radii from the ANW reflect degeneration of the ANS.

2. *Reflexive fibres* Swollen or vascularized (pink) reflexive fibres in the brain or spinal areas, sense organs or adrenals will directly indicate hyperactivity or irritability of that part of the nervous system.

3. *Inherent weakness lacunae:* Whenever connective tissue is weaker, particularly where it allows the collection of toxins or where it is directly related to brain areas, sense organs or the adrenal glands, the nervous system will be insufficient.

4. *Pigmentation:* Pigmentation on iris areas relating to any parts of the nervous system will indicate possible insufficiency of that area, although some patients express active symptoms and others may not. The insufficiency may exist only as a potential, to be activated during stress, trauma, shock or old age.

5. *Lymphatic tophi:* The only part of the body which does not have lymphatic fluid is the CNS. However, excess, toxic or deficient lymph in any other part of the body can affect the nervous system. Irritable focus areas which register other indications of nervous weakness will also have lymphatic tophi nearby. In this case it is another indication of the progression of disease as its influence radiates out from the focus.

6. *Defect marks:* These small but potentially potent marks are activated during shock or low mental and emotional states, especially depression or hopelessness. The marks affect the ANS because they sit on and break through the ANW in the iris. Communication is broken at that point.

7. *Bowel pockets:* Because bowel pockets affect the quality of the ANW (nerve connections being an integral part of bowel wall tissue) they can greatly inhibit nerve function and even cause deterioration of nerve tissue. Other parts of the body can also be affected by reflex communication and the spread of toxins via circulation of the blood and lymph.

CENTRAL NERVOUS SYSTEM (CNS)

Brain zones in the iris

Vitality or life force zone

This brain zone encompasses the hypothalamus discriminating activities, the cortex, pituitary and subtle psychic energy and spiritual

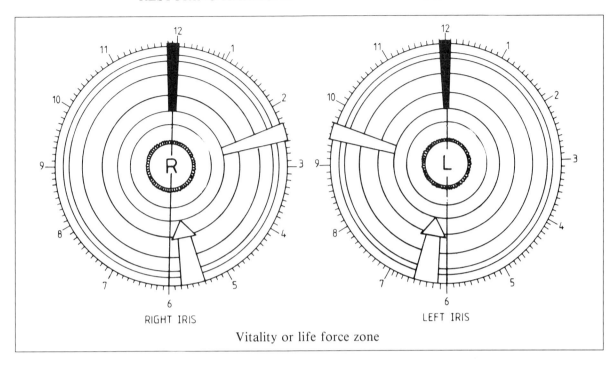

RIGHT IRIS

LEFT IRIS

Vitality or life force zone

centres. Hyperactivity is recognized by whitening of the area, which may be accompanied by headaches or a hot head. Depletion is measured by varying shades of darkness in lacunae, radii soleris, psora, lymphatic tophi, defects and ballooned bowel pockets. Reflexive fibres and nerve rings also denote irritation. Observe whether there is a marking opposite at 6 o'clock which would give a reading on polarity relationships of grounding one's life energies. The Sodium Ring and/or Arcus Senilis or the Anaemia Ring would diminish vitality levels, as well as memory and concentration.

Observe both right and left irides to relate the markings to each other.

Markings on one side only would be related on the right iris to outgoing activities and attitudes and on the left to inner ones. One could almost say that the right iris relates to the Sympathetic Nervous System activity as it represents outgoing activity. The left iris relates to the Parasympathetic Nervous System because it represents inward responsive attitudes.

When normal activity is evident the balance of vitality and fatigue would be monitored and adjusted daily. Appetite, interest and emotions would be kept in balance. When stimulated beyond normal levels, this area contributes heightened state of exhilaration, vitality and fullness of life. Abnormal hypoactivity leads to obsessive morbid mental states, including melancholia, suicidal tendencies, depression, indifference and deep exhaustion.

The brain area also relates to the will and impulses which create our destiny. It certainly represents the central core where prana and life

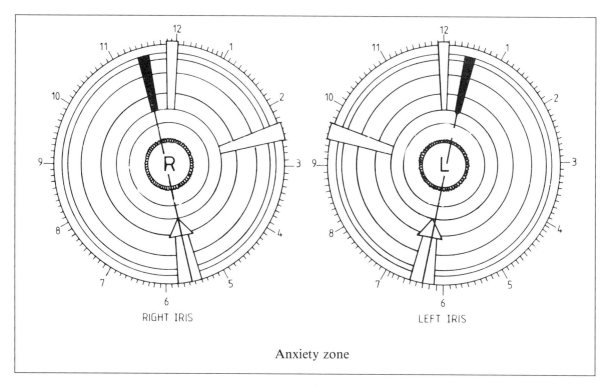

Anxiety zone

energy penetrate the physical body. This is where the young baby has a soft membrane at the top of the skull which eventually closes over. The design of this skull pattern forms the ancient scarab of the Egyptian religious mystical culture.

This is the most important functional area of the brain because it is related to metabolism and energy levels.

Anxiety zone

This brain area is on a radial opposite to the adrenal area. Whether there are markings in both areas or not, the best understanding comes from this potential relationship. Mental and emotional anxiety and conflict patterns accompany negative manifestations of radii, lymphatic tophi, nerve rings, lacunae, bowel pockets, psora, reflexive fibres etc. Whether the problems are obsessions or hallucinations, the result is over-indulgence in conflict and worry, and added stress for the adrenal glands. When the radial is evident in both areas the pattern of behaviour is chronic and compulsive.

An early iridologist, Dr Kritzer, believed that the Right Inherent Mental Area manifested as apprehension. These extreme states of fear and worry were brought about by toxic or inflammatory irritations. The left iris was related to introspection. Mental states of self-analysis and self condemnation, when accompanied by iris lesions, develop into acute melancholia, prolonged brooding and worrying over mistakes which deplete the vital life force and reduce the individual to negative

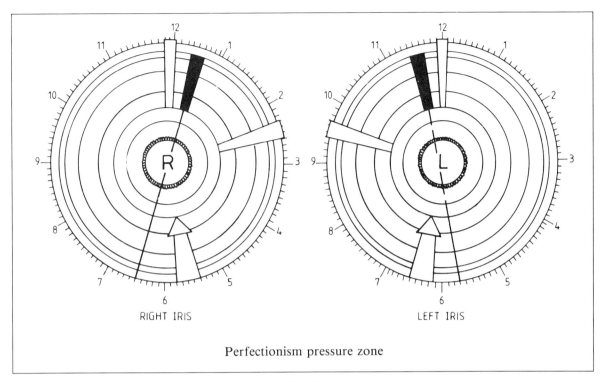

RIGHT IRIS

LEFT IRIS

Perfectionism pressure zone

mental and physical states. The weakened mind becomes receptive to negative impressions and the mind goes over them again and again.

Positive types manifest courage, confidence, optimism and an independent original spirit which enables them to lead successful lives.

Perfectionism pressure zone
This brain area governs blood pressure, regulation, decision-making, psychological stress reactions, sexual activity regulation and ideals and goals, their achievement or non-achievement, and how we pressure ourselves about them. Obviously a lot of mental and emotional energy is invested in ideals and goals. They are the motivating factors in the most worldly activities. One's sense of self and how we pressure ourselves to achieve our dreams is the issue here. The blood pressure relationship is a defence against stress.

In its positive aspect this brain area encourages all the qualities needed to achieve goals and ideals, and bring them into dynamic expression. The radial on the right iris leads to the appendix area. It is well known that most cases of appendicitis occur during times of stress. Extreme pressure can lead to strokes, haemorrhage or blood clots.

When hyper- or hypoactive, the desperate qualities generated by greed, desire or lust manifest. Obsessive, compulsive behaviour and tense, rigid goal directed lifestyles are the result. The individuals are driven by their desires and lose the essence of their achievement because they are unable to enjoy their success.

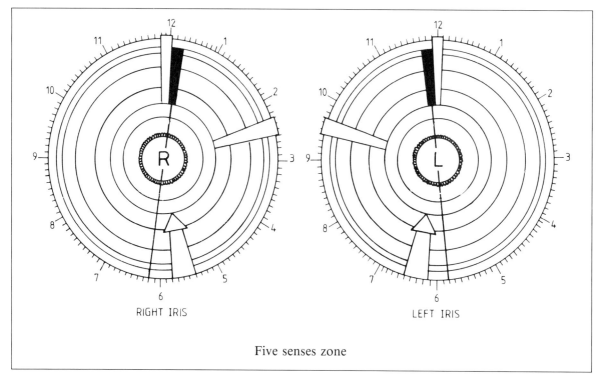

Five senses zone

Five senses zone

This brain area in the cerebral cortex controls normal visual, auditory, olfactory, gustatory and tactile senses. When healthy, the individual enjoys the beauty and fullness of life in colour, sound, smell, touch and taste.

In heightened positive states it augments senses, as with the musician or blind person whose auditory and tactile senses are more acute. When hyperactive it can lead a person to overindulgence and hedonistic practices. Hypoactivity can be the cause of sensory handicaps or impaired sensation, self denial, guilt, severe disciplines and criticism of those who enjoy life. This could lead to anorexia.

Sensory motor zone

This mid cortex sensory motor area coordinates how our senses guide us to stand and move in this world. Therefore it works hand in hand with the five senses zone. This area integrates mental and physical functions and controls movement.

This area influences all the things which guide us to know where we are, sensations of heat, cold, pain, touch, pressure, movement, tension, etc. It also affects the more subtle functions of perception and reactions to sound or light. Muscle coordination, strength and fatigue levels are also governed by this area.

When abnormal, the person suffers from lack of coordination and inhibited movements. The mental state is fear, uncertainty and lack of confidence.

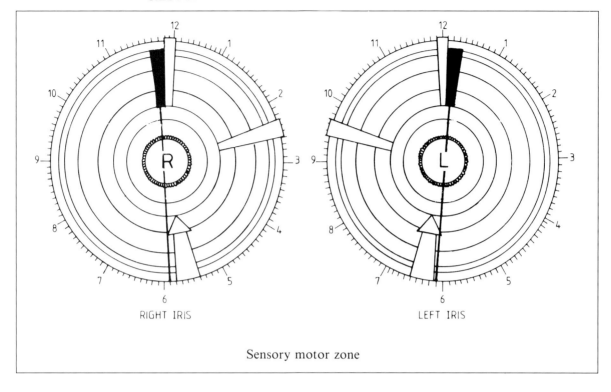

RIGHT IRIS

LEFT IRIS

Sensory motor zone

Listening, learning, speaking zone

These brain centres are in the forebrain, the pineal and pituitary, the cerebrum and the thalamus. The zone is the brain's communications centre and combines speech, listening and visual learning approaches.

During normal activity the brain function which accompany speech, language, memory, concentration and their accompanying skills are all active and functioning. This area determines how we function within our family, work and society.

When heightened, many of the finer intellectual capabilities of man manifest themselves. What drives us to communicate is the key here, as well as desire for knowledge and the urge to transcend normal states of being with creative absorption.

Imbalanced function can lead to impairments such as dyslexia, stuttering and inability to concentrate as well as lack of interest and forgetfulness.

White signs indicate that the person has 'the gift of the gab', either positively as a speechmaker and teacher, or negatively when the person endlessly talks about nothing, or gossips, whether people wish to listen or not.

Lesions show that stress load has been too much. This often means that after a normal day's activity the person may be too tired to talk. Dark fogs indicate a closed mind that blocks seeing, hearing and speaking. Sodium rings inhibit learning because of poor memory, tiredness, lack of concentration and the ability to persevere.

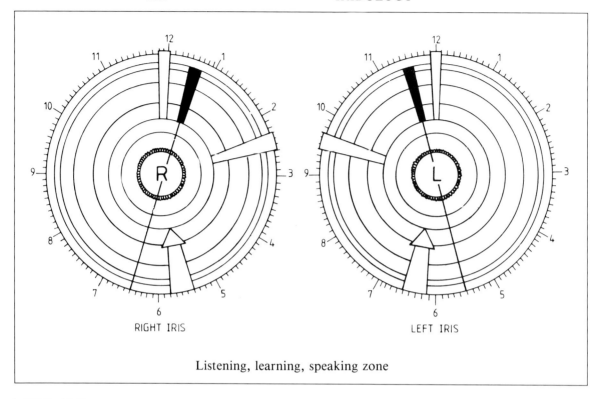

RIGHT IRIS

LEFT IRIS

Listening, learning, speaking zone

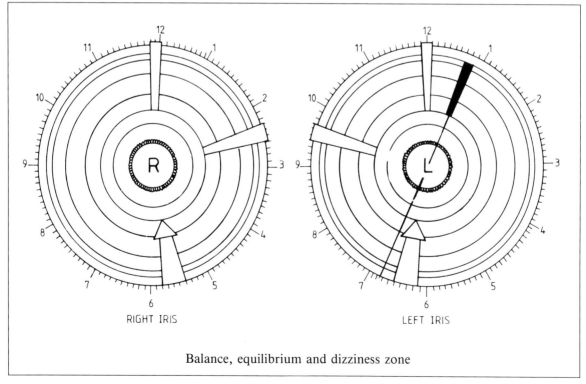

RIGHT IRIS

LEFT IRIS

Balance, equilibrium and dizziness zone

Balance, equilibrium and dizziness zone

Contained in the cerebellum, this brain area governs equilibrium in its physical, mental and emotional aspects. Epilepsy is indicated by black radial lines suggesting severe grand mal, dark radial lines showing milder, less frequent attacks, while dark spots denote petit mal or nocturnal epilepsy. Injury is marked by small black spots.

When heightened it manifests qualities of higher mind and well-being such as discrimination, balance, stability and security – in short what we all seek; the balanced centre within oneself.

When hyper- or hypoactive physical symptoms can be acute and may include multiple sclerosis, epilepsy, dizziness and inability to stand up straight. Also look to the inner ear when these problems occur. Radials connect to the uterus/prostate/vagina/anus/rectum areas. It is interesting to note that epileptic seizures are relieved by enemas and the relaxation of the anal sphincter.

Creative intelligence zone

This brain area is in the prefrontal and frontal lobes.

When normal it encourages intelligence, logic, reasoning, memory and will power. It also affects voluntary movement.

Many fine, creative, intelligent, clever, critical, exact and sensitive qualities thrive in this brain area during heightened activity. A plenitude of creative and artistic abilities are included here.

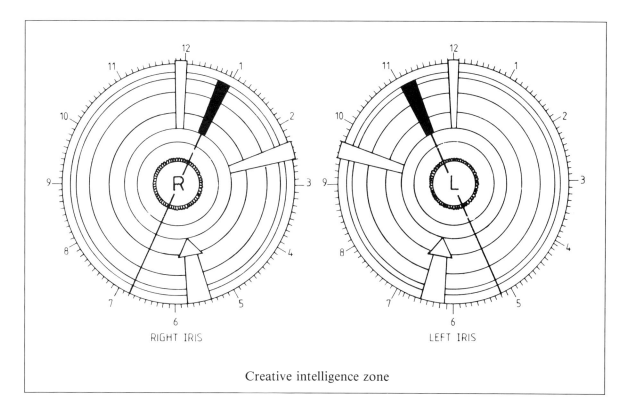

Creative intelligence zone

When out of balance inspiration is blocked, tension dominates mental processes, negativity takes root, and perverse tendencies are encouraged.

White signs occur when students are cramming for exams or they can indicate the mentally active 'quick to learn' types. Radii Soleris reveal that one's abilities are inhibited and there is a lack of perseverance. Students never finish studies and they are doomed to failure. Similar markings will keep a person in a low job without hope of advancement.

Dark signs indicate suffering from mental frustrations and dissatisfactions because they have been stuck in jobs below their potential for so long that apathy, sluggishness and negativity have taken over. Lesions develop if these conditions reach chronic stress levels. Sodium rings indicate that the person is functioning at a lower capacity than their potential and brain functions are inhibited because of lack of circulation.

The radial relationship between the mental ability zone and the pelvis reflects the choice between the dominance of either mental or physical life. Some individuals can achieve a balance between the two with effort, but most succumb to either sexual life and its attendant responsibilites, or the intellectual or spiritual life.

In Polarity Therapy the 'six pointed star' pattern represents the male energy which has its base in the pelvis and its peak in the forehead. The forehead point is this mental ability area, showing the relationship between the positive and the negative aspects of this polarity balance of

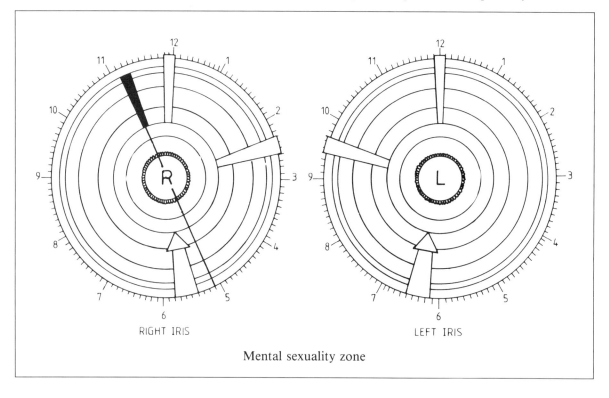

RIGHT IRIS

LEFT IRIS

Mental sexuality zone

the mental as opposed or balanced by one's choice over sexual life.

Mental sexuality zone

Located in the pituitary gland, the cerebrum, hypothalamus and limbic system, this brain zone governs sexual attraction, repulsion, responsiveness, preservation of the race and reproduction.

When heightened it can amplify sexual relationships with fantasy, excitement, creative imagination and bring out many fine, high and noble states of mind.

When abnormal, sexual obsessions, perversions, indulgence and competition take hold. Natural instincts and sweet loving relationships are forgotten in the manifestation of negative states of mind. Sex is either used as a battlefield or there is complete apathy and disinterest.

White signs indicate overactive mental states of fantasy and imagination. Yellow/brown signs show that the individual is overcompensating for not accepting their honest sex drives, therefore they live in a false reality of delusions, hallucinations and fantasies which do not become reality. Lesions show weakness where women are ruled by their sex drives, producing baby after baby, or men making conquest after conquest are unable to control their impulses. The sex area is also affected by the adjacent inherent mental area where anxiety and fear can override sexual feelings and inhibit natural love and caring.

Sexual excesses lead to mental insufficiency. Constructive or creative thought depends largely on taking care of one's vital force, not wasting it. Control over sex impulses frees the energy to develop other areas of being. When there are lesions showing that creative sex or mental force lack vigour, it could be regained by return to proper living. Perversions include stealing, kleptomania, rape, murder etc. or masochistic-sadistic relationships where natural love is replaced by hate, jealousy, hurt and relationships based on dominance. Whenever hallucinations occur they can affect or relate to any of the five senses, so it is important to check those areas as well, both the five sense brain area and the local areas for ears, eyes, tongue, nose and touch.

Radials point the way to strong illusions and delusions, and whether the line is white or dark will help determine more specifically how the person is affected. The radial to the uterus/prostate/vagina reflects the choice or drive of the individual to discriminate and control sex impulses.

Medulla

The medulla at the top of the brain stem is known as the 'respiratory brain' which controls respiration, coughing, hiccoughs, sneezes, swallowing, vomiting and salivation, The heart and vasomotor centre are also affected. The diaphragm is important because of its involvement in breathing, sneezing, hiccoughing, vomiting, and coughing. All these functions are survival and balancing mechanisms aimed at the preservation of vital functions.

White signs indicate a well controlled individual, that the head is telling the body what to do. Perhaps the control may be too great,

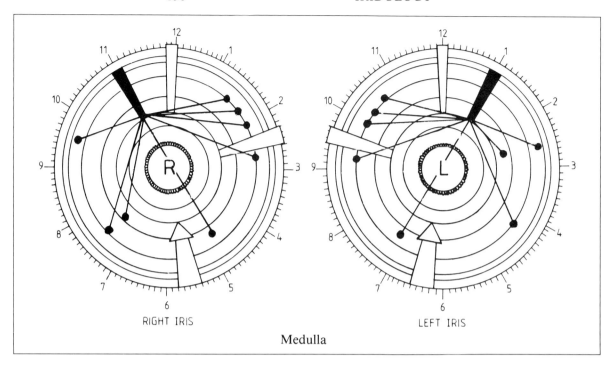

RIGHT IRIS

LEFT IRIS

Medulla

therefore tension occurs. Yellow/brown signs warn that there is a fault in the system, and that the signals to the body are low in power. The body is ruling the head. Cervical adjustment can help to stimulate the medulla, but purification is also essential. Alexander technique will improve posture and muscle tone, and rejuvenation with diet and herbs will help to rebuild the area. Lesions are a result of inherent weakness, or compression, physical trauma and stress. Stretch the neck out to release and free the area.

Medulla/bladder radials indicate that medulla pressure or insufficiency has affected bladder functions. Radials from pupil or ANW to the medulla area indicate involvement of the nervous system and bowel toxins spreading via the lymph and circulation.

When abnormal, many physiological symptoms can occur affecting the above function. Look at the medulla whenever there are iris signs in the lungs, chest and bronchials. The medulla is often damaged in difficult births. Osteopathy, chiropractic and Alexander technique can complement internal treatment guided by iridology.

Sense organs **Treatment of the five senses**
Whenever there are symptomatic problems with one or more of the sense organs, after checking out the 'Five Senses' in the brain zone, look at the specific iris areas (eye, ear, nose, tongue and skin) and consider their condition based on the display of any of the following markings: radii soleris, lacunae or lesions, reflexive fibres, lymph tophi, defect marks, nerve rings, bowel pockets, psora.

The key to all treatment is to work at cleansing and balancing the eliminative channels and the weakest major body systems. This will reduce the irritation and allow the body to adjust itself. With each of the four senses in the head area, adjustment of cervical vertebrae will activate and free the nerves to carry their impulses and reduce venous congestion. Also, it is essential that circulation of blood and lymph to the brain area is adequate. Proper intake of vital foods, minerals and vitamins is also important.

Eyes

The eye wash is an excellent stimulant, healer and nutrient. Make an infusion of eyebright, golden seal, bayberry and red raspberry with one eighth part of cayenne. Poultices of cucumber will also soothe irritated eyes. Eyebright tincture is a convenient eyewash to brighten and refresh the eyes. Stimulate the energy by working on the foot reflexology points. The eyes (Aries energy) are the positive pole of the digestive fire (Leo) particularly the Liver, and will reflect digestive problems. Local treatment is not enough. Release the body from the poison of accumulated toxins, and give it superior nutrition. It will heal to the highest level possible, when it is given the support it needs. Use foods high in vitamin A.

Ears

Whether the problem is lack of hearing, pain, inflammation or discharges, the treatment with mullein and garlic drops is very effective. The mullein gets absorbed into the lymphatic glands, and stimulates them to deal with the infection, and the garlic is antiseptic. If poor hearing is the result of the hardening of the body, improvement will only come as a result of the systemic treatment. Again, foot reflexology is useful, especially of the two small toes.

Nose

Blocked nose, polyps, sinus congestion, mucus and catarrh must be dealt with at the systemic level. When the nose becomes an eliminative channel, congestion has reached unacceptable levels. During a healing crisis it may register as a white marking. Take rose hip tea, vitamin C and garlic. Treat the lymph system as well as toxic digestive congestion.

Tongue

Whenever the sensation of taste is gone, or the person suffers from dry mouth or excessive salivation, systemic treatment is required. Imbalances of this sort are signs of the progress towards chronic disease.

Touch

The peripheral nervous system on the outside edge of the body is purely functional in terms of the nerves themselves and the brain centres. Loss of touch is due to strokes and paralysis. Treatment to restore sensation has to be intensive, encompassing all aspects of water cure, massage, physiotherapy, as well as accompanying treatment such as acupuncture. Dr Christopher talks about cases such as these in his pamphlet, 'The Incurables'.

Ability to touch and feel is strongly dependent on vitality, enthusiasm and activity of five senses zone. Tension levels, fear and shyness also inhibit one's ability to feel, accept and enjoy touch.

Pupillary margin

The pupillary margin represents the CNS because it is a sphincter muscle made up of posterior pigment cells, from the embryonic development of the CNS. The degenerated condition of this pupillary margin signifies the deterioration of the CNS. The darker and wider the ring appears the more advanced the deterioration of the CNS. This is also known as the Pupillary Zone, Stomach Ruff, Neurasthenic Ring, Assimilation Ring or the Pars Iridica Retinae.

While this pupillary edge has a lot of different names given by iridologists in different ages and countries, the basic facts are the same.

Its normal colour is a reddish brown. The narrower the ring, the healthier it is. Ideally it should be a thin even line in a smooth circle. Psychologically, the pupillary border represents our inner world which reacts to emotions. Disturbed markings indicate that we do not have control over our emotions, or that we are obsessed with mood fluctuations. Radii Minoris start at the pupillary edge indicating CNS weakness, and end at the ANW. Radii Majoris break through the ANW and the ANS is affected. When they go to the brain areas they indicate cerebral weakness.

Hypofunction of this stomach margin is indicated by flattening down and pulling back of this pupillary ruff, exposing the darker lower iris layers. When the margin is rough and uneven the condition is even more advanced.

Pupillary margin colour indications:

1. A light white raised border indicates excess HCl.
2. A light brown border suggests active inflammation.
3. A dark muddy brown colour is the result of a chronic lack of HCl and suggests a toughened, hard scarred, inactive stomach which has been affected by poor food and drugs.
4. Black indicates a degenerated CNS and chronic hypofunction of the stomach.

AUTONOMIC NERVOUS SYSTEM (ANS)

This dual nervous system requires active participation of both parts to provide balanced function so that the individual can both function effectively, and relax - enjoy leisure, rest and sleep well. The balance of both inner and outer realities is dealt with by the ANS. Some individuals are better at interactions with the world and others have greater

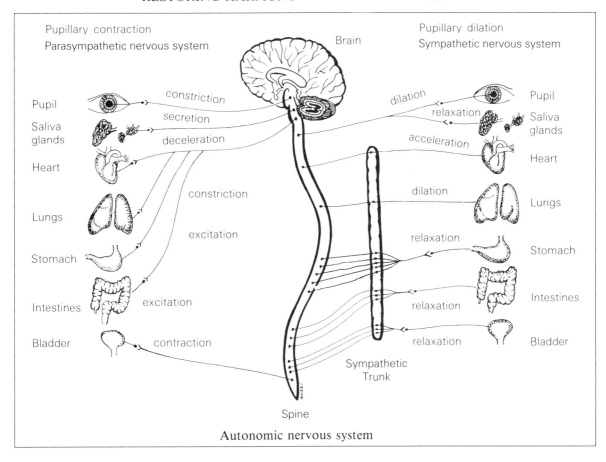

Autonomic nervous system

communion with the inner life. The balance of both, and a healthy functioning ANS is most desirable.

The above figure shows how the SNS dilates the pupil and how the PNS contracts it. As well as this dynamic opening and closing of the pupil, the iris receives impulses which have passed through the thalamus from the various organs and tissues of the body to the hypothalamus. His discriminating centre or control station receives, responds and then acts upon the information as it seeks to maintain the equilibrium of function, homeostasis. Then the nerve impulses travel to the irides via the Edinger-Westphal nucleus and the oculomotor nucleus where the information is thrown up on the iris screen, thereby indicating the condition of the tissues in the various systems, organs and tissues of the body. The selective markings reveal whether the area is normal, inflammatory, toxic or degenerative, as well as the strength or weakness of the connective tissue. The nerve impulses stimulate reflex frequencies which result in the variations of any abnormal markings and colours which appear over the basic eye colour.

Sympathetic and parasympathetic nervous systems (SNS and PSN)

Sympathetic nervous system (SNS)

We are constantly bombarded by stimuli (climate, weather, people, events, work, etc). Our interest and response is determined by the ability of the SNS to deal with this stimulation. Young babies and children who are learning about the world and who enjoy full interaction every waking moment exist for a few years in sympathetic dominance. As long as they can cut off and enjoy deep sleep and rest they will remain balanced, but if not they become hyperactive. If the overactivity continues for too long they run the risk of exhaustion, adrenal weakness and hypoactivity. A white ANW indicates hyperactivity and degrees of exhaustion and hypoactivity are determined by ever darkening shades of yellow, orange, and brown in blue eyes. It is harder to read this in brown eyes, but pupil size also reveals valuable information on the condition of the SNS.

The SNS as revealed in the irides consists of the adrenals, nerve rings, pupil size, zig-zag fibres, ciliary fringe, the ANW and Radii Soleris which break through the ANW.

Parasympathetic nervous system (PSNS)

Aside from the ANS and the pupil dynamics the parasympathetic nervous system can be interpreted from nerve rings. The more nerve rings there are and the deeper they are the less the PSNS has been able to relax tense muscles and restore balance.

Autonomic nerve wreath in the iris Because the wreath contains both sympathetic and parasympathetic nervous systems, we need to look at all the areas to determine the sympathetic signs. However, breaks in the ANW due to radii soleris, defect markings, lacunae and bowel pockets definitely indicate impairment of sympathetic function. Look to the specific areas and the overall pattern of relationships before making your assessment.

The ANW is a self regulating control system which monitors body functions without the need for conscious command. It is a transfer point where two sets of fibres meet, one coming from the pupil and the other

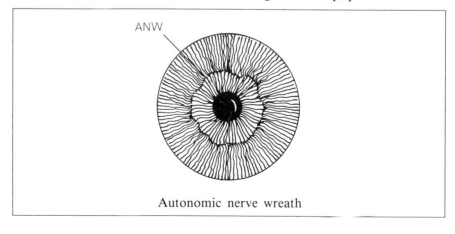

Autonomic nerve wreath

from the iris periphery. The relationship of these sets of fibres is determined by several things: the dynamics of dilation and contraction of the SNS and the PSNS, toxins, inherent weaknesses, inflammatory conditions and specific stress areas.

All the above causes of the shape and condition of the ANW are intermingled due to their integrated relationships. Toxins and inherent weaknesses diminish the efficiency of the ANS response. Inflammation causes irritability and hyperactivity which overstimulates the ANW response. Stress results in SNS dominance. The adrenals are hyperactive until they become exhausted. The individual runs on their nerves, going at high speed due to the activation of the flight or fight syndrome. If we make conscious efforts to balance activity with rest, relaxation, meditation, exercise, sleep and moderate living we can develop a strong PSNS which will balance even the most active SNS. On the other hand, exhaustion, apathy, and depression can cause PSNS dominance. The individual is at the mercy of their body weaknesses because they cannot motivate response to outer stimuli.

The basic shape of the ANW is the result of the rupture of the pupillary membrane which takes place in the last few weeks before birth. At that time the pattern is set, although adaptive variations may occur during the person's life due to constipation, stress and trauma.

The relationship of the ANW to the spinal column is important. It is essential to have free vertebrae movement so that nerve messages are not inhibited. The iridologist will recognize the need for chiropractic or osteopathic treatment.

The relationship of the ANW to the bowel wall is very close because it rings around the bowel on the iris chart. After relating the parts of the ANW to the correct spinal vertebrae you also relate each part of the bowel to the vertebrae. All this information will point the way to accurate analysis and effective treatment.

Adrenal glands

Markings in the adrenal areas on both right and left irides will show us whether these important stress glands are working efficiently. Look for radii, lacunae, psora, reflexive fibres, defect markings, bowel pockets, and also evaluate colours. Notice markings on right or left adrenals and their influence over right activity or left-sided receptivity. Review the section on right/left irides for further clarification of this point.

Nerve rings

Nerve rings reveal valuable information about mental stress, physical tensions, emotional life, pupillary reactions, shocks, accidents, irritation (both chemical and psychological) and mental and emotional patterns formed by the mother and father which help form one's basic attitudes towards life. Nerve rings form a variety of patterns, of varying widths, lengths, depths, colours and distances between the pupillary and ciliary edges. They can stop and start at any place in the iris.

Causes of nerve rings

1. Irritation from toxins, drugs, acids or adjacent areas. Look at the beginning and the end of the nerve ring to trace the cause.
2. Hyperactivity, inflammation and overacidity accompany acute white nerve rings which manifest themselves when an individual is on the verge of a nervous breakdown. At that time rings are more than three or four deep and they are very strong. Sometimes they are close together and sometimes they are spaced according to the circular zones.
3. Lack of iodine in the thyroid produces hypertension, excessive emotional states and nerve rings from the head to neck areas.
4. Poor eating habits and abdominal tension can cause nerve rings in the intestinal tract.
5. Lack of proper exercise inhibits nerve supply and function, due to insufficient nutrition caused by poor circulation of blood and lymphatic fluids.
6. Excessive pupil dilation deepens nerve rings.
7. Injuries, operations, radium treatments and prolonged pain produce nerve rings which radiate out from the focus.
8. Posture and bodily tension. A common nerve ring pattern runs from shoulder to groin.
9. Strong and prolonged mental and emotional anxieties, frustrations, longings and fears produce nerve ring patterns which run down from the appropriate brain areas.

Sources of irritation causing nerve rings

1. Inherited conditions.
2. Drugs.
3. Psora markings.
4. Inorganic minerals from pollution, foods and drinks.
5. Radiation from treatment or exposure.
6. Operations.
7. Hyperactivity, inflammation and pain.
8. Acidic or toxic secretions from a diseased organ.
9. Hypoactivity, toxins, degeneration.

What to look for

Nerve rings follow the same concentric patterns and circular shape as the pupil and iris circles. These rings are the physical manifestation of mental and emotional patterns as well as the results of toxic deposits and injured areas. They always indicate the source and/or the result of irritation in the nervous system and how that affects the body and organ tissues. Accordingly, the iridologist should observe the following:

1. Where the nerve rings stop and start and any other markings at that focus.
2. How deep and light they are and whether toxins have settled in that area.

3. Whether the pupil is large or small as that affects the depth of the nerve rings.
4. How many there are (more than three or four indicate severe tensions).
5. Whether they are stronger or deeper on either the left or the right iris.
6. How close the nerve rings are to the edge of the iris or how far in towards the pupil. The deeper they are the more they affect the workings of the internal organs. Exterior ciliary edge nerve rings affect the function of capillary blood flow, superficial lymphatic fluid flow, and the function of the skin. They can also affect how we interact with the world and other people.
7. More than three nerve rings indicate nerve depletion.
8. Nerve rings in the circulation zone denote nerve enervation.
9. White nerve rings display hyperactivity and inflammation.
10. Dark nerve rings display toxic irritation.
11. Nerve rings at the thyroid reveal hypertension.
12. Nerve rings combined with acute inflammation may suggest muscular spasms.

Nerve ring zones
The iris is divided into seven circular zones. The four outer rings form five zones when divided by four nerve rings. See page 264.

White and black nerve rings
White nerve rings indicate an irritated, overstimulated condition of the CNS, the approach or present activity of a healing crisis or hyperactivity of the brain accompanied by nervous conditions and insomnia. When this condition continues over long periods of time the nerve rings, a reflection of a numb, semi-paralysed state, settle into an atonic state. When this happens the nerve rings darken to grey and eventually black. When the brain nerve rings are white this suggests hyperactivity, irritability, hysteria, insomnia caused by systemic or drug poisons, or mental and emotional imbalances and irritation. Black nerve rings in the brain area manifest after prolonged weakness, prostration, memory loss, numbness, partial paralysis of mental and nervous functions, apathy, regularity or toxicity. These are the unmistakable signs of crystallized mental and physical patterns.

Specific nerve ring patterns

Life force nerve rings When nerve rings radiate downwards from 12 o'clock, the life force brain centre, they indicate mental pressures and anxieties regarding basic vitality. In the right iris the rings would be related to activity, frustration or aggression and in the left iris to fear and lack of trust. Note where they end and correlate the iris interpretations with their psychological patterns.

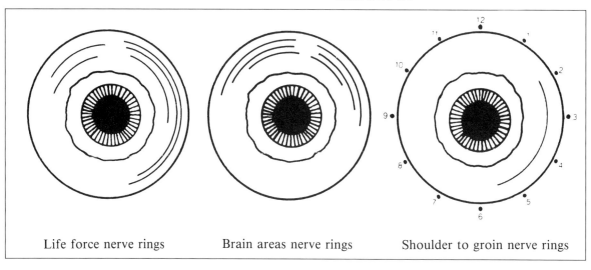

Life force nerve rings   Brain areas nerve rings   Shoulder to groin nerve rings

Brain areas nerve rings Common nerve ring patterns begin in brain zones such as the anxiety, the perfectionism pressure or the balance zone. When extreme these nerve rings can show the cause focus of hallucinations, hyperactivity, mental illness, and severe prolonged anxiety, fear or worry. Treatment relieves the influence of these markings in the iris and releases the patient from their tyranny. In the Soviet Union mental hospitals using iridology and natural treatment have been honoured by their government due to the long term recovery of their patients.

Shoulder to groin nerve rings These nerve ring patterns show the relationship between neck and shoulder tensions and the rest of the torso. Once you start a tension it radiates out and affects other muscles. The way we move and our posture also contribute to this nerve ring patterns. Look to see whether the nerve rings are on both irides. Both mental and physical tensions require treatment and release.

Left iris nerve rings As the left iris corresponds to the feminine principle, the mother and one's basic ground of love and trust in the world and within the family, any resistance indicated by the nerve rings centres around lack of trust, fear, lack of receptivity and suspicion. This protective resistance cuts one off from spontaneous giving and receiving.

Right iris nerve rings As the right iris corresponds to the masculine principle, the father and to how one sets and achieves goals in the world, imbalances manifest themselves as aggression, frustration at not achieving goals, inability to manifest creative activity or blocks towards success. Excessive right-sided activity can also reflect an inability to relax and enjoy leisure.

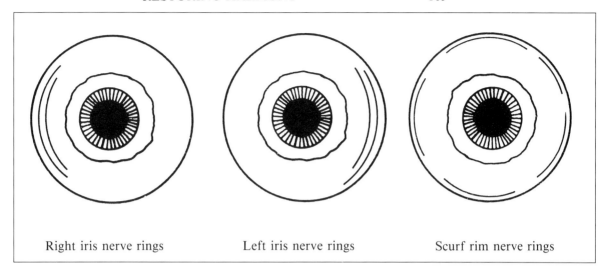

Right iris nerve rings   Left iris nerve rings   Scurf rim nerve rings

Scurf rim nerve rings Whenever nerve rings crowd the ciliary edge of the iris and interfere with the movement of capillary and lymphatic fluids and inhibit the flow of perspiration, it also affects the person's relationship to the environment and social and family contacts. Note whether the edge of the iris is hard or soft. Observe their personality. Are they afraid of touch or do they welcome it and need it? There is much that can be learned from interpreting the scurf rim area in terms of both physical and psychological interaction.

Lymph zone nerve rings The lymph zone functions can be inhibited by superficial muscular tensions indicated by nerve rings. This can cause buildup of toxins, excess weight and fluids. Diminished skin function accompanied by disturbances on the skin itself can also occur. Toxic levels contained within the nerve rings lessen as the system is relieved by increased elimination combined with high levels of nutrient.

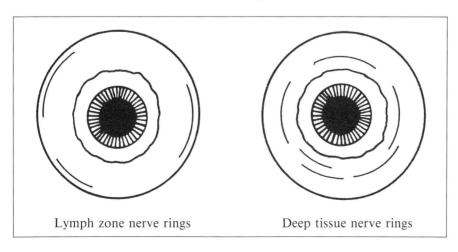

Lymph zone nerve rings   Deep tissue nerve rings

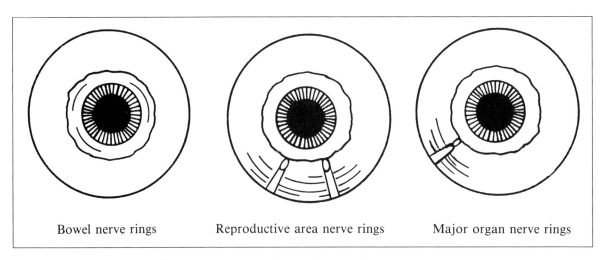

Bowel nerve rings   Reproductive area nerve rings   Major organ nerve rings

Deep tissue nerve rings When tensions have penetrated more deeply into internal muscular tissues, and the nerve weakness is more chronic, nerve rings appear in the inner circular zones. Here, the nerve rings are so much a part of a person's sense of being that they may not even be aware of the tension. Their influence is lessened during systemic treatment and as they diminish the person evolves new patterns of behaviour.

Bowel nerve rings These manifest when irritation from colitis or muscular spasms has reached acute levels of distress. Here the nervous and digestive systems are interlinked and they affect each other profoundly. When these single nerve rings appear within the ANW they are usually quite short. There are excellent charts in Kriege's book, *Iridiagnosis,* which help determine exactly which part of the stomach and intestines are affected.

Reproductive area nerve rings Whether in the breast, ovary, uterus, or prostate, penis iris areas. Nerve rings which point to and accentuate these areas suggest either the tendency to or manifestation of toxicity, tumours, cysts, inflammation and pain. Whenever radiation treatment has focused on an ovary, short nerve rings can point to the area indicating high levels of stress. These fade out as the tissues recover. The chart, above centre, shows nerve rings at the ovary and vagina areas.

Major organ nerve rings When nerve rings stop and start at major organs regard them as serious indications for primary treatment. Only years of experience and a harmonious interaction of scientific and intuitive faculties will enable the iridologist to take the mental leaps necessary to correlate physical with mental and emotional patterns. Each organ has correlations to mental and emotional qualities in addition to their obvious physical functions. The accompanying chart shows nerve rings at the liver area (above right).

If you look at the black markings that I have drawn on the right iris 'A' below, you will see that fibres which come from the pupillary margin meet fibres which come from the ciliary margin. The pupillary fibres meet the ciliary fibres at the ANW. Both the SNS and PSNS are involved. There is a dynamic relationship between them which results in a reflex action. Whenever there is a breakdown of fibres within the pupillary area there is a corresponding breakdown of fibres in the related areas outside the wreath. If the fibres are contracted within the ANW, this pulls the fibres further outside the ANW, and vice versa.

The ANW responds to these inherent weak areas, to toxic bowel pockets, to radii soleris, to tensions, etc. by changing its shape. It either bows out or pulls inward. All these variations in the shape of the wreath must be carefully observed and related to the organs and areas that they point to or away from.

Often only a part of the ANW is dilated or contracted, resulting in an uneven ANW shape. These specific pulls towards the pupil or the ciliary edge are the result of tension, irritation, lack of muscle tone and weak recuperative ability. They are also the result of shock and trauma. The relationship of the bowel wall to the shape of the ANW is integral.

Squaring the ANW indicates that chronic disease is reaching degenerative stages. Severe squaring of all the corners on both eyes can be a sign of approaching death. In many chronic conditions one or more corners are squared.

Whenever the wreath above the transverse colon falls lower than it should, this represents a prolapse of the transverse colon which affects

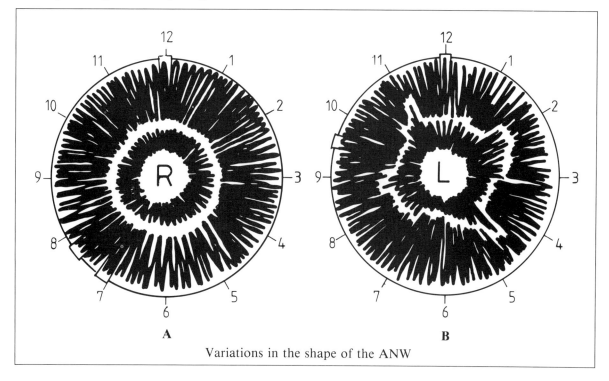

Variations in the shape of the ANW

the brain areas and creates pressure in the lower abdomen and reproductive areas.

Wherever a strong radii soleris breaks through the ANW, coming from the bowel or the stomach, this indicates a breakdown in the function of the ANW. If this break occurs at the 12 o'clock animation life line it could seriously affect the energy level and will of the person. It is also important to correlate the break in the wreath with the vertebrae (i.e. life force at 12 o'clock relates to cervical vertebrae), so that structural causes can be treated.

The PSNS contracts and the SNS dilates the pupil. The sphincter muscle contracts the pupil under direction of the SNS and is supplied by the oculo-motor after excision of the sympathetic urge to dilate. The dilator muscle dilates the pupil under direction of the SNS and is supplied by the cervical sympathetic and trigeminus after paralysis of the oculo-motor. The pupil, which normally rests at 3-6 mm diameter, responds to sympathetic/parasympathetic stimulation with its two antagonistic muscles of accommodation.

The dynamic pulls of the two sides on the ANW determine the irregular shapes that occur in the wreath. The pupillary side reflects the unconscious emotional functions or the will, and the ciliary side is more in response to outer stimuli from the world, i.e. other people, climate etc. In health there is an established harmony and balance between the two. If the wreath is very contracted it means that we are attempting to control body processes with our will and we live in a state of tension, unable to relax. If it is too relaxed then we do not have enough control, and exhaustion, weakness and susceptibility to toxins is the result.

The pupil dilation and contraction affects the size and shape of the ANW and the depth and number of nerve contraction rings. When the pupil is larger, contraction rings are deeper. When the pupil is small nerve contraction rings are pulled straight as they are drawn towards the pupil. When the pupil is large it often obscures the digestive area in the iris, making it difficult to read and interpret the stomach and bowel areas.

The size of the pupil varies when it is exposed to light and darkness, and accommodates itself to tensions, personality, mind and emotions. The pupil size is also influenced by age, when the person may draw away from the world into inward dreaming due to lack of interest in the present and their surroundings. They are larger in youth because of the intense interest in and interaction with the environment.

A weak SNS results in the small tight pupil, the result of dominant parasympathetic control from within. A pulsing pupil, one that tries to adjust pupil size but cannot hold it for long, accompanies a sympathetic nature which is over responsive to the needs and feelings of others.

A large pupil indicates sympathetic dominance, in that stimulation, stress and hyperactivity over long periods has caused atrophy of the PSNS. It can no longer compensate and adjust the pupil back to normal size.

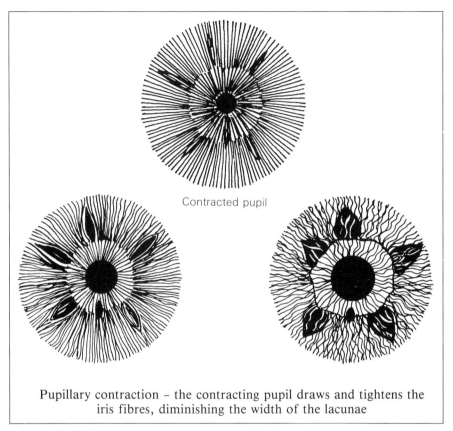

Contracted pupil

Pupillary contraction – the contracting pupil draws and tightens the
iris fibres, diminishing the width of the lacunae

Dilated pupil
The SNS dilates the pupil as a part of the flight and fight syndrome.
When this continues during a long period of fear, pain or stress it leads
to exhaustion of the SNS. This results in a permanently large pupil, a
condition called *vagotonia*. When both pupils are dilated symmetrically
the condition is called *mydriasis*. This sympathetic dominance is related
to adrenal hyper- and eventual hypofunction. This iris condition makes
nerve rings appear deeper because the large pupil pushes the iris towards
the ciliary edge.

Pupils dilate in response to darkness, pain, focus on distant objects,
childbirth, loud noises, diptheria, before epileptic fits, in the later stages
of poisoning, fright, extreme emotion, low mental development,
vomiting, brain anaemia and exhaustion. Short-sighted individuals have
larger pupils.

Contracted pupil
The PSNS contracts the pupil as a part of its function to restore and
relax the body after activity and SNS response. A rigid small pupil
which no longer expands in response to outer stimuli indicates a PSNS
dominance where inner attitudes prevent normal activation and
response because the SNS is weak. This pupil contraction diminishes

nerve rings because they are straightened by the muscles that contract the pupil. Always consider that nerve rings are more serious than they appear when they are accompanied by small pupils. A permanently small pupil is called *miosis* when both pupils are symmetrically contracted.

Pupils contract in response to bright lights, focus on close objects, drugs, chloroform, alcohol, congestion of the iris, venous obstruction, fevers, plethora, paralysis and tension. Far-sighted individuals have smaller pupils.

Anisocoria refers to the condition where pupils display unequal sizes. One pupil could be contracted and the other dilated, or they could alternate in their size differentiation. This is a serious indication which accompanies hereditary venereal disease, diptheria or meningitis. Both Kritzer and Von Graefe associate this iris sign with insanity.

Fluctuating pupils, which pulse large to small to large in alternate dilation and contraction, are due to nervous weakness, past or present trauma and a sympathetic nature which is extremely responsive to the feelings of other people and their sufferings.

Solar plexus
The solar plexus plays a key role in transmitting emotional impulses to the digestive system. In *The Healing Secret of the Ages* Catherine Ponder refers to the solar plexus as a mirror upon which man's deepest, strongest thought impulses are reflected. We experience physical tensions such as butterflies, nausea, sinking feelings and indigestion, but the influence is greater. It is sometimes referred to it as the 'emotional brain' or the 'body brain' because it looks more like the brain than any other part of the body.

Shocks also have a strong inpact on the solar plexus region and unless released will affect changes in digestion which may become permanent. Through the SNS, the solar plexus connects the stomach with the heart and mind, thus acting as a vital receiving and distribution centre. The solar plexus is also connected here via the SNS to the adrenal endocrine glands. Strong emotions are felt in the stomach, and the body reacts to adrenal stimulus. The Chinese regard this area, which they call the 'Dandien', as the centre of 'Chi'. Their systems of exercise, martial arts, acupuncture and philosophy works to strengthen this power centre.

The stomach region, which includes the solar plexus, is the physical reflection of discriminatory brain centres, where we decide what we will accept into our being. The physical functions of selection, digestion and assimilation are a reflection of these mental processes of discrimination. As the Chinese say, the pure is separated from the impure.

This emotional brain is part of the SNS which reacts to fear, stress new experiences or exams. This is often felt as 'butterflies', a 'knot' in the stomach or tension. Before meetings or appearances the person may have diarrhoea or be forced to move their bowels or pass water several times. The relation of the SNS triggers can be quite dramatic.

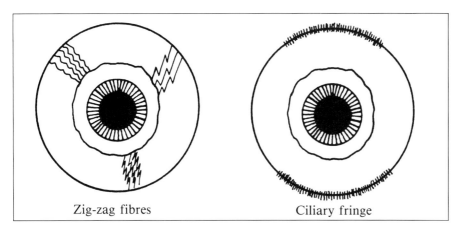

Zig-zag fibres   Ciliary fringe

Zig-zag fibres

Zig-zag constitutional fibres reveal a low tolerance for frustration. These people do not have the strength to fight against oppression or domination from others. They give in outwardly but suffer deeply inside. Their SNS's ability to fight or escape is impaired. They correspond to the Bach flower remedy type 'Centaury' because they find it hard to say no. Instead they give in and give up their own needs. These people need supportive companions around them who are considerate of their needs. They are often attracted to communities for this reason.

Ciliary fringe

Whenever this fringe appears at the head or foot zone it indicates sensitive attunement and vulnerability, or even psychic openness. The SNS needs to be strong to protect the individual from potential invasion. The Bach flower remedy 'Walnut' is useful to increase protection.

The peripheral nervous system

The vast network of peripheral nerves is constantly relating data to the CNS. Disturbances in body fluids, lymph congestion, capillaries, toxins, the scurf rim and the skin zone would impair proper function. The peripheral nervous system is in the iris skin zone.

Right/left iris relationships

When you observe the difference between right and left irides, valuable information is revealed about physical conditions, and related psychological, mental and emotional conditions.

The duality of right and left manifest in the physical body as a result of the pineal and pituitary glands. These glands in the hermaphrodite brain are the first separation into masculine and feminine.

The Chinese see the pineal as the tiger force of will, soul or the pure creative action of the holy man, the focal point for the positive masculine energy of spirit. It finds its outward expression through the right eye and represents the upper brain, and the masculine force.

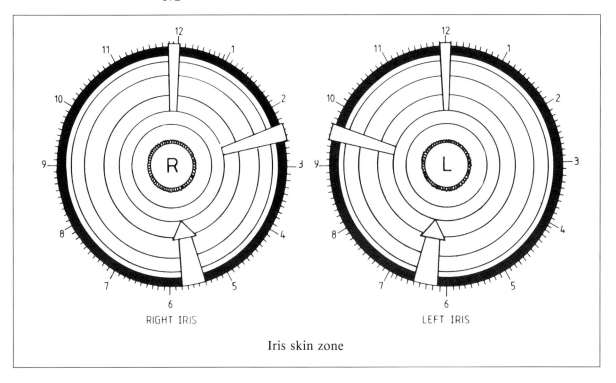

Iris skin zone

The pituitary gland represents the dragon energy, or the feminine personality force as balanced creativity inspired by idealism and imagination. It finds its outward expression in the left eye and represents the lower brain.

The marriage of the tiger and the dragon forces, the pineal and pituitary, results in the harmonious union which is symbolized by the third eye or the birth of Christ conciousness.

The step down of these masculine and feminine energies carried through the right and left irides reflect the qualities and attributes of these primal masculine and feminine forces.

Many humanistic psychology and treatment systems utilize this quality of right and left variables. The feminine left is in harness with masculine right, the two at odds, striving for equilibrium and harmony. The interior masculine/feminine dynamics emerge out of the archetypal male/female energies, our relationships with our father and mother, and control our relationships with men and women in our lives.

Kinesiologists consider the right/left interaction of integral value to harmonious function. The left logic brain governs the right masculine side which reaches out into the world, and the right brain the left intuitive side that receives what the world offers. Muscle testing and exercise like the cross crawl try to balance right and left function so that they cooperate in harmonious balance.

Now that we have established a background we will look at the iris taking all this into consideration:

Right Iris	**Left Iris**
Yang	Yin
Rajas	Tamas
Outward	*Inward*
SUN	MOON
Pineal	Pituitary
Masculine	Feminine
Day	Night
Light	Dark
Outgoing	Receptive
Male	Female
Father	Mother
Worldly relationships	Family relationships
Strength	Weakness
Order	Confusion
Motion	Rest
Cheerfulness	Depression
Life	Death
Fullness	Emptiness
Growth	Retarding
Hardness	Softness
Rising	Falling
Expanding	Contracting
Ambition	Possessiveness
Logic	Intuition
Responsibility	Dependence
Sympathetic nervous system	Parasympathetic nervous system
Creative	Maintaining
Doing	Waiting
Control	Manipulation
Taking	Holding on
Lust	Frigidity
Power	Selfishness
Greed	Apathy
Competition	Passivity, inertia
Aggression	Submission
War	Defence, protection
Letting go	Acceptance
Attacker	Victim
Destruction	Preservation
Activity	Relaxation
Spending	Saving
Hot	Cold
Rage	Lack of anger
Courage	Fear
Fecundating, sowing the seed	Breeding and giving birth

Sattvic balance between right and left irides creates:

Love	Contentment	Harmony	Integration
Communication	Completion	Fulfilment	Synthesis
Health	Understanding	Illumination	Truth
Balance	Being	Knowledge	Communion
Enlightenment	Self realization	Wisdom	Insight

Right-left irides

While it is true that we have the potential for all manifestations of male and female within us, it is clear that various aspects of the masculine or feminine are dominant and recessive in each of us. It is rare to meet a person fully developed in both right and left sides and manifesting a balance of all appropriate qualities. As we polarize masculine and feminine within ourself, they will also manifest as projections on the outside. Thus an aggressive warlike male will seek to conquer and subdue the feminine, depriving himself within and without from satisfying, human relationships. However, it is possible he could meet a magnificent woman with a potent masculine side who could challenge his aggression and tame his nature so that he could enjoy fulfilment of the subtler, more inner side of his life. The interaction of masculine and feminine in relationships often resembles war.

When we look at the irides and see that either the right or the left iris has extensive nerve rings and the other does not, this is an indication of an imbalance of right and left energies. The first time I noticed this I was looking in the eyes of a very successful businessman. He had a cultivated appearance and manner yet one could sense the driving tension of his aggressive competitive nature. I asked him how he got along with his father and he replied 'Not at all. Nothing I ever did pleased him.' It was clear to see he was still trying to prove himself to his father. I then asked him what he enjoyed doing on a Sunday afternoon. 'Oh I attack the garden. We've a big place and it takes a lot to keep it under control.' It is amazing how we reveal our deepest selves with our words. The garden represents his feminine side, but it is not a place where he can relax. His garden is a proving ground for a masculine nature that is so unfulfilled it cannot stop even during leisure. Vervain was his Bach remedy type with Holly a close second.

Nerve rings on the right iris can also indicate a negative manifestation of the masculine side, frustration, rather than aggression. An inability to act in the world is as great an imbalance as doing too much. We all need a balance of both masculine and feminine activity and the full interplay of the sympathetic and parasympathetic side of our nervous system.

Nerve rings can appear in both right male and left female eyes, as either right or left imbalances. A woman can also have either her masculine or feminine side dominant, or out of balance. Likewise the left iris for a man.

Considerable numbers of women display strong left nerve rings due to stress around their feminine role. While many may have had a difficult relationship with their mother, others did not. Their problems might centre around acceptance or fear of their own femininity, fear of having children or fear of men. Left side nerve rings on men's irides indicate a difficult relationship with their mother, death of their mother, fear of women's dominance and lack of trust.

When you see these signs a few simple non-invasive questions will usually bring out the information to reveal the hidden psychology. Sample questions are:

1.   What was your relationship like with your mother (left iris), father (right iris)?
2.   How comfortable are you when you are attracted to someone of the opposite sex? Do you go up to them or do you shy away?
3.   How do you feel about having children?
4.   What was your early family life like? Did your mother and father get on with one another?
5.   Right dominant: What do you do for relaxation?
6.   Left dominant: What are you like at achieving goals?

It is interesting that the liver and gall bladder on the right side of the body are organs which are affected by aggressive strong emotions which increase the production of bile.

The left side holds the spleen which is the receptor for pranic energy and nutrient. The heart also relates to the inner emotional life and the finer nobler qualities represented by the nurturing and caring of the feminine principle.

Always evaluate the left and right organs along with any left/right nerve ring imbalance.

Careful observation may also reveal imbalances in other dual organs and glands. Check both sides:

Dual organs and glands

Right	*Left*
Pineal	Pineal
Pituitary	Pituitary
Eyes, ears, nose,	Eyes, ears, nose
Parathyroid/Thyroid	Parathyroid/Thyroid
Lungs	Lungs
Breast	Breast
Ovaries/Testes	Ovaries/Testes
Adrenals	Adrenals
Kidneys	Kidneys
+ arms	+ arms
+ legs	+ legs

The general systems such as lymph, circulation, digestive, respiratory, urinary, muscular and skeletal may also reveal differences in right and left irides.

Treatment of the nervous system

The restoration and rejuvenation of the nervous system requires the coordinated forms of nutritive, herbal and naturopathic treatment. Often this needs to be accompanied by complementary treatment such as osteopathy, chiropractic, massage, or acupuncture. So many aspects of the person's life must be taken into consideration. Often, life habits, work, family, even climatic situations may require major changes. As strength and balance are the aim of treatment, the patient has to be prepared to leave negative patterns behind.

The daily diet must include adequate nutrient to feed the nervous system, such as foods high in vitamins A, B complex, B1, B2, B6, niacin, C, D, G, as well as calcium, iodine, magnesium, manganese, phosphorus and sulphur. Useful herbs are oat straw, valerian, vervain, skullcap, lavender, peppermint, passion flower, lady's slipper, hops and chamomile.

Foods which overstimulate and exhaust the adrenals, such as excessive amounts of coffee, tea, sugar, alcohol, and drugs must be avoided.

The person must be willing to adopt a moderate lifestyle, which means sufficient sleep, reasonable working hours and the relaxed enjoyment of leisure time. Excessive indulgences of any kind must be avoided.

Herbal treatment provides potent superior nutrient to restore the nervous system. However, this must take place as a part of a total programme of eliminative and systemic treatment so that the body is brought up to a level of proper function. Only then will treatment provide lasting results.

Use the nerve, nerve vitalizer, nerve rejuvenator, sweet sleep, lady's slipper, lady's slipper/valerian formulae as well as serenitea and nervine or wild lettuce/valerian tinctures.

Naturopathic treatments are an excellent way of restoring nerve power. These include: Kneipp water cure, cold packs, aromatherapy baths, massages, herbal baths, deep breathing, yoga, Tai Chi, meditation and jogging. A good way of giving the system a rest and to release tension and fatigue is to take a holiday – not a nightclubbing indulgent holiday but a rest on the sea, in the mountains or at health spas or hot springs. Use the holiday to relax, exercise and purify your body and mind.

If patients are on tranquillizing or anti-depressant drugs they can still take herbal and natural treatment. However drugs can only be diminished by the patients themselves (in cooperation with their doctor) when they begin to feel better. Gradually the need for the drug will be less.

Bach flower remedies are also an excellent means to restore balance to the nervous system when it is the result of mental and emotional irritation, shock, trauma or their constitutional personality.

DIGESTIVE SYSTEM

**The digestive system
in the iris**

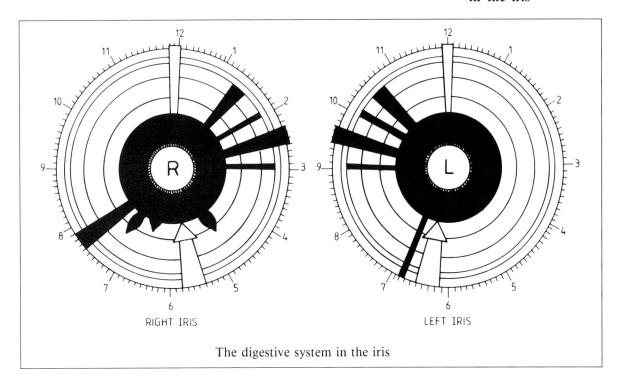

The digestive system in the iris

Mouth, tongue, lower jaw
Tonsils, larynx, pharynx
Vocal chords, trachea (thyroid)
Oesophagus
Pupillary ruff
Stomach ring
Duodenum
Gall bladder, liver
Pancreas, spleen
Small intestines, peyer's patches
Caecum/ileocaecal valve
Appendix
Ascending colon
Transverse colon
Decending colon
Sigmoid
Rectum
Anus
** closely related influences   Medulla
                                     Autonomic nervous system

As you can see in the iris chart, everything radiates out from the
digestion and affects every part of the body via the circulation,
lymphatic fluids and nervous system. As well as problems within the

various parts of the digestive system, the state of the chemistry of the digestion affects the entire body by the balance of acid alkaline and the assimilation of nutrient which becomes a part of the blood stream and is circulated through the liver to every part of the body. Local troubles such as bowel pockets, diverticuli, strictures, etc. send toxins to reflex areas via the lymph and blood, along with nutrients.

Although one could correctly say that the gastro-intestinal tract passes through the body, but is not part of its internal environment, it remains the cause of most disease. This sensitive and integral relationship where the inner and outer worlds meet is a major key to purification and regeneration. Change this influence and the whole body responds. Here, the outer world passes through the body and is transformed. This is why fasting, cleansing, and nutritive diets profoundly influence the body. Toxins are removed, nutrients given, and the balance is restored.

This system also involves two important functions/decisions which have ramifications on all levels of being, mental, emotional, spiritual. One involves the choice of what we take into our bodies, and the other the elimination of what is not needed. Although these are basic functions of human life, they become surrounded by emotions and attitudes of all kinds, from the Ghandi fast that controlled an entire country, to the child who refuses to use the potty, choosing instead to mess his pants in an effort to control his parents. Do we see consciously what we need and eat it in a balanced way? Are we at the mercy of our desires? Do we eat amidst family quarrels? The possibilities are practically infinite, but it is essential that the practitioner tunes into the patterns of each patient so that they can begin to see the stresses that they have accumulated around the basic acts of eating and eliminating.

These same attitudes are reflected in other areas of their being. For instance, a constipated fearful person who holds on to faeces as long as possible may be unconscious about the connection. It may be easier for them to see that they are possessive with relationships or material things and that they hold on tightly long after they are good for them. The Bach flower remedy Chicory is helpful for this state of mind. Strong emotions and shocks also make lasting effects on the gut, and unless released, will form the foundation of future digestive troubles.

Iris signs   **Mouth, teeth, tongue, lower jaw**
Iris signs in these areas will range from the white acute inflammatory radials, flares or lymphatic tophi to the radials and toxic deposits of the grey, brown and black markings. Psora would indicate a block on normal function. This area often suffers from an overlay of central heterachromia, sometimes related to catarrhal settlements in the sinus cavities. It is significant when a radial from this area is also balanced by a radial on the right iris to the liver area, showing that how the hand feeds the mouth affects the digestion. Compulsive eaters often have an inflammatory radial showing the hyperactivity of the mouth and the related digestive area in the liver. Bowel pockets also toxify the area,

which becomes sluggish and eventually diseased.

Tonsils, larynx, pharynx, thyroid
Here, where the lymphatic involvement of the mucous membranes is so significant, pay particular attention to white, yellowish or brown tophi, each colouring a guide to the level of toxicity. Bowel pockets and toxins often congest the area and when combined with a lesion or inherently weak structure the pattern can indicate a chronic condition. Adjacent iris signs from the thyroid such as nerve rings, radials, hyper- or hypo-activity can affect this area also.

Trachea and oesophagus
There is a close relationship here with the respiratory system. Any markings from the bowel must pass through the bronchials. Also any radial relationships would be opposite in the lung areas. Whether white inflammatory or toxic dark markings are present, cleansing and regenerative therapies will prepare the ground for the healing forces of the body to normalize function.

Pupillary ruff
It is important to observe the size and colour of the pupillary margin to learn further of the condition of the stomach lining, the assimilation and the central nervous system. (Refer to the information on the pupillary ruff in this chapter, under the Nervous System). The wider and darker the margin, the more chronic the condition.

Stomach ring (halo)
Here, markings tend to manifest as either white or dark, either acid or toxic, or hyperactive or hypoactive.

In blue eyes the colour of the stomach halo can appear anywhere from white, through grey, brown, yellow, orange, to black. In brown eyes, the differentiation is much less, and shades of brown to black are observed, sometimes with overlays of pale white, or yellow to rust colours, indicating chemical or mineral deposits. The stomach halo can be correlated with HCl secretions.

1. white stomach halo represents the acid stomach of excess HCl.
2. grey stomach halo indicates the sub-acute stomach of insufficient HCl.
3. grey/brown/black indicates the chronic stomach which lacks HCl.

As the stomach halo progresses towards malfunction small grey/black lines begin to fill up the space, until the whole circle is dark.

Duodenum
This iris mark should break through the ANW. It is often the site of a single outstanding mark, indicating digestive trouble in that area where the bile and pancreatic enzymes mix with the food released by the initial stages of digestion in the stomach.

1. white marks – hyperactivity, acidity
2. brown over white – ulceration
3. dark brown marks – ulcers
4. yellowish – sluggishness
5. check out gall bladder and pancreas marking

Gall bladder
Often the duodenum mark continues out into the gall bladder area, or the whole area is covered by a lesion/bowel pocket which indicates toxic congestion or degeneration, depending on the colour. Gall stones, as such, are not indicated by iris signs, only a predisposition to them. Cholecystitis may show as an inflammatory white or yellow-white cloud. A strong radial coming from the pupil will indicate a chronic condition affecting the central nervous system, and if the radial comes from the ANW it is affecting the ANS. Chronic signs like these require the full gall bladder cleanse.

Liver
The liver area may show a continuation of a radial which has covered the duodenum and gall bladder, indicating the serious and chronic nature of the toxicity, weakness and insufficiency. However, often liver signs show in the lymphatic zone, where they may be white, greyish white, yellowish and yellow-brown, the colour indicating the degree of severity. You will also see bowel pockets or inherent weaknesses which will guide you towards the proper treatment.

Small intestines
White signs in the small intestines indicate hyperactivity, governed by thyroid metabolism. This means that the food is moving too quickly through the small intestines for proper absorption of nutrients to take place. If the ileo-caecal valve is also weakened, this can also cause severe diarrhoea as the liquid food passes too quickly into the large intestine.

In some irides the small intestines stand out clearly as a dark grey colour, indicating sluggish activity which contributes to overweight when malnutrition causes hunger and overeating. Toxic small intestines means a more toxic blood stream.

Take notice of the condition of the peyer's patches area of the small intestines on both irides. When congested, fevers are stimulated as a part of the response of the lymphatic system of defence. When inflammatory this would be indicated by white markings.

Ileocaecal valve
Brown flares in this area indicate sluggish activity which allows toxins to collect in the area, leading to pelvis disorders as the toxins spread to the uterus/prostate/vagina areas. White markings would relate to the overactivity of diarrhoea and pain.

Caecum/appendix

This is commonly the site for a bowel pocket laden with toxins, which might lead to appendicitis. Radials often run through this area also, sometimes coupled with the opposite radial showing the relationship of stress in the perfectionism pressure brain area. White would signify pain and inflammation. Other colours which spill over from the bowel, such as yellows, rusts and browns from drugs, minerals, and inherited toxins, would all make their influence and contribute to impaired function. Brown flares mean that peristalsis has slowed at that spot, and this can be referred to as a 'grumbling appendix'.

Large intestines

The bowel shows a variety of structural types, from the contracted tight bowel controlled by the mind, to loose net and flower petal structures indicating lack of tone. Refer back to all the implications of the structure types in earlier chapters. Within these various structures the most common signs are the bowel pockets, diverticuli, radials, and strictures or balloons in the shape of the bowel. The true iris colour may be overlaid with white, grey, brown or black indicating the stage of inflammation or toxins. Also the bowel is often coloured with yellow rusts, browns or central heterochromia which we have discussed in earlier chapters. The bowel is the hub. The condition of the bowel influences every part of the body. It is also one of the prime eliminative channels. There is no true cure unless toxic or inflammatory bowels are healed.

Other significant colours are:

1. white – hyperactivity
2. psoric spot – blocked function, inefficiency, resisting peristalsis
3. reddish brown – medication for ulcers, cramps, indigestion, etc.
4. yellow – sulphur settled in the digestive area
5. black dots – intestinal parasites.

Sigmoid

Officially part of the large intestine, it is prone to pockets and ballooning due to faeces being held too long. All the same iris signs apply as for the large intestine, and toxins there affect the ovary and groin on the right side.

Rectum/anus

This area is commonly affected by haemorrhoids caused by the pressure of hard faeces and blood congestion. Iris signs range from the white of pain and inflammation, either in the lymphatic zone or as reflex radials, to the darker greys and browns of more sluggish conditions. Once again, look to the structure of the irides for keys to muscle tone.

Mouth, teeth, tongue, lower jaw and tonsils, oesophagus.

Problems in these areas are caused by inadequate nutrition, nerve inflammation and infections and are often associated with eliminative functions of the lymphatic system in the mucous membranes. After examining the iris signs, treat systemically and then also consider specific treatment for conditions such as pyorrhea, falling teeth, tonsillitis, cold sores, etc. I will mention a few safe general treatments under each category, with the understanding that in-depth treatments of great variety are to be found in diploma training courses and excellent reference works.

1. Tincture of myrrh, rubbed on gums, is excellent for healing any infection.
2. Nutritive foods and formulae are necessary to rebuild bone and teeth, such as the body building formula and the calcium formulae. Also, seaweeds, alfalfa, etc.
3. For sore throats and tonsillitis drink thyme tea whch is antiseptic, and make an effective syrup of hot water, lemon, honey, garlic, apple cider vinegar, cayenne, and ginger. Simmer. Sip and gargle.
4. Cleanse the bowels and stomach.
5. Dysphagia is a condition where natural swallowing movements are not possible. Look for causes in the muscular and nervous systems and use potent nutritional treatment both inwardly and locally.

Stomach

Acute, acid hyperactive stomach conditions Often difficult digestion problems require soothing, healing and alkalinizing treatment to relieve the pain, belching and heartburn. It is essential, also, in conditions of this nature to consider the nervous and emotional background and the causes which lead to the problems both in living and diet.

1. Useful diets are the mono diet (one food for a meal), alkaline diet, juice fasts and care with food combinations.
2. An excellent stomach acidity formula is equal parts of dandelion root, slippery elm, calamus, meadowsweet, irish moss and iceland moss.
3. Excellent teas are meadowsweet (balances HCl secretions in the stomach) wood betony (most reminiscent of regular tea) and peppermint.
4. Slippery elm also makes a soothing healing drink. Liquidize one teaspoon in a cup of soya milk and add honey to taste. Add wild yam root if there is flatulence (equal parts).
5. Regular drinks of aloe vera cactus will ease the pain of ulcers and stomach cancer. Cayenne stops bleeding of ulcers.
6. Drinks of apple cider vinegar, water and honey are a popular folk remedy to aid stomach alkalinizing and improve digestion.
7. Ginger is a kitchen carminative which aids digestion and relieves flatulence.
8. Golden seal is a potent remedy for the entire gastrointestinal tract.
9. Regular intake of fresh garlic disinfects the system thus avoiding gastrointestinal infections, colds, flus, etc.

Liver/gall bladder/duodenum

The radial in the right eye reveals the condition of this digestive area. The liver secretes alkaline bile which is held in the gall bladder until it is needed in the duodenum. These organs are particularly susceptible to negative emotions such as anger, bitterness, jealousy, resentment, etc. The liver is also a blood-purifying and nutrient-distributing organ system through the hepatic portal system which absorbs nutrients from the small intestine.

Treatment must begin with causes of the problem, which may be bowel toxins, inactive lymphatic system, poor nutrition, nervous stress or emotional disturbances, etc.

Pancreas

The pancreas secretes enzymes, as regulated by hormones and the vagus nerves, into the duodenum to prepare proteins, fats and carbohydrates for digestion and absorption in the small intestines. In the iris one often sees a diamond-shaped organ lacuna in the pancreas area, often related to a bowel pocket. When it is white, it indicates hyperactivity. After treating the whole body, its weakest eliminative and body systems, the pancreas is best aided by the following treatment:

1. Pancreas formula
2. Reflexology foot massage
3. Natural insulin is found in Elecampane; drink decoction regularly
4. Counselling and treatments to relieve negative emotions affecting the digestive system
5. Useful treatments for diabetes in addition to the above:
    a) cranesbill and golden seal
    b) red raspberry, myrrh and cayenne
    c) infusion of sumach berries

Small intestines

This area of the bowel, where blood assimilates nutrient and draws liquid from the chyme as it passes through, responds to natural therapeutics, particularly simplification of diet, cleansing, bowel formula and general purification of the pelvic area through such methods of the castor oil pack and poultices as needed. There is a close relationship of the small intestines to the nervous system via the solar plexus. It is also important to consider the thyroid, as the rate of metabolism determines the speed with which food passes through the intestines. Of course the composition and chemistry of the food by this time has been determined by each of the previous steps of digestion such as chewing, saliva, stomach acids, mixture of bile and pancreatic enzymes in the duodenum. Common problems in this area are diarrhoea, wind, flatulence, constipation, colic enteritus, gastro-intestinal flus, etc.

Treatments: 1. cramps and colic are relieved by wild yam root and cramp bark
                      2. thyroid rate of metabolism by kelp or thyroid formula

3. gastrointestinal flu – evening primrose root decoction
4. see diarrhoea treatment in Chapter 4
5. castor oil packs are very effective here, for absorption problems, relaxation and softening the faeces.

Caecum and ileocaecal valve

This area of the body can become tense and congested, allowing faeces to collect. Also the ileocaecal valve plays an important role where the small intestines open into the large intestine, at the bottom of the ascending colon. Often tension, sluggish bowels, constipation, etc. cause this important valve to lose its tone, or to become spastic and throb with pain. Treatment aiming at both the digestive and nervous systems, together with local relief of muscular tension, will help to relieve the congestion and sluggishness and restore normal function. Also, the bowel walls stretch and form pockets once the muscles have lost their tone.

Treatments: 1. Bowel tonic
                2. Castor oil pack
                3. Deep massage
                4. Slippery elm/lobelia poultice
                5. Reflexology massage

Appendix

Although part of the lymphatic system, the appendix secretes both antiseptic and lubricant solutions which aid bowel function, by stimulating peristalsis and protecting the tissues against infection. When inflamed, it acts as a warning device against high levels of infection.

Treatments: 1. cleanse the bowel with lower bowel tonic
                2. castor oil packs
                3. slippery elm/lobelia poultice

Bowels, colon and sigmoid

Almost every patient requires lower bowel cleansing. Iridology shows how important this is. The bowel and the small intestines are the hub from which nutrient is distributed throughout the body. Refer to Chapter 4.

Rectum/anus

This area suffers easily from haemorrhoids and piles created by pressure usually caused from constipation and dry faeces. Aside from treating the whole body and the bowels, and improving diet, an effective local treatment is to use regular, frequent applications of iced witch hazel on the area. When the blood has retracted enough so that the swollen area can be pushed inside, make a ovule of soaked cotton and push up inside. Astringent enemas are also very helpful.

Gall bladder treatment (gall stones)

Calcarious stones Dr Shook recommends intensive treatment with hydrangea root decoction (1oz of the herb to 1 pint of distilled water). Taken 4-6 wine glass doses daily until the condition clears.

Frank Roberts' herbal treatment for gall bladder inflammation
2oz fluid extract each of black root, kava and euonymous and 4oz fluid extract of marshmallow root
Dosage: Take a small teaspoonful immediately after every meal, with a
         minimum of 3 doses per day in a wineglassful of tepid water

Holistic herbal treatment
1. Liver/gall bladder formula (3 x day)
2. Calcarious stone formula if needed, with hydrangea root
3. Special diet (avoid fried and greasy foods, spicy foods, pastry)
4. Daily oil and lemon liver flush
5. Reflexology
6. Gentle daily exercise (walking, swimming)

Gall bladder cleanse
TEXTBOOK: *Modern Herbalism for Digestive Disorders* by Frank Roberts

Need:
$\frac{1}{2}$-1 pint cold-pressed high quality pure olive oil
$\frac{1}{2}$ pint fresh squeezed lemon juice (8-9 lemons)
Enema kit
Strainer screen
Ingredients for coffee enema

Rules:
1. Choose a weekend or two days when you do not have any social engagements or commitments (especially for the second day).
2. Do not eat anything after the midday meal on the first day. Eat a light fresh salad lunch (fruit or vegetable) and drink juices and herb teas.
3. Commence treatment about 7p.m.
4. Take 4 tablespoons of the olive oil and immediately take 1 tablespoon of fresh undiluted, unsweetened lemon juice.
5. Repeat every 15 minutes until all the oil is taken. If you need to take an extra tbsp. of lemon juice for any dose, this is all right.
6. Between each dose, lie down, with your head on a pillow lying on your right side, with your knees bent towards your chest.
7. IMPORTANT. If you vomit any oil, continue taking the doses, Sometimes an excess is eliminated this way.
8. The treatment is also successful using only $\frac{1}{2}$ pint of the olive oil when there is not a chronic gall stone condition. As a cleanse in the relatively healthy person, $\frac{1}{2}$ pint is good.

9. If there is a chronic gall stone condition I strongly recommend preparing for the treatment by diet, body work, relaxation. poultices and herbal baths, massage, and Bach flower remedies, before the actual gall bladder cleanse. A tight, tense congested area will make the treatment more uncomfortable than it needs to be. Truly, if a real cure is to take place, all those other dimensions of holistic healing need to be considered.
10. Lie down for 1 hour further after the last dose is taken.
11. Retire early.

Reactions:
1. Nausea – Being quiet and still and lying down will reduce any nauseous effects. If you do vomit some of the oil, don't worry.
2. Wind – rub stomach, take up squat position, gently rocking back and forth.
3. Burning (slight) in bowel means that chemical toxins are being released. Do not worry. Gerson Therapy people have done a lot of work with this and confirm my experience.
4. Sleeplessness – often people experience a happy, high feeling. Some dream a lot. Others are more uncomfortable. If you do this work you will find each time is different, depending on what the body is releasing with the cleanse.
5. If you need to move your bowels, do so. Go into the strainer and then pour water over so you can see what comes out. Many people like to collect all the stones and gravel so they can see the extent of what they have passed. I've even seen small tumorous growths come out. The stones vary in colour and size. The usual colour is a green bile colour. These stones are called biliverdin. On occasion bilirubin stones pass which are red. Usually any calcarious gall stones will not pass with the cleanse. They need to be dissolved from within by such herbs as hydrangea root.
6. The stones will come out up to 48 hours after the cleanse, and as they are exposed to the atmosphere they begin to soften and dissolve, until they are completely gone. In some cases the liquifying takes place before they leave the bowel. In this case the bowel movement is usually very soft and messy (much more oily).
7. Anyone suffering from a chronic gall stone problem should follow through with herbal treatment to relieve the weakness and inflammation in the area.
8. The coffee enema should be given the following morning on rising to stimulate the eliminative process.
9. Often there is up to 1 cup or more of stones passed with a very minimum of discomfort.

Follow up:
1. You may repeat the cleanse in three months if you wish.
2. Pay attention to fatty foods and dairy products, and minimize these in your diet.

3. Do follow-up herbal treatment for inflammation. Gall bladder formula.

4. Explore emotional causes for gall stones; a condition of negative fire emotions; anger, resentment, jealousy, bitterness.

Liver cleansing and strengthening

1. *Liver flush on a purifying diet: Dr Stone*
   Cold pressed olive oil with lemon is a cleanser for the liver, whereas cooked and fried oils are harmful.

Daily Breakfast:
Mix 3–4 tbsp. pure, cold pressed almond, olive or sesame seed oil
   6–8 tbsp. (twice the amount) of fresh squeezed lemon juice
   Fresh ginger juice may be added to taste
   Add fresh grapefruit, orange or tangerine juice to taste
   Liquify with 3–6 cloves of garlic
   Drink and follow with herbal tea containing 2 cupfuls of a mixture of:
      Licorice Root
      Anise   simmer and add peppermint and violet
                             leaves.
      Fennel
      Fenugreek

If constipated: add more licorice root and fresh garlic

If diarrhoea: no licorice, ginger or liver flush *but substitute* cinnamon bark in the tea and use ground cinnamon with baked apples and dates, raisins OR cinnamon cooked with rice and barley and curd.

Also chew citrus seeds, keeping in the mouth for at least 15 minutes to gain the benefit of enzymes, vitamins and minerals. The bitter essence is helpful to the liver. This also helps to relieve the garlic odour, as does chewing parsley or whole cloves.

NO FOOD TO BE TAKEN WITH THIS MORNING CLEANSE!

2. *Liver flush on a health-building diet: Dr Stone*
   Take 1–3 tbsp. of pure, cold-pressed almond or olive oil mixed with $3 \times$ the amount of fresh lime or lemon juice – stir and drink.
   Then take 2 cupfuls of HOT water with the juice of $\frac{1}{2}$ to a whole lime or lemon juice to each cupful.

Or Alternative: Take 1 glass (8oz) fresh orange, grapefruit, pineapple or pomegranate juice with the 1–3 tbsp. oil added in and followed by 2 cupfuls of HOT lemon water as above.

ALSO helps to relieve constipation.
   This health-building liver flush may be followed by fresh fruit with a few almonds and raisins about 15 minutes after the liver flush.

Heavier breakfast: may be taken 1 hour or more after the liver flush. Millet ($\frac{3}{4}$) and fenugreek ($\frac{1}{4}$) steamed porridge with $\frac{1}{2}$ cup of juice containing fresh pressed ginger juice and water in which raisins, dates and/or figs were soaked overnight. Sweet fruit may also be added, like banana, honey, but never a citrus fruit. Also you may have 2 dozen peeled almonds (preferably soaked overnight). Chew well. This is a very substantial breakfast.

Strengthening liver weakness with herbs and diet
1. AVOID alkali medicines completely as they neutralize the substance which sets off the instructions which eventually result in the flow of liver bile.
2. AVOID ALL FRIED AND FATTY FOODS, including dairy products.
3. AVOID all alcohol.
4. AVOID tea, coffee, spices, condiments.

1. Use coffee enemas to stimulate flow of bile and cleanse the liver. How often depends on individual needs.
2. Work on mental, emotional problems and conditions.
3. HERBS: a) Liver/gall bladder mixture
             b) Cleansing the bowel
             c) Normalizing hydrochloric secretions in the stomach (meadowsweet tea is excellent)
             d) Bitter digestive tonics are excellent to stimulate and balance flow of bile (bayberry, dandelion, barberry, etc).
4. When conditions like hepatitis have developed, additional treatment using fomentations and poultices are essential to relieve congestion in the area (slippery elm & lobelia).
5. *Jaundice* formula: restores liver to normal function.
   1 oz. Mandrake root   Mix all powders and place in
   $\frac{1}{2}$ oz. Culver's root   capsules size 0, 1, 3 × daily
   1 oz. Dandelion root
   1 oz. Gentian root
   $\frac{1}{2}$ oz. Golden seal root
   $\frac{1}{4}$ oz. Cayenne
6. *Inflammation* of the liver   Mix powders and take 1 capsule
   formula.   nightly on retiring
   1 tsp. Mandrake root
   2 tsp. Culver's root
   1 tsp. Blood root
   2 tsp. Dandelion root
7. Tissue salt Nat. Phos. – (bladderwrack, fennel, elecampane.)
8. Castor oil packs on liver area are also very helpful in relieving congestion and helping the lymphatic system to clear the area. Softens. Relaxes as well.
9. Liver/gall bladder formula.

10. Gentian root (read Dr Shook).
11. Acupuncture to balance liver/spleen function.
12. Reflexology foot massage
13. $\frac{2}{3}$ lobelia, $\frac{1}{3}$ slippery elm poultice on the liver to relieve congestion – excellent for hepatitis.

The digestive system and the nervous system

The nervous system is dependent on the digestive system for nourishment. If digestion fails, the nervous system draws what it needs from the stomach and intestinal walls and muscles, thus causing problems and weakness in those areas.

The digestive system is intimately connected with the nervous system via the ANS, particularly the cranial nerves, coeliac and solar plexuses and the plexus of Meissner in the duodenum. The climate of our emotional life affects our digestion and the best food can be spoiled by tensions, nerves or upsets. Sight, smell, touch, taste, all increase or decrease the appetite, showing the close relationship with the five senses.

The medulla also plays its part in the digestive system, particularly controlling the vomiting reflex. Also, as previously discussed, the absorption ring of the stomach pupillary margin reveals the relationship of the CNS.

The digestive system and the circulatory system

The digestive system provides the nutrient for the circulatory system to distribute, but if it is toxic, then it is also the means for bowel toxins to be spread throughout the body. A clean bowel is essential for good health. When the circulatory system is severely unbalanced, as for instance, when the sodium ring is apparent in the iris, digestive chemistry is intimately connected. A hyperacidic stomach burns out sodium from the stomach which migrates to the sodium ring, eventually causing a lack of HCl (hypoacidity) and an inability to digest protein. If the causes of the sodium ring are not treated as well, treatment to eliminate the circulatory congestion will not be effective. The digestive organs are often called the blood forming organs; each playing a part in preparing the food for its assimilation and absorption into the blood so that nutrient can be distributed all over the body and transformed into energy and new body cells and tissues.

The liver performs several functions which assist the circulatory system. After nutrient is absorbed by the blood in the small intestines it is carried to the liver, where it goes through chemical processing before it is sent to every part of the body. The liver also raises the temperature of the blood, forms red blood cells in foetal life, destroys red blood cells, stores haematin for maturation of new red cells and manufactures plasma proteins.

The digestive system and the lymphatic system

The lymphatic system is a subtle multi-faceted system which is closely interconnected with the digestive system. In fact, several parts of the digestive system are also parts of the lymphatic system. These parts are the tonsils in the throat, the appendix in the caecum, the peyer's patches and the lacteals in the small intestines. While the tonsils, the appendics and the peyer's patches are part of the warning and defence system, the lacteals are actually involved in the absorption of the nutrient which is taken into the liver via the hepatic portal tributaries or via the cysterni chyli thoracic duct and venous circulation to the liver. The mucous membranes in the throat and mouth are also lymphatic. As well as these major lymphatic centres, the lymph is an integral intercellular fluid which flows through all tissue, distributing nutrient and cleansing toxins, and so is an essential part of all digestive organs, muscles and tissue. The liver also aids the lymphatic system in detoxification of the blood, especially of foreign substances.

The digestive system and the respiratory system
Aside from the obvious function of nourishing the tissues of the respiratory system, the digestive and respiratory systems are most closely connected by the sharing of the mouth and throat passages, and in subtle contributions the digestive system makes in preserving the alkalinity of the blood which helps the medulla to govern respiration. They also function and support each other as eliminative organs; bowels move wastes down and the lung expels wastes upward, back into the air.

The digestive system and the endocrine system
The most intimate connection perhaps is the thyroid gland which governs the basic metabolism of digestion. Also, the adrenals affect the digestive system through the sympathetic nervous system.

The liver also aids the pancreas in its endocrine function by helping to maintain normal blood sugar levels. The liver cells produce glycogen which is stored in liver cells and converted back to glucose when needed.

The digestive system and urinary system
The digestive and the urinary systems are interlinked in that the urinary system becomes responsible for the elimination of most of the fluid taken into the body. Fluids are drawn out of the foods and taken through the liver's chemical factory. There nitrogen is separated from the amino acids in the blood and ammonia is converted into urea which is removed from the blood by the kidneys and excreted into the urine. It is also one of the eliminative channels, working together with the others to keep the body clean and clear.

The digestive system and the reproductive system
The most outstanding relationship is nourishment, particularly with the female, during pregnancy and nursing.

The digestive system and the skeletal system
The skeletal system is completely dependent on the digestive system to build and maintain its strength and flexibility. When nourishment is lacking in the blood, the body draws it from the bones and teeth. The skeletal system supports the digestive system by its structure.

The digestive system and the muscular system

The gastrointestinal tract is one long tube of layered muscles which move in a rhythm called peristalsis. The movement of food down this tube begins with chewing and swallowing. Toxic bowels also reflect on the skin, as the blood throws toxins up as skin troubles. As the skin is also an eliminative channel, holding on to attitudes of not letting go will also reflect as a scurf rim. It is quite common to see the circle of toxic congested bowels together with the circle of a toxic scurf rim.

THE CIRCULATORY SYSTEM

The circulatory and lymphatic system complement each other like night and day, black and white, hot and cool. A strong beating positive heart sends red arterial blood outward (male or yang energy) while the passive spleen is a quiet force, duplicating all the individual functions of its various parts of the lymphatic system.

Lymph is an almost colourless whitish fluid without the strong pathways of arteries, veins or capillaries, more like a sea of fluid in which all the individual cells of our body float. It is a passive, receptive (feminine or yin) energy, moved only by the force of breathing, intestinal pulsations and muscular movements.

The two systems complement each other and support the essential body functions of transport of nutrient and purification (the liver purifies the blood), and they both participate in maintenance, balance

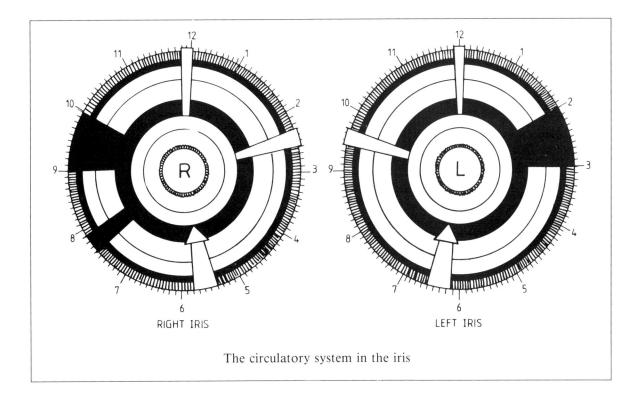

RIGHT IRIS   LEFT IRIS

The circulatory system in the iris

and defence against internal or external forms of disease. Because they work together so closely and our health is dependent on the function and balance of blood and lymph, it is essential to understand how they do so and how we can bring about better bodily function and equilibrium so that the individual can throw off negativity and disease. The heart and the spleen also work together to distribute the subtle energies and prana throughout the body. From the earliest signs of imbalance we should make efforts to regain equilibrium of function. This section will give an understanding of how the lymphatic and circulatory systems work together for the benefit of the body. Most people understand the circulatory system, but few have an understanding of the lymphatic system. These days when so many people are concerned with obesity, water retention, and cellulite, as well as cholesterol buildup, cancer, heart and circulatory disease, it is worthwhile educating patients on how these systems work together.

It is not enough just to read eyes and see that the sodium ring is inhibiting circulation, or that there is anaemia of the brain, or that the lymphatic system is congested; you also need to understand how each system affects the others, otherwise you cannot treat causes. If the patient is not responding to treatment it is because you have not seen the relationship of one area of trouble to another part of body function. Until the weak or disturbed areas of function are brought up together, the treatment will not be successful. To do this we have to understand how the systems work together and support each other.

Strong circulation and a full blood supply is essential for good health. This can be evaluated by iris diagnosis together with details of history and other forms of analysis. One of the first tasks of treatment is to achieve pure fresh blood to all parts of the body, relieving excess where there is congestion and reaching parts that have been deprived. In order to achieve a clean blood stream, strive for a healthy stomach, a clean well functioning bowel, efficient eliminative channels and an efficient liver. Evaluate all these aspects during the iris analysis.

The acid alkaline levels must also be assessed. When the blood becomes acid, red blood cells die, reducing the oxygen carrying capacity of the blood, slowing down metabolism and the capacity of the body to carry off wastes. Iron levels in the blood are also important as the iron atoms collect oxygen in the respiratory system.

David Tansley puts it thus in *Subtle Body*:

'Blood – the mysterious essence. Blood is the bearer of life. Physiologically it carries a continuous supply of nutrients and oxygen to all parts of the body and removes debris and waste gases and other impurities. According to the Vedic teachings the life-principle anchored in the heart of man is able to blend with the blood and thus carry the life-force of prana to all areas of the organism. Prana is the name given to those energizing forces which flow from the sun. The heart, working in conjunction with the spleen, distributes these solar energies to vitalize the physical form. The Rosicrucian Max Hendel wrote that the soul controls the dense physical body by way of the blood which is its particular vehicle. Empedocles in 480 BC states that 'blood is life', and Goethe had Faust say that man's blood is liquid fire. Steiner spoke of the blood as containing a record of the life of the individual, registering every thought and emotion, life being transmitted from the ethers through breath to the lungs and there making its impress on the blood. All mystics agree with Jacob Boehme that the spirit of God moves in the blood of man, and everyone is familiar with the Christian phrase "saved by the blood of Christ". There are of course many interpretations of this and some recognize that it can mean the reorganization of the energies within the individual as the Christ comes to birth within him.

Buddhist texts outline techniques for determining the nature of another's thoughts through the colour of his or her heart-blood, such cognition is produced by developing the power of clairvoyance in order to see the heart-blood. If a person has happy thoughts then the colour seen is red like the ripe banyan fruit, sad thoughts produce a black colour, and neutral thoughts have a colour of clear sesame oil.'

Of course the hormones secreted by the endocrine crystal sets in response to changes in the universe, environment and emotions flow into the blood stream, thus contributing their messages to the overall picture. Also, acupuncturists tell a great deal about the body and emotions by the pulse readings.

Heart

The circulatory system in the iris

Although western iris charts show the heart area only on the left eye, it also appears in the right iris from 9:30–10:00 o'clock. Whenever strong heart signs appear, also check out the right heart signs. The German iridologists make more precise indications. Josef Deck in the recent translation of his *Principles of Iris Diagnosis* differentiates the left heart and the right heart and that maintains 'insufficiency of the heart is indicated by a constitutional marking at 2:30 and at 3:30 on the left. Marking in the zone of 2:00 o'clock on the iris collarette indicates aortic insufficiency. Small markings in the heart zone indicate defects, resolved quiescent infarcts or toxic damage. Markings between 3 and 4 o'clock in the pulmonary sector are sometimes very prominent especially in pulmonary congestion with cardiac insufficiency.' It is important to clearly differentiate between pulmonary and heart markings.

The two genotypes, Cardio-renal syndrome and Cardio-abdominal syndrome are significant considerations in relation to constitutional types, according to Josef Deck.

Cardio-renal syndrome is a constitutional inherent weakness where lacunae appear in both heart and kidney zones; treatment of both weak areas must proceed together, and in relation to their particular constitutional type.

Cardio-abdominal syndrome is shown by a heart lacuna or crypt with or without a defect marking, together with a lacuna in the left colon, often in the sigmoid-colon zone about 5 o'clock. The colon affects the cardiac function not only with gas, congestion, but with toxic impregnation. This is a common syndrome where there is dysentery, starvation, oedema of malnutrition, and is a direct reflection on constitutional weakness.

It is important to consider the heart whenever the constitutional type is neurogenic or anxiety tetanic; strong nerve signs will affect the stability of the heart on the emotional level, and where there is physical weakness or toxicity, stress will penetrate and disturb function.

Thiel makes the comment that the nervous heart affects the pupil size showing the means whereby the emotional life as felt in the heart affects the nervous system and the balance of sympathetic and parasympathetic nervous systems, causing a continuous fluctuation which affects pupil dilation and contraction. Acupuncture is valuable here after cleansing and balancing treatment of the tissues, to balance and protect the heart, both physically and emotionally.

When we examine the heart area of the iris, we need to look for inherent weakness, nerve strength, toxic conditions and reflex effects from other organs. If the ANW is pierced by a radii soleris in the heart area, inherent weakness is noted but not necessarily disease. The radii soleris may refer to weak nerve activity here or toxins draining toward the heart. In all kinds of cardiac pathology we find the ANW is involved, which is a definitive means of distinguishing a cardiac problem from bronchial trouble.

The following factors contribute towards heart disease:

1.   constitutional weakness (lacunae, defects)
2.   toxin overload from the bowel (radii soleris, bowel pockets)
3.   lack of exercise and fresh air
4.   plaquing of arterial and heart walls (too much fat)
5.   emotional stress, love relationships, passions, overexcitement
6.   weak medulla
7.   fermentation in the bowel causing blood and stomach gases
8.   excessive physical exertion
9.   overindulgence (tea, coffee, alcohol, meat, drugs, tobacco, sex)
10. deficiency of blood salts, which are needed by the heart
11. sunstroke
12. anaemic conditions
13. overstressed liver not able to clean blood properly
14. nerve weakness, insufficiency of chest, brain and cardiac nerve
15. lack of chlorine, iodine, iron, calcium, magnesium, lecithin, vitamin E, phosphorus, nerve fats, salts
16. the more toxic the lymphatic system is, the more toxic the blood stream is
17. inefficient function of skin zone also accounts for a heavier burden of toxins in the lymph and blood

Circulation zone (outside ANW)
This iris area immediately outside the bowel and ANW tells about the condition of blood and lymph after it draws nutrient from the intestines.

Here we can see clearly how a toxic bowel affects the quality and purity of blood, when the bowel colours spill over and through the ANW into the first circulation zone. This zone is the interaction field between the digestive process and the circulatory and lymphatic fluids which draw up the nutrient from the chyme in the bowel to move outward for utilization or elimination.

The close relationship of the ANW is integral, as the communicating link of unconscious body function and the emotional life. Here these body systems come together producing the total picture and all affecting the function and quality of each other. Self destructive radii soleris lines break through the ANW from the digestive system, indicating the physical toxic dispersion of bowel wastes at chronic levels, as created by negative attitudes.

Dorothy Hall does not consider the *deep circulation zone* necessary for diagnosis, and interprets congestion close to the ANW as poor or impeded nerve supply to that organ or area.

Lightening of this area signals increases of uric acid in the blood and a tendency to pain, inflammation and the production of mucus. Darkening indicates general circulation and muscle weakness. The spill over of reds, oranges, yellows, browns, etc. from the bowel areas shows the degree to which toxins collecting in the bowel are affecting the blood and are being distributed throughout the body.

Where spill over colours rise upwards from the autonomic nerve wreath into the head areas, particulary when they are yellow, orange or light brown, they are often associated with sinus symptoms.

Disturbances in this zone would represent obstructions to the flow of nutrient, and a diminishing of the quality of the nutrient, so that organs and body areas would therefore become weakened.

German iridologists (e.g. Kriege) consider this zone worthy of accurate mapping.

Circulation & lymphatic zone (inside skin zone)

Blood and lymph moves through the muscular system, into the capillary zone where the circulatory and lymphatic systems interact, the blood being lost from the capillaries and the lymph system collecting it. This zone also represents blood supply to the various organs and areas, and valuable analysis can be made about the organs of transport and utilization as well as purification of the blood and the elimination of its wastes.

Lymphatic rosary

This area can be dominated by a sucession of white, yellowish or brownish lymphatic tophi, indicating the condition of thick, sluggish catarrhal encumbrance. Lymphatic types may have this condition from birth. When it is bright white it indicates a hyperactive lymphatic function with resulting colds, allergies, etc. The sluggish, more toxic colours of yellow and brown indicate lack of ability to fight diseases.

Darkening, especially when accompanied by a dark scurf rim, shows that the toxic levels are chronic. The thickness of a dark zone in an infant shows the degree of inherited toxins, many of which will be eliminated when the body throws them off in childhood diseases.

Black spots indicate chronic toxic deposits and a chronic level of lymphatic stasis and degeneration of tissue.

Note all disturbances in this zone, the areas they relate to, and whether the sign is hyper- or hypoactive. Also, examine an area or organ by checking the circulation zone at both the ANW end and the ciliary end, differentiating between the flow of nutrient at the ANW end and the blood supply at the ciliary end. Inhibition of blood flow at the ciliary end causes nutritive deficiency and poor elimination, affecting the quality and integrity of tissue and function. We must not forget the subtle etheric pranic energies which are also contained in blood and which bring life to every cell and tissue. Blood flow is life flow and is essential to every part of the living body.

Reflexive fibres and *transversals* are more common in this area than anywhere else. These swollen fibres reflect blood conditions (especially when pink or red), indicating congestion, irritation and pain. They are actually swellings of these minute blood vessels in the iris. Refer to the section on reflexive fibres.

Remember to visualize that what has been taken into Zone 1 is now being moved through Zone 2 on its way to utilization and elimination. The iris reflects this vital life process.

Sodium ring or *arcus senilis,* also called the *calcium ring* or the hypercholesterol ring, tells us that there is plaquing of the arterial walls. The heart has to work harder to pump the blood around. Therefore, there is lack of circulation in some areas, and imbalances in body chemistry and endocrine function. The colour, depth and width of this sign together with the other aspects of the individual iris reading reveal the complete picture.

What is called *anaemia of the extremities* is shown in the varying stages of the development of the sodium ring; first a fuzzing over, a greyish cap, which slowly turns to white. This sign may appear in both head and leg/pelvis zones or in just one. The *broom or fringe* pattern added to the *anaemia of the extremities* shows on the physical level that suppression of toxins is penetrating inward together with inhibition of perspiration and skin elimination. Dorothy Hall maintains that this reflects a sensitive nature and tender skin which is easily hurt.

Aorta
Aortic markings occur about 2:30 on the left iris. Interpretation of lesions, radials, reflexive signs, crypts, and colours together with heart and circulatory zone markings will help the iridologist to determine the condition of the tissues and the source of either toxic or inflammatory irritation. It is important to take into consideration an accurate assessment of constitution and muscular tone in these areas and the relationship of the nervous system with its influence through emotions and adrenal response.

Arteries
Sodium ring markings indicate the condition of arterial walls. Assess the balance of the autonomic nervous system, especially in relation to adrenal stimulation, so you can determine the balance of the vasoconstrictors and the vasodilators.

Veins
Examine markings where the major veins drain from the pulmonary and gastric areas, and the liver, spleen, head and lungs. Disturbances in the flow of this drainage would increase toxic congestion in those areas.

Capillaries
These extend and multiply throughout the skin zone, especially in the extremities (head, hands and feet). There is a close relationship between the circulatory and skin zones. Assess the skin tone. Scurf rims indicate that inactive skin is causing a buildup of toxins. Anaemia is revealed by the bluish iris marking, extending over into the sclera. Often dark skin zones accompany congested lymph tophi, or a black skin zone thinly rings the sodium ring, showing that elimination is blocked to a severe degree, affecting the quality of blood.

It is possible to organize an approach to anatomy and physiology by arranging body organs and functions the following way:

Holistic anatomy & physiology

1. Blood-forming organs – stomach, small and large intestines
2. Blood-purifying organs – bronchi and lungs, kidneys, skin, liver, spleen and lymph glands
3. Blood-circulation system – heart, veins, arteries, capillary systems and lymphatic system
4. Blood-utilization systems – organs, bones, tissues (created through nourishment carried by the blood).

The blood flows through seven circuits:

1. Heart
2. Upper extremities
3. Neck and head
4. Thorax
5. Digestive organs, liver
6. Pelvis and lower extremities
7. Kidneys

Treatment of these two systems proceeds together. Everything that improves the blood improves the lymph. When the blood is stimulated and purified, the lymph system is relieved, functions better, further relieving the function of the blood. Once again we see how the two opposites support each other and bring about a balanced function of the whole system.

Treatment of the circulatory and lymphatic systems

   Whether herbs, exercise, massage, diet or water therapy is applied, both circulatory and lymphatic systems are brought up together as purification, stimulation and balancing take place.

Before any treatment of the circulatory or lymphatic systems can take place the bowels must be cleansed, the liver (as the blood purifying organ) must be functioning properly, and the eliminative channels must be doing their jobs. If structural problems or injuries cause impediments to function, these must be adjusted and overcome by additional therapies.

Many of the treatments for the circulatory systems are found in the section on the lymphatic system, on pages 222–30. Treatment for one of these two systems is treatment for the other.

Herbal treatment
Alterative herbs are blood and lymphatic purifying or sweetening herbs. While certain herbs are more strongly one or the other, they both influence blood and lymph function.

Specific herbs for the circulatory system are:

1. *Red clover*: a soothing pleasant tasting herb commonly used as an herbal tea (beneficial for weak children and skin diseases) or as an excellent part of a combined formula.
2. *Burdock*: this herb relieves the skin when impure blood causes boils, psoriasis, etc. also aiding kidneys and balancing fluids.
3. *Chaparral*: potent anti-cancer purifier also aiding urinary system.
4. *Oregon grape root*: blood purifier and liver stimulant which improves digestion and absorption, thereby increasing strength and vitality for healing.
5. *Capsicum*: antiseptic, stimulant, equalizes circulation, warming.

You can also use the following formulae from Appendix I: blood purifying formula, blood circulation formula, bowel formula, and liver/gall bladder formula.

Dietary treatment
Causes in the diet must be altered if any permanent improvement is to be maintained. While iris signs may show up in the circulatory and lymphatic zones as a sodium/calcium hypercholesterol ring this can be associated with a variety of causes and symptoms.

The circulatory system is inhibited in its function by excesses of fats, salt, cholesterol and by imbalances in sodium and calcium. Plaquing of the arterial walls is a chronic condition.

Holistic relationships: interaction with other systems

The circulatory system and the muscular system
Kriege writes, 'The state of the muscular system is shown in the iris by the appearance of the lacunae. If the lacunae appear inside the ANW, then the state of the muscle layers of stomach and intestines is indicated. When small lacunae are observed outside the rim of the iris wreath, then a lability of the circulation is indicated. When the lacunae extend to the

muscle zones, then the muscle fibres of the organs indicated by the particular areas involved are weakened through defective blood supply. If the lacunae extend fully to the iris margin, then it indicates that even the bones and mucous membranes suffer from nutritional disturbances'. This shows clearly how muscular weakness inhibits sufficient supply of nutrition, further weakening that area.

The circulatory system feeds the muscular system. Nutrient is distributed via the blood stream. The level of toxins in the blood affects the condition and function of the skin. Whenever there are injuries in the tissues, extra blood, carrying extra nutrient for healing, is drawn to the area, often producing swelling and pain. If direct feeding by the use of poultices is given to the area, the tissues can heal without depriving other areas of the body. This also happens when infants are teething. If sufficient calcium is available in the normal blood supply there is no need to pull it from other areas, causing irritability and other problems.

The elasticity of the arterial walls influences an increase in blood pressure. If their stretch cannot accommodate so much blood after systole, there is not enough recoil after diastole.

The circulatory system and the digestive system
The circulatory system draws up nutrient from the chyme as it moves through the intestines. How effectively this process works depends on whether the walls of the colon are clean. Fluids from toxic areas of the bowel transport toxins as well as nutrient, creating the foundation for disease. Also, poor circulation or anaemic conditions would impede the flow of nutrient and the cleansing of tissues.

The circulatory system and the nervous system
The amount of oxygen available to the blood via the respiratory system is partly controlled by the medulla. Impeded nerve supply to the heart would diminish proper circulatory function. The nervous system guides and monitors circulatory activity.

Conversely anaemia, or lack of blood supply to the brain areas, affects the function of the nervous system. When the sodium ring or arcus senilis render brain functions slow and ineffective, it is easy to see how one closely affects the other.

Adequate circulation and nutrition during foetal life greatly influences brain development. Dr Jensen makes the point that every conscious experience affects the ANW and the glandular system, resulting in changes in organs, body tissue and circulation of blood. Brain centres affect the state of tension or relaxation, thus affecting blood flow. Pressure of excess fluids on nerves causes pain.

Parasympathetic impulses to the heart pacemaker restrain its action and decrease its excitability. Sympathetic impulses accelerate the action of the heart and increase its excitability. These are opposite effects and both parasympathetic and sympathetic nervous systems are constantly sending messages to balance body responses and needs. Refer to the effects of adrenaline in the circulatory system and the endocrine system — most of these effects can be produced by stimulating sympathetic nerve fibres. The sympathetic dominance of heart activity is felt strongly during times of stress, exercise, excessive heat, etc. When at rest parasympathetic dominance is experienced.

The circulatory system and the urinary system
The more toxic the blood is, the greater the burden on the kidneys to purify the blood. About 25 per cent of left ventricle output of blood is distributed to kidneys for filtration in each cardiac cycle. Urine formation begins with filtration of the blood, and is completed by reabsorption of essential materials back to the blood stream and by secretion and synthesis of other wastes. These systems are intricately connected and affect each other closely.

The circulatory system and the reproductive system
The reproductive system is controlled by hormones which are secreted into the blood by the endocrine glands and then carried to the various parts of the body. The penis fills with blood during erection. During the menstrual cycle, the endometrium grows, filling with blood and mucus which is shed because of constriction of blood vessels in response to hormone directions. Each stage of the menstrual cycle is governed by hormones released into the blood stream.

During pregnancy, after fertilization, the embryo invades the endometrium where chorionic villi from the embryo invade the mother's blood vessels which interlock with mother's tissues and blood, forming what is eventually known as the placenta. Here in the placenta, the chorionic villi dip into maternal blood, allowing diffusion and interchange of materials between the mother and the foetus, but no direct connection. The placenta also secretes hormones into the mother's blood stream which influence the uterus to maintain the full term of pregnancy. Constituents of mother's milk are also derived from blood flowing through the mammary glands.

The circulatory system and the endocrine system
Hormones pass into the blood stream for general circulation and are taken to the part of the body which picks up the messages and acts upon them in body processes of metabolism, growth, inner stability, resistance to stress and reproductive cycles. Each gland has its arterial and venous blood supply. The amounts of thyroid hormones affect the heart, respiration and blood pressure. The parathyroids affect the blood calcium levels.

Adrenal hormones affect blood sugar levels, and the lack of oxygen in the blood stream has a direct effect on the adrenal medulla. When adrenaline stimulates the sympathetic nervous system to prepare the body for reactions to stress, this results in general vasoconstriction (except of coronaries) and a rise in blood pressure. This stimulation also excites cardiac muscle and its rate and force of contraction, cardiac output and dilating coronaries. A better supply of air to alvioli stimulates respiration, causing the release of carbon dioxide (CO_2) from the blood and an increased supply of oxygen. Through the mobilization of muscle and liver glycogen there is an increase in blood sugar, and an increase in the coagulability of the blood.

The osmotic blood pressure affecting the hypothalamus influences the rate of secretion and release of antidiuretic hormone, which migrates along nerve fibres for storage in the posterior pituitary. One of the main effects of these hormone secretions is a constriction of smooth muscle of the blood vessels and a raising of arterial blood pressure.

Aldorsterone secretions from the posterior pituitary stimulate hormones which help the blood volume return to normal after loss of blood or body fluids. Secretions from the islets of Langerhans in the pancreas affect fat deposits in blood vessels and levels of blood sugar in the blood.

The circulatory system and the respiratory system
As blood circulates through the lungs each haemoglobin molecule collects four oxygen molecules, forming oxyhaemoglobin, which is necessary for the body's metabolic processes. When the iris shows a blue anaemia ring this indicates a lack of oxygen and iron together with poor circulation.

Proper and deep breathing combined with exercise is essential for a good healthy blood supply. The more active the respiratory system is in oxygenation and elimination of carbon dioxide, the better the quality of the blood. The right atrium of the heart receives the venous blood returning from body tissues with its diminished oxygen supply and increased CO_2, and passes it into the right ventricle which pumps it around the lungs. Here it releases CO_2 and gathers its fresh supply of oxygen. Then the left atrium receives this revitalized blood and passes it to the left ventricle which pumps it around the body to supply oxygen and collect CO_2. Red blood corpuscles carry the oxygen and CO_2.

The circulatory system and the skeletal system
The bone marrow plays an integral role in the manufacture of the formed elements in the blood stream, which develop from primitive reticular cells chiefly in the red bone marrow. While the skeletal system is the end product of nutrition as are body tissues, they also return the cycle, so to speak, by being involved in the creation of new blood. Once again we see in the body how each cycle is balanced and the flow of energy out is returned. Bone is richly supplied with blood vessels.

THE RESPIRATORY SYSTEM

How we breathe is how we live. Without breath we do not live. The quality and balance of breath determines the purity of our blood and the equilibrium of our nervous system.

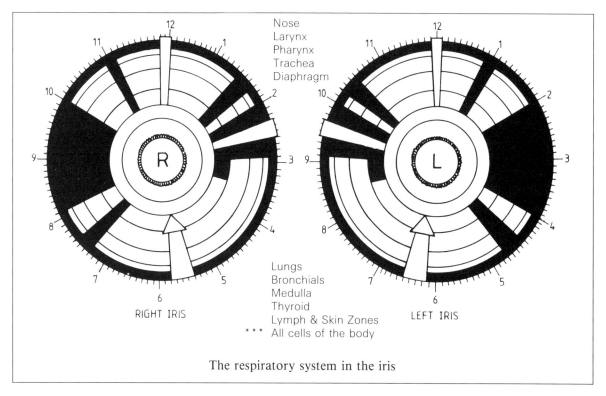

Nose
Larynx
Pharynx
Trachea
Diaphragm

RIGHT IRIS

Lungs
Bronchials
Medulla
Thyroid
Lymph & Skin Zones
*** All cells of the body

LEFT IRIS

The respiratory system in the iris

Types of respiration The body has four different types of respiration.

1. External respiration (breathing).
2. Internal respiration (cellular).
3. Primary respiration (cerebrospinal fluid).
4. Skin respiration.

1. External respiration

When we come into this world we take the first breath of life, and just before we leave it we take our last breath. Our life, every minute, waking or sleeping, is a continuous breathing process. This can be conscious when we put our attention to our breathing rhythms. On the physical level the rate and control of respiration is governed by the respiratory centre in the medulla oblongata. These signals affect the intercostal muscles, causing rhythmical contraction of the diaphragm and the muscles.

It is also important to mention that we have a basic pulsing rhythm, part of the mysterious beat of life, perhaps coming from our higher brain impulses. This pulsing rhythm changes according to our age and consciousness and affects our breathing patterns. When we meditate, or relax and attune to higher centres, our breathing patterns change. When we react to fear or live in stress our breathing pattern is also affected. Yogis gained high levels of consciousness and the powers to perform miracles by governing the breath.

A great living master of this century, Maharaj Sawan Singh Ji, describes the human body thus:

'How skillfully the five elements, earth, water, fire, air and ether, antagonistic to each other in their nature, have mixed together to form the human body. Earth is eaten up by water, water is dried up by fire, fire is consumed by air and air is swallowed up by ether. But how skillfully these five enemies of each other unite in a love embrace to run the body! Does our body move by itself? This body, after death, lies on the ground in the same condition as before, but that which causes motion in it has gone out. What is it that moves it? The pranas, the vital air, you say. Who moves the pranas? The mind. Who enlivens the mind? The soul. Exactly, but the soul receives light and life from that Power-House of Energy, whose secret Hand works all the machines, but is invisible except to the very rare seers, who know the secret. There is no motion or movement in the world without a mover. All movements start from Him.'

This mysterious invisible part of life we cannot see with our outer eyes. We only observe the changes in the physical side. We see a child come from the mother and begin breathing when it starts its individual life. When that life ends it is accompanied by the cessation of breathing, which has been with that person for their entire life. While we are alive, we breathe, and the quality and rhythm of our breath determines the quality of our life.

The alkaline balance must be maintained in the blood. Excesses of acid carbon dioxide stimulate the respiratory centre to quicken breathing so that purification will take place at a quicker rate. Exercises, vigorous work, emotions and extreme changes in temperature will cause sudden deep inspiration. Full and complete breathing is essential to the maintenance of a pure blood stream and the oxygenation and purification of body tissues.

Even though breathing is an automatic process most of the time, we should do all we can to ensure that quality of breathing takes place. We can form habits where we check our breathing at various times during the day. Soon it becomes a part of our living pattern so that our breathing comes into our consciousness on a regular basis. Exercise, singing, deep breathing and regular conscious breathing will all play their part in healing the body. Although one could say that all parts of the body are equal and interdependent, there are two functions which are primary and essential to stimulate the healing process. These are the cleansing of the bowel and restoration of normal breathing. These two together will affect the balance and quality of blood and help return the body to normal as quickly as possible.

It is an interesting observation that in the West when we exclaim with an OH or an AH we do this in an out breath. In the East it is the opposite, exclamations are made on the in breath. This is another indication of the yin and yan and opposites of the east and west, in such a universal process as breathing.

Sound is closely connected with breathing. We harness the energy created by breathing so that we can create sound. The quality and strength of vocal expression is intimately connected with how we breathe and where we breathe from. A rich resonant voice comes from someone who breathes fully. Singers and athletes reach high levels of lung development and breath control as they exercise and train for their performances and competitions.

2.   Internal respiration

Cellular breathing continues the fundamental process of oxygen dispersion and the elimination of the waste products of oxidation. The inhalation of air and pranas makes possible cellular metabolism when it combines with carbon and hydrogen, and carbon dioxide and water are eliminated. The functions of the circulatory and respiratory systems coordinate here as the blood circulating through the lungs becomes saturated with oxygen and carries it through the body. The tissue cells absorb the oxygen from the blood, exchanging their wastes to be carried back to the lungs via the blood stream.

The success of internal respiration depends on the exposure of blood to all cell surfaces. Therefore, wherever circulation is inhibited, cells are deprived and the cellular respiration is diminished, both in terms of oxygen dispersion and the elimination of wastes. Whenever this happens a stagnant condition develops.

A primary goal of treatment is to equalize circulation and carry it to all parts of the body, both in terms of nutrient distribution from food, and oxygen dispersion from respiration. Here balanced function of holistic relationships is essential for good health.

When disease develops, cell respiration slows down. Medical researchers such as Heinrich Jung and P. Seeger have confirmed that degenerative diseases arise from disturbances in cellular respiration, resulting in less energy and serious disturbances in metabolism. Leslie Kenton in her book *Raw Energy* draws our attention to research proving that a raw diet increases the vitality of the whole organism by restoring normal cell respiration and functions which provide immunity against disease.

'Over quite a short time, an all-raw or nearly all-raw diet does several things. It eliminates accumulated wastes and toxins and restores optimal sodium/potassium and acid/alkaline balance. It supplies and/or restores the level of nutrients essential for optimal cell function. It increases the efficiency with which cells take up oxygen, necessary for the release of energy with which to carry out their multivarious activities. With all these desirable and interactive functions to their credit it is hardly surprising that raw foods have proved effective against cancer.'

3.   Primary breathing

Primary breathing is a pulsation coming from the lateral ventricle of the brain around the hypothalamus, stimulating the movement of cerebrospinal fluid (CSF) in cycles of 8–14 seconds down the spine between the meninges to the sacrum. It is essential to have a soft supple movement which is not inhibited by locked muscles. It has been discovered recently that retarded children have locked sacrums which inhibit this essential flow of fluid to and from the brain to its polar opposite, the sacrum.

There are three diaphragms, which work together to achieve the proper flow of CSF. These are:

1. the occiput, just under the back of the skull
2. the perineal muscles at the floor of the pelvis
3. the diaphragm, the neutral centre in the middle

Body work and exercise will free the muscles and allow full expression of primary breathing. It is significant to notice holistic relationships here as the parasympathetic nervous system sends its nerves both to the top and the bottom of the spine. The PSNS focus of relaxation, rest and receptivity encourages full movement to primary breathing, so easily inhibited by tension and locked muscles.

Consider also the pulsing rhythm from the higher centres which will also affect the rate, rhythm and quality of primary breathing.

Primary breathing bathes the brain in CSF and sends it pulsing downward to the opposite pole, the sacrum, creating a field of energy like a magnet. In the past it was thought that the fluid was contained within its own system, but evidence has been found recently that there is seepage at the sacrum pole into the body system.

Pulsing as it does from the higher brain centres to the opposite pole of the central nervous system one can visualize this process as similar to a magnet. Both the top of the spine and the base of the spine send out pulsing radiations of fluid and are connected via the spinal cord. The brain pulsations send the fluid downward and sacral movements send it back. The ebb and flow of this pulsing creates a communicating link between the two poles.

Cranial osteopaths tune into the dynamic process of the curling and uncurling of the central nervous system and the spine. Treatments will help to restore normal functions. The rhythm pulses at 12–14 times per minute. Due to this primary respiration tissues are always in dynamic motion. There is never true stillness in the body. Lung breathing and primary respiration, together with the heart beat and digestion, keeps the body in perpetual motion.

CSF is a clear, colourless fluid with a pH of about 7.4. There are not more than 5 lymphocytes per cubic ml. CSF contains very little protein, but has a high chloride content. It is formed by the choroid plexuses from blood plasma both by secretion and by ultrafiltration at a rate of 0.3 ml per minute, or 430 ml per 24 hours. The whole of the CSF is exchanged every 6–8 hours. It maintains a constant composition, differing from plasma or plasma filtrate, and the pressure remains constant. Production must be balanced by an equal reabsorption of fluid into the venous blood stream via the arachnoid villi, which project into venous sinuses, or by diffusion where the interstitial fluid of brain tissue is added to CSF. It is also reabsorbed into the venous system along the roots of spinal nerves into spinal veins, though the choroid plexuses themselves, and by the reabsorption into the blood stream favoured by the colloid osmatic pressure of plasma protein, since CSF contains very little protein. Some CSF also escapes into the lymph system, although there is no lymph in the CSF itself.

The CSF acts as a cushion between soft and delicate brain substance and the rigid cranium. It supports the weight of the brain and distributes the force of any blows to the head. Constant adjustments take place to maintain equilibrium. It probably also has metabolic functions, but these are not yet clearly known. One suggestion is that it takes the place of absent lymphatics. It obviously also acts as a communicating fluid between the two ends of the central nervous systems.

It is also important to note that there is a selective blood brain barrier so that most substances cannot pass into the CSF. However this barrier does not exist at birth, and takes about a week to develop. Water passes freely into the CSF.

Movement of the CSF is influenced by arterial pulsations, respiration, changes in venous pressure together with pulsing rhythms from one's higher centres, and blockages creating lack of response and movements on the physical tissue level.

4. Skin respiration

Our skin is more than just a body wrapping. It is the largest organ of our body, and good health depends on the skin performing its two-fold duties of respiration and excretion. If it is not performing these duties, the kidneys, liver and lymph have to compensate.

Skin inactivity is due to several causes or a combination of them, from poor and irregular bathing habits, to wearing of synthetic fabrics and lack of exercise. Inactivity of the skin is one of the main causes of all skin diseases, combined with poor eating habits. Any person who wishes to cure any physical problem, or enjoy an excellent standard of health, must apply therapeutic means to re-establish normal skin function.

Our skin is an organ of respiration and excretion. It absorbs oxygen (and water) and exhales poisonous gases. The skin also absorbs whatever lotions, creams or oils we put on the body. The rule should be that we should never use anything on the skin that we would not eat, as the body must assimilate, metabolize and eliminate such lotions as it would any food. Mineral oil cannot be absorbed and clogs the pores. Pure vegetable oils or natural organic creams would not only be readily absorbed by the body, but would also contribute to positive improvement by feeding the skin and providing the necessary moisture and nourishment for suppleness and tone.

The skin has millions of pores from which a constant stream of poisons should flow. If these pores are blocked, the poisons collect and are held in the skin and lymph, or try to return to the liver, thus forcing extra work on an active major organ. Bathing and brushing the skin is important so that dead dry skin is shed, allowing fresh skin to breathe and eliminate without inhibition. Hot and cold alternating temperatures in bathing, showering, saunas and packs, etc. give exercise to the skin, and increase and equalize the circulation, so that each part of the body receives its equal share of life-giving blood. The cold water contracts blood vessels and lessens the amount of blood, and the hot water draws the blood back, thus stimulating the blood, giving relief to the organs under the skin, as it breaks up any congestion.

Good bathing and cleansing habits are essential for good health. We have heard many times that 'Cleanliness is next to Godliness'. Prophets have guided their followers to be scrupulously clean. Plants appear fresher and brighter, refreshed after a shower, and birds and animals do not neglect their daily bath. Similarly, for us, a daily bath is ideal, and should not be less than three times a week. The pores open during baths and toxins are eliminated.

The skin also regulates the body temperature. Usually it is non-conducting and dense, preventing the escape of body heat, but in fevers and heat, the skin sweats and lets heat escape. Drinks of water and bathing the body with cool cloths, will aid this process. When water surrounds the body it influences the nervous system through the skin, as the skin is also the organ of touch, closely connected with all the great nerve centres. Openings into the body are also lined with mucous membranes which resemble the skin in structure. These membranes also secrete and excrete. The skin also helps us by storing large quantities of water and salts, resisting the invasion of germs, and absorbing gases and fatty substances. It is richly supplied with blood vessels. The sebaceous glands secrete a greasy substance which keeps the skin supple.

Radials

The respiratory system in the iris

It is interesting to see that the nose/jaw radial is opposite the diaphragm area on the iris chart. Here reflexes link sneezing and coughing, which clears the head and nose. Do we breathe through our nose or mouth? Look in these areas for disturbances in colour, weak connective tissue, and nerve rings which will contribute to evaluation.

The lung throat radial reveals the close connection of the passages of inhalation and exhalation through the throat, as breath moves from the throat via the bronchials into the lungs.

The medulla to sacrum radials reveal the connection between the two ends of the central nervous system, the parasympathetic nervous system and primary breathing. Here the law 'as above so below', applies. Posture of the skeletal frame and strength and quality of the muscles affect the position of the spine. Mental disease and retardation is associated with a frozen sacrum, which affects the flow of CSF.

Inherent weaknesses

An inherent weakness in the medulla would indicate weak governing function to the respiratory system. Lacunae in the lung areas would suggest weak connective tissue together with lack of nutrient and inefficient eliminative processes in lung and bronchial tissue. It is important to evaluate the level of tissue in these areas and determine whether acute to chronic processes are taking place. I have seen many cases of inherent weakness in the lung areas, when they suffered severe whooping cough during childhood. We do not know whether the weakness was there before the whooping cough or whether it came as a result of severe prolonged coughing. It would be valuable research to be able to take case histories before and after whooping cough. Large lacunae in medial and/or lateral areas of one or both irides also relate to the psychological life as the TB miasm (Hall) or heart/nurturing issues (Johnson).

B3 bulge and scurf rim
The common bulging out of watery grey colour from the lung areas into the sclera, at 3 and 9 o'clock on one or both eyes, indicates (according to Dorothy Hall) a lack of B3 in the digestive process. Niacin affects both circulation and assimilation of nutrient. According to turn of the century pioneer iridologists this also indicates suppression of illness together with a high level of inherited toxins. As I have found this mark to clear up during purification and regeneration treatment, as circulation and body processes normalize, I imagine this to reflect the collection of fluids and toxins together with sluggish and inactive skin, circulation and lymph functions. Thick scurf rims indicate toxins collected in the lung areas.

Acute to chronic colours
As the respiratory system is an eliminative channel one or more of its parts may experience exudative release of acute elimination during disease or healing crises. Whenever reflexive fibres register large and swollen, especially when accompanied by lymphatic tophi, one can assume inflammatory conditions are taking place or are about to take place.

When dark colours indicate hypofunction of any of these areas, one has to evaluate the function of the entire body and begin treatment with weakest systems and organs and eliminative channels.

Always pay special attention to any signs which might indicate that there may be an elimination from the lungs at some stage. It is wise to prepare the person for this eventuality so that the patient will not think it is an ordinary flu and suppress it with aspirins or antibiotics. I always tell my patients to ring me if they get a flu or cold during treatment for support and guidance.

Treatment of the respiratory system — the eliminative channels
As the lungs are in the *heart centre*, negative emotions, fear, selfishness, inability to give or love, possessiveness, etc. will cause restriction of the muscles, affect breathing and inhibit the function of the thymus. Lobelia packs, osteopathy, meditation, counselling, body work and Bach flower remedies will all contribute to the release of these life patterns.

Collapsed shoulders (as a reflection of over-concern, fear, excess feelings of responsibility and protectiveness) will also inhibit full breathing potential. Alexander technique is excellent to restore proper posture and give the skills to maintain posture during daily life. Bach remedies will help to restore positive expression of life attitudes.

Solar plexus tensions will inhibit diaphragmatic movements which contribute to full and deep breathing. Shock will freeze the diaphragm, and as it is the valve between the emotional brain and the expression centres, any repression of emotions will cause tensing and hardening of the diaphragm. Body work, bowel cleansing, nourishing of the nervous system, emotional counselling and Bach flower remedies will help to soften and release the diaphragm. The castor oil pack is also excellent to soften and relax the area.

Treatment for asthma

Although this is a complex chronic condition and requires individual assessment and treatment of basic weakness and the eliminative channels, we have found that the following treatment (once balanced normal functions of the above are restored) to be excellent. We have had cases where the patient has been on several drugs and inhalants and has been able to completely stop the drugs and live a normal life. The general treatment is: asthma tea, respiratory formula, lobelia tincture for spasms, lobelia poultices, mullein and lobelia smoking mix and the antibiotic herbal formulae. It is not possible to apply the above treatment except within the framework of an individual assessment.

Herbal replacements for cortisone are possible with the regular intake of wild yam root and licorice over a period of weeks together with gradual decreases in the drugs. Eventually the patient will be able to come off the drug altogether, but it is only the patient who can monitor the treatment. The practitioner can never suggest this. It must of course take place within the framework of a complete individual treatment programme.

Breathing exercise

This exercise builds up the medulla and improve the quality of breathing. Take in strong, quick inhalations until the lungs are full, then tense the fists, feeling the lungs expand, then release the tension slowly. After taking about four normal breaths repeat the same exercise.

The diaphragm is a unique muscle which like breathing, continues its movements all through each person's life. It is that which brings what is up, down, and what is down, up. The power or weakness of the diaphragm influences the quality of blood, because it draws air into the lungs, and stagnant blood up from the lower limbs into the pelvis.

Respiratory system and the lymphatic system

The lymphatic endocrine gland sits between the two lungs in the heart centre offering its protective influence. The entire respiratory system is richly endowed with lymphatics. The more effective the respiratory

Holistic relationships: interaction with other systems

system is in cleansing the blood and oxygenating the system, the more it aids the lymph to do its job of purification. As they are both eliminative channels, the function of one closely affects the function of the other. They support each other closely. When lymphatic tophi show in the respiratory system, this indicates that catarrh has collected and a sluggish system is inhibiting normal functions. Whenever adenoids are congested they inhibit breathing processes.

Respiratory system and the endocrine system
The thymus gland rests between the two lungs. The thyroids and parathyroids sit on either side of the neck, governing the rate of metabolism and the balance of calcium in the blood. Thyroid would also affect respiratory processes because of its effect on metabolic rate. It is not hard to imagine that the movement of air throughout the throat must affect the function of these glands, as would the sounds of the voice.

Respiratory system and the reproductive system
The mother's respiratory system maintains functions for the baby while it is in the womb. The exchanges of blood taking place in the placenta provides the foetus with all its requirements. Obviously the quality of the mother's respiration processes directly affects those of the foetus.

Respiratory system and the urinary system
Both eliminative channels work together to purify and balance the blood. If the respiratory system is not functioning adequately the kidneys take on a greater burden, and vice versa.

Respiratory system and the muscular system
One strong lifetime muscle, the diaphragm, is a constant part of the constantly dynamic external respiration, as are the lungs themselves. Also the respiratory system carries the oxygen to all the tissues and the cells of the muscular system to participate in internal respiration.

Respiratory system and the skeletal system
It is very important that the skeletal system supports the lungs so that they can function properly. Incorrect posture where the shoulders move forward and down will inhibit breathing because the lungs cannot expand fully. The medulla can also be restricted and weakened by improper placement of the skull and position of the cervical vertebrae. Accidents and birth injuries to the spine can both affect medulla and lung function.

Respiratory system and the nervous system
The medulla brain and nerve centre controls the activity of the chest and all its functions. Breathing stops when the nervous system is cut off from the medulla. A weak medulla means weak lungs, because it is the chest brain governing all parts of the respiratory system.

In the nervous system we also have to consider that the sympathetic nervous system dilates the lungs and bronchi and the parasympathetic nervous system constricts them. When we need more energy and a quick response, we need more oxygen and a quicker breathing rate.

Respiratory system and the digestive system

Nutrition affects the lungs. Mucus foods cause catarrh to collect, which provides a feeding ground for viruses and the development of inflammation and infection. Adequate nutrition is also essential for keeping the medulla in optimum function. The digestive system and the respiratory system both share the same mouth and throat passages. The respiratory system provides the oxygen which is necessary for cellular metabolism. Constipation and tense spastic muscles in the digestive system may affect the function of the diaphragm, causing it to become rigid or hindered in its movements, thus affecting breathing quality. The production of gases in the digestive system may also cause blockages in the tissues, affecting proper respiration. It is also necessary to drink enough so that water is available for the elimination of wastes via the respiratory system.

Respiratory system and the circulatory system

These two systems are closely intertwined. The drawing together of air from the outside to meet blood from the inside so that oxygen can be absorbed and transported throughout the body, and the subsequent return of wastes for the exchange of fresh oxygen, shows that communication and harmony of both systems is essential to health and well-being. The heart and lungs are both governed by the medulla, again a coordinating factor in their close relationship. When the medulla is cut off the heart stops and the lungs cease breathing.

THE LYMPHATIC SYSTEM

Each cell of the body floats in a sea of clear fluid, each cell like an island surrounded by tides of movement and pressure. Like the weather, the fluid changes direction, quality and viscosity. Wherever movement of the fluid is inhibited by tension, excess collects the fluid causing insufficiency in another, resulting in congestion. Fluid is denied access to these islands of tension, inhibiting the flow of life. Visualization helps one to gain an understanding of this invisible mysterious body system, the lymphatic system.

For many years if you asked anyone what the lymphatic system is they would never know. Some might reply, lymph glands, others with more knowledge, the immune system, yet this system has many different parts and functions absolutely indispensable for our health and well-being. Perhaps it is a good thing that we have been forced to learn about this system because of the spread of auto-immune diseases as it is the key to our survival in this toxic age.

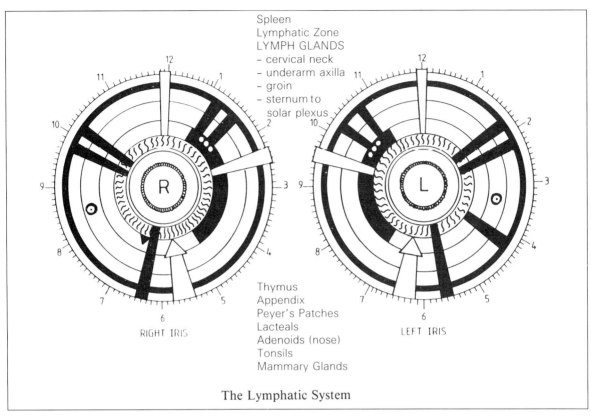

The Lymphatic System

How the lymphatic system works   The lymphatic system, with all its many and varied parts, provides many different functions, all essential to our health and well-being. Perhaps one of the most important functions is that it acts as a drainage system for all the body tissues of the byproducts of metabolism and waste materials. That is why it is so important that the lymph flows equally through all the tissues. Once it is denied access, wastes collect and auto-intoxication begins. As it moves about the body the lymph also carries nourishment and hormones. A collector of spent blood flow that seeps from the capillaries, the lymph purifies itself and returns to the blood from the main lymph channels near the heart. At least half of the blood protein lost in the circulation is retrieved and restored by the lymphatic system as a part of this process.

Many of the functions centre around its role as a warning and defence system. The most important warning devices are the appendix, tonsils, peyer's patches in the small intestines and the adenoids. The removal of these warning devices when they become infected leaves the body defenceless before the increase of auto-intoxication. The cause of the infection needs to be removed, not the warning device itself. The lymph nodes filter the lymph fluids and remove dangerous impurities, such as dyes, chemicals, old red blood cells and debris-laden white cells. They also manufacture antibodies to fight infection, and in the lung area the lymph nodes filter out soot from the air.

It is very interesting how the main lymph areas centre around the neck, the arms and the top of the arms and legs, where we have most movement in the body to aid lymph flow. Once the fluid is purified by the lymph nodes it joins the main lymph channels and is then returned to the blood and body as required. Every part of the body, except the central nervous system, has its own lymph system to keep the tissues clean and to protect the area from invasion, whether by toxic materials or viruses.

The lymph system also has an important function in the intestines, where the lacteals absorb fats, and then lets them seep slowly into the blood stream in safe amounts.

Anything that we bathe in or put on our skin is absorbed quickly and directly into the lymphatic system. If we use chemical cosmetics, lotions, bath oils, cleaners, etc, the lymphatic system must work to purify and eliminate them. It is important to realize this so that we choose wisely and follow the rule that we would not put anything on our body that we would not eat. This helps to explain the effectiveness of treatments such as aromatherapy, poultices, baths and fomentations, and to appreciate the stories where we hear that people are kept alive by soaking them in special baths and rubbing oils on their body.

The work of the lymphatic drainage system is tireless. It is working constantly to reduce excess catarrh, mucus secretions and waste. In this capacity it acts as a channel of elimination. When the lymphatic system is not functioning properly due to high levels of toxicity and a sluggish metabolism, or a long period of sedentary or bedridden illness, other eliminative channels have to work harder to compensate, such as the kidneys or the skin, and vice-versa. The five eliminative channels work in ecological concert, the function of one affecting the function of the others, and each one helping to compensate for lack of function in any of the others. Any assessment of the lymphatic system must be made in relation to the function of the other eliminative channels. The function of the lymph is particularly close to that of the kidneys in that they retrieve and eliminate toxins.

What does the lymphatic system contain?

The lymphatic system contains approximately two gallons of white, colourless, clear interstitial tissue fluids, twice to three times more than the volume of blood. This is a slightly alkaline fluid which is kept in balance by the normal production of HCl in the stomach. When it goes out of balance, normal salts are excreted in perspiration, air, urine and faeces and the body becomes deficient, eventually resulting in acidosis or alkalosis. This helps us to understand why auto-urine therapy is so effective in chronic disease. The lost salts are returned and the body is helped to return to balance. Another result of any imbalanced constituency of the lymph fluids is that calcium is deposited in the joints. Lymphatic constitutions have a predisposition to arthritis and rheumatism.

How does the lymph move?

Every movement in our body stimulates the lymph. The pulsations of our intestines during the process of digestion, breathing, eating, as well as the more obvious muscular movements all help to move the lymph fluid forward along their tiny pearl like strands, each one a valve so that once the lymph is moved forward, it cannot move back, until it reaches the main lymph channels where it is returned to the blood, purified and sterile. The pressure behind the valves forces the lymph forward and upward through the nodes to the main channels. Rebounding, aerobics and running stimulate lymphatic movement. The lymph nodes act like thousands of tiny hearts, pumping lymph up from the extremities towards the neck where it enters the venous circulation. These spontaneous pumping contractions are a result of the stretching caused by the buildup of lymph – a process called frequency stabilization. Movement is life and the movement of lymph results in quality of life, another reason to make sure that exercise is an important part of your life.

Blockages in the lymphatic system

Blockages which inhibit the flow of lymph and their essential bodily processes are caused in several different ways:

1. *Mechanical blockages* result after physical strain, long periods of inactivity, childbirth difficulties, structural problems and vocational posture. Continued blockage begins the process of degeneration which sets the foundation for illness.

2. *Infectious diseases* cause blockages which must be cleared so that the person can completely recover from the illness and not set the stage for chronic disease.

3. *Serious injuries* such as burns, exposure to extreme hot or cold weather, accidents and broken bones can cause inflammation and eventually lasting malfunction to lymph glands.

4. *Abrasions and small injuries* need healing in local areas which require lymphatic participation. The areas furthest away from vaso-motor distribution and activity can be deficient if the body is not working at optimum efficiency. The longer the healing takes to accomplish, the more the body is disturbed and affected.

It is important to remember that blockages in one area can cause symptoms in other remote areas. It is essential to keep the main terminals clear in the neck, under the arms and in the groin, otherwise colds and flus result as the body attempts to clear them by manifesting acute elimination. Exercise is important as well as drinking sufficient fluids.

When the blockages become chronic, lymph stasis, the precursor of cancer, manifests. This congestion is a significant factor in obesity, oedema, anaemia, angina and many other chronic conditions. As the congestion increases due to the blocked lymph flow, there is a shortage of lymph fluid inside the area where regular body functions have ceased.

The tissues do not receive nourishment and elimination, and outside, excess fluids denied access to the area create congestion, inflammation and increased tension due to unequal blood and fluid pressures. The oxygen supply is decreased and waste toxins are retained. The nerve endings become impaired in function and in some areas the excess fluids press on the nerve endings, causing pain. Eventually there is a loss of control over cell proliferation and a predisposition to tumour formation and abnormal cell growth.

The lymphatic system may also be regarded as the negative pole of the water principle flowing in the body, the positive being the firey hot red blood which beats the tune of our life from a large central heart. As a negative pole the lymph is slow, cold and heavy. Its natural tendency is to settle, so we must move to make it flow. This correlates to the emotional aspects of the feminine nature, as defined by the moon. Whenever lymph collects, so does negativity, whether in the form of toxic waste or unfinished emotions. It is essential to realize that negative emotions also affect the flow of the lymph. When we tense our body and hold on to things we also inhibit the flow of life processes. The result is that all carcinomas are the result of local lymph obstruction.

When the lymph system is diseased a number of changes take place. The first thing to happen is that the lymph glands become swollen. This is comparable to clogged drains. If this continues for too long it begins to affect the tissues in the area, preventing such basic functions as the circulation of nutrition from taking place. Disordered lymph function can cause anaemia. Imbalanced nutrition causes the blood to be alkaline which makes iron move into the lymph. It is still in the body but it is not available to the blood stream for distribution. An unbalanced lymph system can alter leucocyte production causing excess or insufficiency, disturbing our immunity. It can also cause variations in blood pressure, body temperature and the body's ability to heal. It is extremely important that the lymph system maintains the correct acid/alkaline balance, because an over-alkaline body produces acids, and an over-acid body produces alkalines as the body attempts to restore balance, both situations putting undue stress on the lymphatic system which should always be kept at prime levels for defence and all its other important and necessary functions.

The subtle lymph system
According to David Tansley, author of *The Subtle Body*, 'The spleen chakra's role is to supply vital energy to all the chakras on all levels of the personality or lower self. It is not directly related to major chakras. Its role is to vitalize the etheric body.'

The spleen is such a mysterious organ that it is easier to understand the importance of its subtle functions, because its physical functions are so varied and indefinable.

Through the ages metaphysicians, healers and mystics have written

The spleen

about the subtle functions of the spleen. In *The Secret Doctrine* Madame Blavatsky says that the physical spleen is only a cover for the real spleen. The spleen acts as the distributing centre for prana (life vitality) coming into the body.

Acupuncturists view the spleen as an organ in which yin and yang are most balanced as it is neither full nor empty. They consider the most important functions of the spleen as the distribution of nourishment throughout the body and the governing of will, concentration and memory. In the five elements school of acupuncture they regard the spleen as the centre. When the spleen is sick the entire body is fundamentally sick. It is a 'ki' disease, 'ki' being the force of the universe which circulates throughout the body and animating it. When this force is prevented from circulating properly, disease begins.

Dr Randolph Stone, creator of Polarity Therapy and author of *The Mystic Bible,* believes that when the spleen is malfunctioning food is not distributed. When the spleen over-works it attempts to balance the body, and excess periods and a lack of discrimination can result. Relationships also become unbalanced as one cannot distribute oneself evenly on any level, physically, mentally or emotionally. In *The Mystic Bible* he talks about the spleen as a psychic door where we are connected with the finer energy regions. When our sensory (umbilical cord) and our motor energy (end of the spinal cord in the back) are linked, the spleen acts as a real door for finer energies and as an etheric exchange centre for these functions. Aside from the more obvious physical functions, the spleen centre absorbs and distributes prana and vitality to our etheric and physical bodies. It also brings down into physical consciousness whatever inherent qualities are in the corresponding astral centre. This relationship between etheric energies and moral qualities are not spiritual energies, but qualities of higher mind.

In David Tansley's *Radionics and the Subtle Anatomy of Man*, the *etheric* body is seen as a receiver, assimilator and transmitter of prana. These energies streaming in from the sun are absorbed by the etheric body through a series of small force centres and then passed on to the spleen, where the vital essence of the sun is subjected to a process of intensification or devitalization according to the condition of the organism before being circulated to vitalize the physical body. The etheric body of man has therefore been described as negative or receptive in respect to solar radiations, and as positive or expulsive in respect to the physical body.

Auryavedic medicine holds the function of the spleen to be very important, as its pyramid shape contacts many other organs, the diaphragm, stomach, left kidney, colon and pancreas, thus connecting all the elements of air, fire, water and earth in the body. Because of this unique position the spleen has intimate association with all three doshas or energies in the body, which we can loosely describe as wind, bile and mucus. The spleen unites the physical and subtle bodies and communicates and distributes the elements and energies in the body.

Vitality globules from the subtle body are first drawn into the spleen centre and then broken up into seven component atoms. Each atom is charged with one of the seven prana varieties and then caught up and spun around the appropriate chakra. The seven prana varieties are correlated to colours, which relate to colours on the higher levels of causal, mental and astral bodies. The pranic colours are: violet, blue, green, yellow, orange, dark red and rose red. Indigo is divided between violet and blue, and red is divided into dark red and rose red.

The seventh colour, rose pink, is despatched through the hub or centre of the spleen and distributed over the whole of the nervous system as the life of the nervous system. The atoms grow paler as they sweep along the nerves, parting with their pranic content until they are eventually discharged from the body through the pores of the skin forming what is called the health aura, a pale bluish white emanation. A healthy person has an excess of prana charged particles which are discharged from the body in all directions through the health aura, along with particles from which the prana has been extracted. Someone like this is a source of health and strength to those around them as they shed vitality. Healers have this energy in great abundance. The astral centres corresponding to the spleen also have the function of vitalizing the whole astral abody.

David Tansley, in *Subtle Body*, describes the spleen as the physical organ which is an externalization of a subtle force centre which is directly responsible for absorbing the solar or pranic forces from the sun and distributing their vitalizing qualities to the physical body by way of the etheric body.

Paracelsus's descriptions of the closeness of the animal body and the sidereal body, and their interaction, supports the theory of the spleen acting as a doorway and distributing centre of the life energy which comes from the sidereal body into the animal body. The sidereal body consists of fire and air while the animal body is made up of fire, air, earth and water.

In acupuncture the spleen and liver have a balancing relationship. They are on opposite sides of the body, the spleen secreting acids into the duodenum and the liver secreting alkalines. The spleen is also recognized as the organ which digests and assimilates nutrient.

When the spleen is inactive or removed some of the spleen functions are carried on by lymph nodes and the bone marrow. In acute spleen disease the spleen is soft and flabby whereas chronic spleen conditions result in a hard spleen.

Functions of the spleen
The spleen has many and varied functions, some of them only activated when another part of the immune system becomes hypoactive. The spleen seems to communicate with, balance and compensate for all the other parts of the lymphatic system. While it can be removed without causing death, quality of life and protective functions are impaired, as well as vibrant energy levels reduced.

The spleen acts as a detoxicant and helps to remove dead cells. It filters as it maintains the composition of circulatory blood and is involved in the manufacture of blood cells. Whenever infection occurs it forms antibodies and anti-toxins and manufactures lymphocytes and monocytes for export, and is active in immune response to antigens. The spleen helps to remove debris from the blood and breaks down aged red blood corpuscles. It also acts as minimal storage for red blood corpuscles. The spleen is responsible for converting the *haem* portions of haemoglobin molecules indirectly to bilirubin, which goes to the liver and helps to manufacture bile, causing the yellow colour. Excessive bilirubin results in jaundice.

When diseased the spleen may cause severe anaemia, typhoid, typhus, malaria, brain malfunction, lack of concentration, hyperacidity, acidosis, and toxaemia.

The spleen is a purple, concave delicate structure which sits at the tip of the pancreatic tongue. This passive heart of the lymph system repeats all the functions of all the parts of the lymphatic system. It stands in for or supports any part of the system which breaks down or becomes overloaded and assists generally in the functions of blood production, defence, transport of nutrient and hormones, body purification and storage of blood. It also functions most significantly in the subtle energy bodies.

The spleen in the iris
The spleen appears in the iris in the left eye at 4:15 to 4:30. Toxins from the bowel can affect the spleen, and cause darkening in the iris, and often insomnia results. When feverish illness occurs check out the markings in the peyer's patches in the small intestines. Black spots in the spleen area may indicate tumours.

Lightening of the spleen area indicates splenitis (inflammation of the spleen) and is related to disease of the stomach and intestines. Acute splenitis may manifest white, pink or red reflective fibres or transversals.

The spleen–heart transversal is a well known iris marking which should be taken as an indication for immediate treatment.

Lymphatic congestion in the spleen area shows up in the outer lymphatic ring as white, yellowish or brown lymphatic tophi. Lacunae suggest weak connective tissue. The radial opposite to the spleen is the lower jaw, and on the right eye the jaw reflexes to the liver, indicating once again the close connection to the liver. Both liver and spleen disturbances result in eye swelling and itching.

When the spleen is enlarged, the iris area can also be larger. The ANW may point outwards into the spleen area drawing our attention to nerve involvement and stress. Nerve rings may also circled inwards close to the ANW. Psora would indicate insufficiency on the physical level and issues with anger and resentment on emotional levels.

The lymphatic rosary in the iris
The Hydrogenoid Constitutional type manifests the lymphatic rosary in the lymphatic zone in the iris. The tophi may completely circle the iris or

may only appear in certain places. It is important to observe whether the tophi appear in significant areas, like the liver, spleen or kidney. Variations of colouring reveal the level of toxic encumbrance or exudative activity.

Whenever lymph collects toxicity results both on physical and mental-emotional levels. Thickening and slowing of these lymphatic fluids and functions represents a diminishment of one of our most self protective forces. In this age of pollution we fear cancer and spend millions on research to try to find a cure. It is better for each person to take the responsibility to clear their bodies of waste, and activate their own immune system.

Lymphatic or lymph glands

The lymphatic system has many different types of glands appearing in different parts of the body acting as warning devices and warriors for defence. They produce white blood cells, leucocytes, which are like police patrols or refuse disposal for the body, removing rubbish and filtering lymph, removing the fertile ground for infection.

Adenoids are placed at the back of the nose to act as warning devices whenever infection, catarrhal encumbrance and mucus exudations occur.

Appendix in the lower ascending colon, where the caecum empties through the ileocaecal valve, secrete lubricant to aid the passage of bowel matter up the colon and an antiseptic solution to prevent infection. Inflammation begins when constipation retains faecal matter in the colon. The removal of the appendix leaves the area without protection, thus allowing further degeneration into seriously chronic conditions.

Cervical lymph glands in the throat swell up when toxins from the head, neck, throat and shoulders create infection, as they attempt to purify the area.

Inguinal glands purify toxins from the pelvis, groin and legs.

Axillary lymph glands purify toxins from the body trunk and breasts, lungs and chest under the arms.

Lacteals are small intestinal lymphatics that absorb fat slowly from the chyme and pass it into the lymph system by way of the thoracic duct to the blood stream.

Peyer's patches in the small intestines, near the distal ileum, stimulate fevers to overcome infection whenever digestive conditions, viruses, parasites, worms, etc. take hold. They act as the centre within the digestive system to create antibodies against the invasion of micro-organisms. The body's natural fevers kill the infection by raising the temperatures. Excessive fevers over long periods of time can damage the ability of the peyer's patches to protect the body from digestive infection.

Thymus is the endocrine member of the lymphatic system. It is very active during infancy and youth, defending the child against infection. It seeds the other lymphatic organs and glands with potential 'T' lymphocytes which secrete a substance that attacks the proteins of tumour cells, foreign cells, and invaders of all kinds. It produces thymosin hormone that enhances the development of 'T' lymphocytes.

Tonsils act as a warning device in the throat. They become inflamed when toxic encumbrance produces infections. Removing them damages the protective system of the throat area.

Lymphatic glands in the iris
When assessing the lymphatic glands in the iris, pay particular attention to lymphatic tophi if they appear in the neck, underarm or groin areas where the major lymph glands are placed to purify the body, especially during fevers, infections and when there are swollen glands. Acute eliminations, whether during a healing or disease crisis, will register as white exudations. It is important to determine whether bowel toxins are adding to the problem. Check out the spleen reading and determine whether other eliminative channels are involved. Look for tiny black spots which may signify chronic toxic levels and ineffective leucocyte functions.

Thymus This endocrine gland is rarely shown on iris charts. As it is in the centre of the body in the bronchial, lung areas, look for hypoactive signs when this the body's protective system is not working properly. This gland is becoming the subject for research as we learn more about its importance in immune defence.

The thymus is responsible for immunological surveillance. After the lymphocytes have formed in the bone marrow, they travel to the thymus gland where they mature and then move on to the lymph nodes and spleen. Here they reside as 'T' cells (thymus derived cells) which respond to thymus hormones travelling through the blood stream. Continued stress depletes the gland of its 'T' cells, so that when they are really needed there is an insufficient supply to ward off the disease. Conversely, the parasympathetic state of relaxation, together with a calm mind and quiet emotions, will keep the thymus operating at peak levels.

John Diamond, MD, and president of the International Academy of Preventive Medicine and recipient of the Naughton-Manning Prize for Psychiatry states 'I have never seen a patient with a chronic degenerative illness who did not have an underactive thymus gland .... I believe that it is the thymus weakness, or underactivity, that is the original cause of the illness. All illnesses start with a diminuation of the life energy. Should this decrease continue, some organ of the body will be the target for the illness.'

It is most significant that this gland is in the heart centre or chakra. Here, we either express love, and warmth which enables the thymus gland to flourish and protect us, or inhibit love and caring which contracts our thymus into inactivity. It used to be accepted as normal that the thymus shrivelled and became redundant. This is not natural or right. Children rejoice in an open heart centre but if life closes down our heart centre we are the ones to suffer. If we restore our capacity to love and open our heart centre the thymus benefits and provides us with the protection we need.

The thymus gland is the first organ to be affected by stress, therefore it is an important link between mind and body. The six factors which strongly affect the thymus are stress, emotional attitudes, posture, food, social environment and the physical environment. Smoking and depressive mental states also weaken the thymus. It is called the gland of love, youth and enthusiasm, and reflects the person's outlook and attitude to life. It also holds the sex expression in abeyance, the opposite of the adrenals which accelerate it. Where self destructive illnesses have taken hold, improvement in life attitudes will help to activate this essential gland for defence against disease.

Catherine Ponder in *The Healing Secret of the Ages* says

'Metaphysically, the thymus gland, being closely situated to the heart, is associated with man's love nature. A malfunction in this area, whether heart, chest, lungs or breast, indicates a malfunction of the mind power of love located in that area.'

Appendix

Lacunae (muscle weakness) in this area and bowel pockets are commonly associated with toxic conditions. White signs indicate acute inflammation and dark signs reveal toxins and hypofunction. If the ascending colon has become swollen due to sluggish bowel movement the ileo-caecal valve is often involved. Here the lymphatic warning device works as a part of the digestive system where good muscle tone is necessary to move faeces upward.

Peyer's patches

In acute fevers this area appears white. In chronic diseases when the ability for the acute fever reaction is lost, this area appears dark and hyperactive. Bowel pockets and markings affecting the ANW are also important considerations.

Lacteals

These appear all throughout the small intestines, there is no actual place in the iris where they can be assessed except as a part of the digestive and assimilative process.

Adenoids

Trouble here would appear as part of a sinus congestion rising up to the head above the transverse colon and in the nose zone, particularly the lymphatic end of that zone.

Tonsils

The tonsil, larynx and pharynx zone indicate congestion in the back of the throat when lymphatic signs appear in the outer circulation zone. When there is active infection and inflammation these signs would be white.

Mammary glands

Lymphatic drainage here is significant, both to drain the fat portion of milk produced during lactation and as a vehicle to transfer infected material or cancer cells from the breast to distant parts. Once again, this area is part of the heart centre, where as we discussed in the section on the thymus, one's attitude to life and one's ability to love affects the function of physical tissue. Here, the breasts are the symbol of loving nourishment and nurturing. Inhibition and congestion reveals the struggles taking place in this love centre of the body.

Treatment for lymphatic system

Specific herbs for the lymphatic system

1.   *Echinacea:* This prime lymphatic herb is known as the *herbal antibiotic.* In America it was called 'Prairie doctor' because it was such a beneficial herb. It promotes the production of white blood cells which then destroy invading bacteria, microbes and virus infections. Echinacea also neutralizes acid conditions of the blood associated with stagnation of lymphatic fluids and increases the body's resistance to infection.

Dosage: Powder in capsules: 2 every half hour in acute conditions for 2 hours, then decrease to 2 every hour for 2 hours, and then maintain dose 2–4 times a day until the condition is clear. This treatment is ineffective unless accompanied by thorough bowel cleansing, rest, juice and fruit diet and baths to stimulate the flow of perspiration. Non-toxic herbal medicines will never knock out a virus, but will effectively increase the action of the immune system.

2.   *Mullein:* relieves lymphatic congestion in swollen glands, earaches, toothaches, haemorrhoids. Poultice: $\frac{2}{3}$ mullein, $\frac{1}{3}$ lobelia.

3.   *Poke root* reduces inflammation of lymph glands, especially of tonsillitis, mumps, mastitis (caution: not over 1 g per day).

4.   *Yellow dock:* high in iron, nourishes spleen, aids lymph functions.

5.   *Herbs for injections:* any one or combination of: plantain, black walnut, golden seal, bugle weed, marshmallow root, lobelia, garlic, parsley, watercress, rosemary, rose hips.

6.   *Lobelia:* the herb of equilibrium; restores balance of congestion or depletion. This herb reflects the quality of the lymph and restores communication between the circulatory and lymphatic systems.

Formulae

Lymph formula: (equal parts echinacea, lobelia, mullein, poke root, burdock, cayenne, chaparral).

Antibiotics naturally: (equal parts of golden seal, burdock, lobelia, mullein, $1\frac{1}{2}$ parts echinacea, $\frac{1}{2}$ parts cloves, garlic, thyme).

Chronic purifier: (Dr Shook) (40g mimosa gum, 120g echinacea, 40g blue flag, 120g comfrey root, 40g irish moss, 40g cloves).

Heavy metal purifier: 300g yellow dock root, 300g bugle weed, 75g lobelia and 300g chaparral (must take daily Epsom salt baths) and the kidney formula.

Diuretics: Because the lymphatic system and the urinary system have a close relationship when it comes to water balance and fluid retention, diuretics also work to reduce lymphatic swellings and obesity. The most common and effective herbs for this purpose are marestail, parsley, uva ursi, clivers, buchu, nettles.

It is also a great help to drink purifying teas on a regular basis such as red clover, violet leaves, red raspberry etc. These are pleasant tasting and over time will improve function.

It is very important to read good herbal books like those of Dr Shook, Dr Christopher and Michael Tierra to get a good understanding of each herb. Read about alternative and lymphatic herbs. This will also help you to understand the formulae.

Begin treating the eliminative channels and progress slowly towards more intense purification. One might use the lymph and blood purifying formulae in the beginning and then proceed to the chronic purifier. Only after the body is really working very well would one proceed to the heavy metal purifier. Each eliminative channel must be working very well before strong purification can proceed safely without aggravation.

As purification will mean that toxins will also pass out of the body at a higher rate, weak systems and organs have to be supported. If there is any sign of hypofunction in the kidneys use the kidney/bladder formula and/or diuretic herbal teas and make sure the patient is taking in an adequate amount of fluids. This will eliminate any chance of headaches and fatigue due to too many toxins in the blood stream.

Poultices and packs

Castor oil packs feed directly into the lymph system. See Appendix III.

Poultices and fomentations: Direct herbal feeding into the area of need. Herbal properties are absorbed directly into the skin, moving into the blood and lymph to supply tissues with what is needed to fight infection and regenerate cells.

Poultices: Local lymph obstruction, swelling and congested glands can be helped immediately by poultices of mullein and one third lobelia. Put the herbs in a gauze, pour just enough boiling water on to saturate. After it has cooled enough to put it on, cover with plastic wrap, and leave on. If you do not have mullein and lobelia, use comfrey, slippery elm, golden seal or poke root. Onions, potatoes and carrots, grated and semi-cooked, will help to relieve congestions.

Emetics: Cleansing the stomach of morbid matter and fermentation will diminish the body's need to produce a healing or disease crises, and so relieve the lymphatic system.

Water of life: From the earliest dawn of man's history in the Auryavedic teachings man has recommended drinking one's own urine. In modern terms it is as though you are drinking your own homeopathic potentized water, replacing the balance of what an unhealthy body is eliminating in the urine.

Sore throats: whenever the lymphatic system is draining poisons via the mucous membranes of the throat and tonsils, drink and gargle a mixture of cider vinegar, hot water, pressed garlic, cayenne, honey and lemon. This combined mixture blends nicely, neutralizing the strong taste of some of the individual ingredients. Thyme tea is also an excellent antiseptic tea.

Homeopathy
While these remedies are highly regarded lymphatic remedies the prescription would of course be based on regular homeopathic analysis: nat. mur., calc. carb., echinacea, ceanothus, calc. iod., veratrum alb., hepar. sulph.

Aromatherapy
Injection or absorption into the skin is injection directly into the lymphatic system. The use of specific aromatherapy oils, in massage or baths which affect the lymphatic system, will greatly enhance the healing process. Use the following oils:

1. *Spleen tonic:* black pepper, chamomile, fennel, lavender, rose.
2. *Antibacterial:* (does what antibiotics do) cinnamon, eucalyptus, origanum, sandalwood, thyme, tea tree oil.
3. *Internal toxic congestion:* peppermint.
4. *Oedema:* pennyroyal, pachouli, juniper.
5. *Stimulate leucocytes:* bergamot, lemon.
6. *Scrofula:* (TB of lymphatic system) frankincense.

In aromatherapy, as in iridology, there is a lymphatic type characterized by a weak spleen, which suffers from imbalances in emotions. One aspect is an excess of wonder and compassion, being too kind, always wanting to help, with a tendency to gullibility. The other aspect is lethargy, melancholy, lack of interest and grief. Rosemary, juniper and sage are used to restore balance.

Madame Maury explains: 'This diffusion of aromatherapy oils takes place by exchanges between the extra-cellular and lacunary liquids (contained between pleura and lung, peritoneum and all other fluids) and the blood, lymph and the tissues. The elements introduced are carried by these liquids to the organs and retained selectively by the latter.' Dispersion takes three to six hours in a healthy person, six to twelve hours in a congested body, and even shorter time for transparent and diaphanous natures. When applied over specific areas, oils penetrate directly to the organ or area in need.

Recommended reading
Art of Aromatherapy Tisserand.

Water and water therapy

It is essential for proper quality and movement of fluids that sufficient fluids be drunk on a regular daily basis. Every person must drink enough fluids to flush the toxins out of the body and to allow the proper viscosity of blood, lymph and urinary fluids. The general rule is that each person should drink half their body weight in ounces daily. Therefore, an average adult could drink 40 oz daily and children 20 oz. The ideal intake is about $\frac{1}{2}$ cup per hour so that the fluids spread evenly and regularly into the body and an increase to 1 cup per hour will flush the cells, aiding purification.

Fluids move nutrients and act as a transport system for hormones, nutrients, wastes, leucocytes and natural medicines. Fluids increase oxygen dispersion. There is one water molecule for every other molecule carrying nutrients. The osmotic pressure changes when there are high amounts of fluid, sodium is diluted and the system is flushed.

The hypothalamus signals to the pituitary, regulates water reabsorption and the adrenals regulate salt absorption.

Water cure is an old respected form of natural medicine, practised from the earliest times to the present day. We all know the stimulating force of a cold shower or bath, and the comfort and relaxation from a warm bath, as well as the stimulation of perspiration from hot air or baths. This was organized into water cure by Father Kneipp, a priest in Austria in the 18th century.

The main principle of water cure is based around alternation of hot and cold water, the hot drawing the blood and lymph to the surface of the body, and the cold sending it back to the centre. This is exercise for the fluids, and the movement disperses congestion and restores circulation to areas which were difficient. Between the opposites lies the path, the balance, or health and a feeling of well-being. This expansion and contraction process moves the blood and lymph, stimulating it and aiding elimination through skin, kidneys, bowel and lymph and lungs.

For specific treatments, read Kneipp Water Cure books.

It is necessary to visualize two forces of circulation, one coming from the centre outwards and the other returning to the centre. The heart beats and sends out red arterial flow from the centre outwards, and passive blue venous blood and lymph fluids are moved back to the centre by muscular movement, activity, seepage and the pulsations of internal organs.

Possibilities for imbalances of these two fluid flows include:

1. Excess of blood at the centre, lack at the periphery.
2. Excess of blood at the periphery, lack at the centre.

3.   Excess of blood in trunk of body, lack in extremities.
4.   Excess of blood in pelvis and legs, shortage in upper body and brain.

The power of alternate hot and cold treatments when they are balanced is that the blood is sent in and out, like exercise, bathing the tissues, overcoming obstructions and reaching every part of the body.

HOT water expands blood outwards toward the periphery; also pores open and release toxic perspiration, encouraging elimination. (Alkaline force of expansion.)

COLD water contracts blood flow and sends it back to the centre; pores are closed and elimination stopped. (Acid force of contraction.)

The combination of the two in balanced contrast clears stagnant areas and brings fresh blood to every part of the body, so that the negative and positive, yin, yang relationship between the outward and the inward fluid flows is equalized in harmony.

The following simple treatments will accomplish this effectively:

1.   Turkish baths - equal time in steam room and cold plunge. Do not be afraid of the cold water, go in again and again until you glow and feel clear and light.
2.   Saunas - must be balanced by cold showers or plunges. Be brave!
3.   Hot baths alternated with cold baths (let cold water run in while you are still in the bath, then let water run out as more cold water comes in, splashing all over you). It is also helpful to walk around cooling down before you put clothes on again.
4.   Alternate hot and cold foot baths will prevent swelling and inflammation after sprains, reduce oedema, stimulate and relieve lymphatic swelling in the lower limbs and increase circulation. Three minutes in the hot and one minute in the cold.
5.   When you have warm weather, lie in a large pan of cold water while the sun toasts the other side, and then alternate, reversing the hot and cold to front and back of the body. Change every five to six seconds.

The addition of herbs to baths also increases their effectiveness.

Stimulating baths: Make a paste of 1 tbsp. each of mustard, ginger and cayenne pepper. Take a HOT bath for 20–30 minutes, then wrap up thoroughly under quilts to encourage perspiration. This will diminish the onset of cold and flu if taken at the earliest signs.

Relaxing baths: Make a strong decoction of lobelia, catnip or chamomile and soak at least 20 minutes.

Dr Christopher's Cold Sheet Treatment: See 'The Incurables' for his powerful all inclusive treatment to relieve healing and disease crises.

Aromatherapy baths: The same principles apply. Use 6/12 drops of oil on their own or in combination with others according to instructions in the aromatherapy books.

Foot and hand baths: Maurice Messegue pioneered this method of healing and quick and efficient results can be obtained by this absorption directly into the capillaries of the hands and feet. Herbal properties move quickly through the blood and lymph without having to go through the longer process of digestion.

Exercise

Exercise stimulates the movements of fluids throughout the body and increases the oxygenation of the blood. There is enough written about this today so nothing needs to be repeated. Whenever illness causes the patient to be bedridden, it is necessary to compensate for the slowing and stagnation of the body by massage, lymph drainage massage and skin rolling, foot reflexology and alternating hot and cold water therapy. Herbal formulae taken internally will also relieve the system, and the bowels must be kept clean and active.

Any exercise which pumps the thighs will drive the lymphatic fluids throughout the body. Likewise movement of the arms will move the lymph towards the axilla. Circular movements of legs, arms and neck will move the fluids through those terminal glands. The following exercises may be particularly beneficial.

1. *Squats* – moving up and down out of a squatting position will stimulate lymphatic fluids, and warmth. Use 'HA' breath.

2. *Woodchopper* – hold something (like an axe) high above head with legs apart. Bring the axe downwards and as you come down, move into a squat, with the axe far between the legs.

3. Drain the *arches* by leaning against the wall and raising up and down on the arches.

4. Yogic postures which involve lifting the legs over the body to the floor while lying on your back are excellent for draining and flushing the *spinal column*.

5. *Sacroiliac drainage* – lying on back, lift bent legs up until the knees rest on the abdomen. Wrap arms around the legs, pulling them in towards the abdomen. Hold and then let go suddenly. Do on both sides, repeating fives times on each side.

6. *Head and neck* – hold your neck in the occiput area, with fingers meeting in the middle around the back. Using repetitive movements, drain from the centre outwards. When you start to move from the centre the head is forward. As you start to drain to the side, move the head back. When the head is right back, bring the fingers down the neck and drain into the scapula area.

Emotional counselling

As the water principle of the body is directly connected with the emotional life, holistic treatment must consider clearing and releasing past and present conflicts, both by Bach flower remedies and counselling. Clearing of past shocks and traumas will release the physical congestion.

Massage

Any massage will improve circulation of both blood and lymphatic fluids. If the aim is directed towards this, certain techniques will accomplish this more swiftly. Massage towards the heart working from the periphery to the centre. Using lymphatic massage techniques, drain the main lymph channels.

The application of simple techniques such as the *liver press,* the *spleen pump,* and the *aorta press* are simple to master. Stand to the side of the head and press down firmly over the liver, spleen or above the heart, then release suddenly. The *liver or spleen press* is done in a regular rhythm for up to three minutes and the *aorta press* is done 20 times per minute. A good Swedish massage will clear congestion and help to equalize circulation. The addition of aromatic oils which absorb directly into the lymphatic system will travel and circulate quickly to accomplish positive effects in the shortest time possible. These presses which move lymphatic fluids through lymph nodes increase the defence power as the fluid emerging from the lymph gland will contain many more antibodies than when the lymph entered the node.

Reflexology

A much more complete lymphatic foot drainage can be accomplished with reflexology. In the original Ingham method, each system can be worked with individually, and the lymphatic system can be stimulated and drained in the following way:

1. *Groin reflex area:* Work the lymph area from ankle to ankle on each foot with whatever technique suits you, either with thumbs or fingers. Also, holding the ankle in one hand and the toes in the other, rotate the foot several times in each direction.
2. *Breast reflex area:* Starting at the base of each toe, work up the top of the foot through the lung and breast areas.
3. *Tonsils and adenoids:* Working in the first one third of the large toe from the base of the toe, in the neck area, will stimulate the tonsils and adenoids. Support by working the two small toes.
4. *Thymus:* Located in the body below the thyroid, in the centre of the sternum, find the foot reflex below the thyroid reflex and beside the upper thoracic spinal area. Start the massage at the diaphragm line and work up to the base of the toes, and repeat.

Whenever local or systemic infections cause fever, swelling, congested lymph glands, etc., massage to clear and drain those areas. Understand your lymph system and work with it. Give it the support that it needs so that it can do its job to protect you, as your system of immunity and defence.

Try the following drainage techniques:

Clear *scapula and shoulder* congestion by asking someone to lift up your scapula, and press their fingers inside, massaging and freeing the area. When this is done, massage around the scapula, drawing the lymph in towards the centre of the spinal column.

Ask someone to press their hands over the *liver* area, with the fingers pointing to the apex of the ribs. Ask the patient to exhale, and then as they inhale, push the left hand up into the apex, while the right hand presses in the opposite direction so that the natural function of squeezing the liver is accentuated and supported. Repeat four times. If the liver is tender use light pressure.

The *cysterna chyli* is the main large deep lymph channel above the umbilicus. You can drain this yourself or ask someone to do it in this manner. Start in the centre of the abdomen, just above the pubis, press inwards and move upwards till you pass the umbilicus. Repeat five times. This is excellent to do at the end of a treatment, when the lymph has collected in the chyli and you want it to disperse into the bowel.

You can reach backwards to the kidneys and press inwards towards the spine with the fingers, breaking up congestion and stimulating lymph flow.

Manipulative therapies

Never underestimate the effect of correct posture and structural adjustments to clear energy flow and relieve muscular tension. Adjustment of the third dorsal ganglion relieves any stagnation in the pineal gland, thus increasing communication between the psychic body and the lymph system.

Diet

The lymphatic system is more affected (when it shows as a congested rosary or tophi) by mucus forming foods, such as dairy products, sugar, white processed flour products and processed foods, aspirins etc. Heavily acid forming diets will take their toll on both systems.

Diets to improve these conditions must be both purifying and mucus-free, in the beginning and then proceed to regeneration with easily digested and assimilated nutrition such as seaweeds, spirulina, soy protein and organic fruits and vegetables, grains, nuts and seeds. The Purification Diet (page 322) is an ideal diet to purify the lymphatic fluid and still feel reasonably well and strong.

Chronic disease therapy programmes such as the Gerson Therapy insist on high levels of fresh juices and distilled water to support the purification of blood, lymph and tissues. A main focus of their treatment is the support and generation of the liver. This accomplishes the elimination of high amounts of toxins so that cell growth is restored to a higher proportion than cell death.

HCl as a nutritional supplement will alleviate lymph stasis because it enters the lymphatic vessel and helps to break down toxic congestion, eliminate lactic, carbonic and other acids and lowers the pH reaction in congested tissues. In health, enough HCl should be secreted by gastric mucosa which would be absorbed in regular doses by the lymph from the intestinal walls. Extra feeding of HCl, potassium and mineral salts will aid the lymphatic system.

The lymphatic system and the muscular system

One of the main ways the lymph moves throughout the body is through muscular movement and the effect of blood pulsations. The skin is closely connected with lymphatic function, first because whatever you put on the skin is directly absorbed into the lymph system, and second, if the skin is not eliminating properly, this causes toxic buildup in the lymph zone.

The lymphatic system both feeds and drains the muscular system, maintaining the nutrient levels for tissue regeneration and the elimination of cell waste. The lymph carries fat to deposit in muscle and skin areas. Whenever injuries occur, the lymph is drawn to that area to support healing by raising the levels of nutrient and leucocytes, and increasing elimination. If infections take hold, the lymphatic defense system, the leucocytes, are stimulated to resist invasion and multiplication of bacteria and minimize inflammation.

The lymphatic system and the digestive system

The lacteals in the small intestines absorb fats from the chyme and release them in slow safe amounts into the blood. Wherever proteins are lost by the blood, the lymph picks them up and returns them.

Intestinal pulsations help to move the lymph along. Peyer's patches in the small intestines protect the body from infection and invasion by germs by producing fevers. The appendix aids the digestive process where the caecum changes into the ascending colon. This is a potentially sluggish area where faecal matter will have to move against gravity, and the appendix, as well as acting as a warning device when it becomes inflamed due to high levels of toxins collecting, also secretes an antiseptic lubricant to help maintain the area and encourage upward motion.

The tonsils in the throat also act as a warning device for mucus congestion in the throat and mouth areas. Unless very overloaded, the tonsils secrete toxic waste which goes into the gastrointestinal tract to be eliminated from the body. The main lymph channels down the front of the body also drain waste lymph into the bowels after lymph massage. The lymph glands in the groin work to purify the pelvic digestive areas.

The lymphatic system and the nervous system

The central nervous system is the only part of the body which does not require servicing by the lymphatic system and contains no lymph vessels of fluid.

The lymphatic system and the urinary system

Toxic lymph creates a further burden for the urinary system. The kidneys have their own lymph system to maintain tissue health. They are both eliminative channels and if one is not working properly the other has to work harder to compensate.

The lymphatic system and the reproductive system
The lymphatic system contributes to the nourishment of the reproductive system as well as the drainage of wastes, and the protection of tissues from infection and inflammation.

The lymphatic system and the endocrine system
Each part of the endocrine system receives nourishment, drainage and protection from the lymphatic system. The lymph also carries hormones.

The lymphatic system and the respiratory system
The lymph carries fat molecules necessary for respiration. Lymph is also moved around the body by respiratory breathing.

The lymphatic system and the skeletal system
There is a high proportion of cells in the bone marrow which are a part of the lymphatic reticulo-endothelial system for ingesting foreign particles and bacteria.

The red bone marrow is the birth place of both white and red blood cells. In infant life this process takes place in the spleen, and can be duplicated there if the bone marrow doesn't manufacture enough later on in life.

THE ENDOCRINE AND REPRODUCTIVE SYSTEMS

The endocrine and reproductive systems are closely intertwined in that the reproductive system is largely triggered by hormones secreted by the endocrine system into the blood stream.

Our growth as a male or female, and the various stages of maturation, are triggered by impulses stimulated by the secretions of the glands. The pineal, the pituitary and the thyroid set the other glands in motion.

Anatomy and Physiology of the endocrine and reproductive systems

The seven major endocrine glands are also aligned with the seven yogic chakras or the seven roses on the Rosy Cross of the Rosicrucian Order who call the endocrine glands the 'Invisible Guardians' or 'the controllers and guardians of life who determine the equilibrium of spiritual and physical forces in man.'

The word 'hormone' actually comes from a Greek word which means 'to set in motion, to arouse'. These hormones are secreted from the seven major gland centres, but are also related to the etheric chakras of yogic and mystic teachings.

Vera Stanley Alder in *The Fifth Dimension* calls the two endocrine glands in the brain, male and female aspects of the hemaphrodite brain. When these two glands blend harmoniously, the third eye comes into being and the individual attains direct perception and wisdom which is

The subtle mystical endocrine system – seven chakras or seven roses

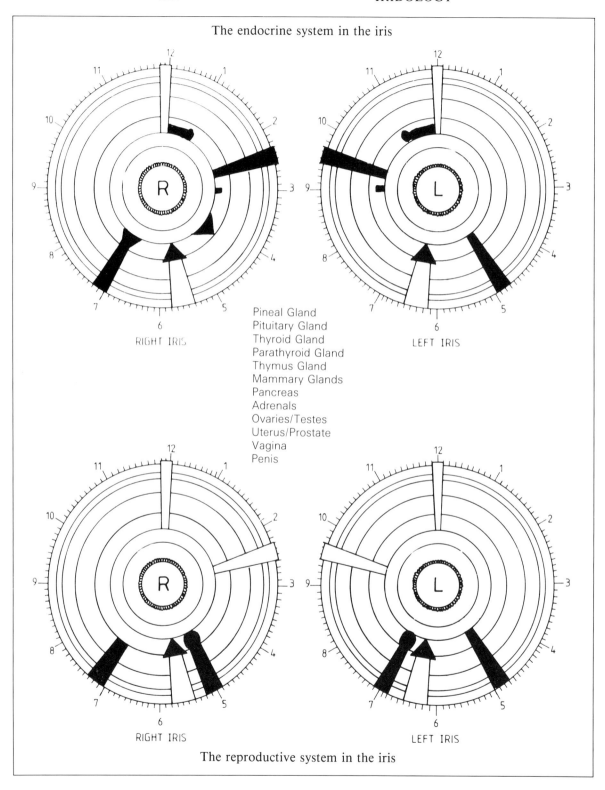

The endocrine system in the iris

RIGHT IRIS

LEFT IRIS

Pineal Gland
Pituitary Gland
Thyroid Gland
Parathyroid Gland
Thymus Gland
Mammary Glands
Pancreas
Adrenals
Ovaries/Testes
Uterus/Prostate
Vagina
Penis

RIGHT IRIS

LEFT IRIS

The reproductive system in the iris

not dependent on the five senses. In other words the marriage of pineal and pituitary, the male and female forces, result in the birth of 'Christ consciousness'.

The pineal was thought by Galen to be a regulator of thought. The Greeks claimed that the soul was anchored here. The Gordian knot is the web of mind and soul in unconsciousness. The Chinese liken the pineal to the tiger force which copulates with the pituitary dragon force. It represents WILL, the spiritual will to be, SOUL, the primal yang power of heaven, the pure creative action of the holy man as idealized by the six yang lines of the I Ching and the focal point for positive masculine energy of spirit. The pineal releases spiritual essence into man when the dross has been burnt away from the personality. It is the male crown chakra which finds its outward expression through the right eye, and the upper brain.

The pituitary or brow chakra represents the dragon, feminine, creative personality force as balanced creativity inspired by idealism and imagination. It finds its expression through the left eye and represents the lower brain. Here energies gather momentum in preparation for union with the spirit in the pineal. It is the controller, or conductor of the endocrine orchestra, and when hyperactive, the individual is successful, and enthusiastic. The gland rests in sattvic balance when the blood stream is correctly tuned and homeostasis reigns. However, when changes produce imbalances, the pituitary secretes a trophic hormone to stimulate the underactive glands to restore balance.

In the throat centre the male and female principles divide into left and right, in the dual thyroids and parathyroids, in this area of active intelligence and expression. The thyroid is the focal point for higher creative energies to disperse into the body and the world, and it is also the polar opposite of the gonads, the sexual reproductive glands. Here, duality appears and the separation of male and female into right and left sides continues down the body, as it began in the right and left eyes, the expression of the male pineal and female pituitary forces.

David Tansley says the thymus is 'related to the life thread anchored in the heart, in this chakra of LOVE in the Heart Centre. Here the higher the consciousness and the more illuminated one's love consciousness the more effective is the protective immune centre. When children are loving and open, this centre functions well, and when we close down in adult life, the gland atrophies and loses its ability to protect.'

The pancreas rests in the ark and cauldron of the solar plexus centre. It is also centred where the diaphragm valve releases or holds the volcano emotions, allowing natural expression and cleansing, or damaging suppression where one's vital energies are drained by the energies required to hold the emotions down. Here, positive firey digestive functions through the naval plexus provide the earthly foundation for the mental and spiritual life.

The adrenals represent the physical will-to-be, providing the extra energy to deal with stress and overcome obstacles.

The gonads manifest the active counterpart of pineal or pituitary, whether the person becomes dominant male or female, and concerns itself with sexual reproduction and of the species preservation. If energies are concentrated unduly in lust, loss of mental and spiritual consciousness results, and the person becomes burdened with the physical life, to the detriment of developing the higher centres. This energy is also related to the will-to-create on the physical plane, closely linked to thyroid control.

The endocrine and reproductive systems in the iris

Pineal gland

This iris area is most often affected by problems associated with the *transverse colon*. Radials, whether from the pupil or the ANW, pass through this brain area. Also bowel pockets send toxins to this area and when there are lesions the toxins collect because that body area does not have the energy and the strength to throw off the toxins. Whenever the circulatory and lymphatic zone outside the ANW is coloured (rust, yellow, browns, etc.) this affects the sinus cavities; the glandular function is also inhibited. Toxins in this gland area indicate that the spirit is weak due to lack of will combined with an invasion of the psyche. The pineal takes up excess iodine as a backup for the thyroid.

Pituitary gland

This gland, adjacent to the pineal in the iris, is exposed to the same influences via the transverse colon. Because the pituitary seeks to balance the endocrine orchestra by the secretions of its various hormones, any troubles here, and in the pineal area, affect the function of the whole body. I once had a patient, a Cypriot female about 28 years old, who was in great nervous distress, and after she described her complex of symptoms, she announced that she had been medically diagnosed for something quite serious and wanted to know what I saw in her iris. Immediately on examination, two huge dark lesions were evident, reaching from the ANW of the transverse and encompassing a large brain area including the pineal and pituitary glands. I asked her if the diagnosis was to do with severe pituitary weakness and she was amazed, saying that the doctors diagnosed a pituitary tumour. She also had very long arms and short legs with small feet. Although only the right thyroid showed a diamond shaped lesion, it was evident there were imbalances in growth hormones. Both adrenals were also covered with deep bowel pockets and lesions. Very slowly she responded to cleansing programmes and in time her desperation eased. Great efforts were made to relieve her of self consciousness of her appearance, which one actually only noticed after she mentioned it. Her last letter to me after five months of herbs said that she was getting better and she thanked me for 'all the help and patience' shown to her.

Thyroid

Here attention should be focused on left and right balance, and whether both or one are hypo- or hyperactive. Lesions denote weakness, and of course any problems here affect the function of basic metabolism, speed of digestion, nutrient assimilation, weight, warmth etc. White denotes acute hyperactivity and the grey/black darkness of toxins denotes the hypoactive state. Psora indicates inhibited function and radials, the severity of the toxic discharge and the depth of the chronic malfunction. Because hypothyroidism slows down the healing process, it is essential to clear this area and return it to the acute hyperthyroidism stage so that the healing crisis can take place. It is often said that over-emotional personalities are prone to thyroid problems. The throat is the area of voice expression, and is easily affected either by excessive expression or repression of strong emotions.

If we think of hormones as crystals circulating throughout the body, carrying vibratory rhythms that are picked up by the various glands and interpreted in terms of the required function, we can imagine the fine tuning and balancing that is constantly taking place. Radio sets were made with crystals to pick up and interpret the radio waves – the principles are similar.

Parathyroids
The parathyroids nestle near the thyroid in the neck. Although the iris sign area is tiny, one can see that in most cases where the thyroid is affected by bowel pockets, radials, lesions and toxic or inflammatory catarrhal circulatory zones outside the ANW, the parathyroids are also affected. In some cases it would be clear that small pockets, etc., would be affecting the parathyroids, but not the thyroid. Lymph tophi nearer the periphery would indicate malfunction of the lymph glands in and around the thyroid and parathyroids.

Thymus gland
For some time men have thought the thymus gland naturally atrophied in adult life because this was true of many cases. However this does not mean that this is the true and right condition of such a valuable part of the body's immune system. Because the gland is in the heart centre, it reflects both the positive and the negative condition of love and its attributes of enthusiasm, warmth, generosity, etc. or selfishness, apathy and inability to love. Although the main role of the gland seems to be during childhood, it is called into action whenever invaders threaten the body in adult life. As it is placed in the centre of the body, between the upper part of the sternum, it is logical to assume signs could also be found on both eyes where the bronchials meet the lung breast line at either 9 pm on the right eye, or 3 pm on the left eye. Whenever patients cannot seem to recover from glandular fever infections, viruses, etc. check out this area. Radials and psora would relate to the emotional side of this gland, explaining the negative personalities we see carrying diseased bodies and living unhappy marginal existences. If a child has been suffering from continuous infectious conditions check the causes of the toxins and also the marks in the thymus area to guide your cleansing and balancing treatments.

Mammary glands

This area commonly shows grey shadows or lesions, radials from bowel pockets, or lymphatic tophi indicating the congestion in the area. Acute conditions manifest as white reflexive fibres. Severe psora spots and changes of tissue structure have accompanied diagnosed breast cancer patients.

Pancreas

This area often displays a diamond-shaped lesion together with a bowel pocket showing that toxins have seeped into this area causing inhibition of function. Less commonly, one sees radials, and white reflexive signs indicating acute conditions. Many cases show the lesion in the gall bladder and appendix areas as well, indicating general digestive breakdown.

Adrenals

Adrenals manifest lines, both white and dark, and lesions separately or as a part of a marking which also encompasses the kidney. Bowel pockets press out from caecum and sigmoid, polluting the areas and causing toxic seepage. When the ANW is white and hyperactive this is usually matched in the adrenal area. Reflexive radials indicate irritation.

Ovaries

Here we have dual right/left glands so when either one or both of the ovaries have problems they can be similar or different. Women ovulate from one ovary at a time, and painful periods often come alternately, just from one ovary. Here it is important to look at the ovary in each eye and correlate the information about both. The same applies to the testes in the male. Nerve rings leading up to the ovaries indicate the level of tension and restriction in the area. They have also been caused by radium treatment on the ovary.

Uterus/prostate

This is another area commonly affected by bowel pockets, and lesions coming out from the bowel. Strands of several reflexive fibres waving out indicate hyperactive irritation associated with inflammation and pain.

Vagina/penis

All the above uterus/prostate signs apply, as the signs extend further to the vagina/penis area. Nerve rings stop and start here indicating irritation.

Treatment of the endocrine system and reproductive systems

The essential foundation for treatment of the endocrine system is purification. Sources of irritation are removed so that when superior nutrition is offered, the best healing level possible is achieved.

1. Hormone formula.
2. Thyroid formula.
3. Twelve kelp tablets daily help to balance thyroid function.
4. Natural hormones are available in herbs and plants: Genitstein from soybeans, Prunetin from prunes species, Diadzein from soybeans, Formononetin from red clover, Coumarin from alfalfa, Estriol from willow catkins. Female hormones are also found in carrots, soybeans, oats, licorice root and blessed thistle herb. Other sources of female hormones are wheat, barley, potatoes, apple, cherry plums, garlic, wheat germ and rice bran.
5. Progesterone and testosterone are both found in sarsaparilla root and ginseng.
6. It is said that high amounts of bromine (found in melons and celery) influence the pituitary and therefore fertility and harmonious life attitudes. Cultures such as that of Hawaii had high bromine levels in their foods.
7. The effect of yoga, meditation, exercise, sun and air on the balanced function of the endocrine system should never be underestimated.

Mammary glands
Swelling, pain, congestion, etc. of the mammary glands is closely related to both the emotional life and the lymphatic system. After foundation treatment, local treatment may be applied:

1. poke root poultices
2. castor oil packs
3. lymph massage
4. comfrey poultice
5. saw palmetto tincture
6. clivers juice on breasts and nipples
7. poultice of marshmallow root, chamomile and poppy heads for mastitis

Breast milk
Holy thistle and/or marshmallow infusions stimulate breast milk, while sage tea stops the flow. To help the breasts reduce when it is necessary to stop breast feeding, bathe the breasts with witch hazel tea and wrap them in cloths soaked in the same. Also a crushed cucumber poultice is effective.

Pancreas
See the section on the digestive system, page 183. Licorice tea (6 cups daily) helps to balance hypoglycaemia.

Adrenals
Parsley root and herb is a specific for adrenal treatment. Drink several glasses daily. Licorice root is an energizer for the adrenals. Vitamin B complex and vitamin C help restore adrenals after stressful periods.

Pelvic reproductive organs

Here the importance of clean bowels is emphasized even more clearly because of the close proximity of the organs, all pressed closely together. Toxins seep into vital organs causing much distress. Tensions radiating out from the solar plexus into muscles and tissues further inhibit the flow and movement of peristalsis, and blood and lymph circulation. No treatment can be successful unless bowel toxins are removed.

Uterus/vagina

Cramp Bark is an excellent female relaxant and regulator, helping to prevent spontaneous abortions; relieves pains from abdominal and uterine cramps.

Vaginal ovule treatment

The ovule is an internal poultice which is inserted into the vagina or the rectum to draw out toxic poisons and offer superior healing agents and nutrition to an area of need. It is used whenever women have problems such as cysts, tumours, infections, sores and toxic conditions in the pelvic/abdominal area. The ovule spreads its influence through the mucous membranes of the vagina, via lymph and circulatory channels, into the bowel, urinary and genital areas.

The formula contains equal parts squaw vine, slippery elm, yellow dock root, comfrey root, marshmallow root, chickweed, golden seal root and mullein, all in powdered form. Add this formula to the same amount of slippery elm. Mix well.

Melt solid coconut oil butter (over hot water) until you can mix it freely with the powder and obtain a doughy paste which you can form into finger size rolls. Then refrigerate so the rolls will solidify. It is useful to place the paste on a plastic bag, then roll inside the plastic, for a smooth finish as well as clean hands. Each day you insert the ovules, you will put in three one-inch long rolls.

Often it is necessary to plug the opening with cotton or a homemade tampon made of natural sea sponge. You can sew in a thread for easy removal if you like. It is easy to prepare a month's supply at once and keep them ready in the refrigerator. As you will be using a fresh supply every two days, three times a week, you would need nine one-inch rolls per week.

Dosage and treatment

Monday	a.m.	Insert three one-inch ovules into the vagina and leave in *two days*.
Tuesday	p.m.	Douche well with 1 cup of yellow dock or burdock tea. Insert a further three one-inch ovules into the vagina and leave in a further *two days*.
Thurs.	p.m.	Repeat procedure as above.
Sat.	p.m.	Repeat procedure of the douche but do not insert another ovule until the Monday morning. 1 day of rest.

If possible continue through periods. If not, count off the days, and continue with the same weekly schedule when the flow is light enough. Discharges, odours, etc. will occur naturally during cleansing.

Use the female reproductive and women's period pains formulae to complement treatment.

Dr Christopher's book, *School of Natural Healing*, is an excellent and invaluable aid to any practice. Whether it is prolapse, pain, inflammation, venereal disease, etc. these treatments combined with purification and regeneration will help rebuild the most chronic weak organs and tissues.

Prostate/testes/penis
The male reproductive organs are subject to the same influences from toxins spreading through the pelvic cavity. After foundation treatment the following are useful:

1. Prostate formula.

2. Vaginal ovule is inserted into the rectum for male patients. The procedure is otherwise exactly the same. Best during a cleanse where bowel movements are minimal.

3. Chickweed is excellent for swollen testicles. Also for burning and itching genitals. Bathe with strong decoction and use chickweed ointment.

It is interesting to note that 80 per cent of sexual secretions are composed of lecithin, another reason why excessive sexual activity depletes mental energy and activity.

Over the years I have treated many hopeless cases with severe symptoms. Have the faith to apply the principles of treatment and then use specific treatment after that. Make good use of reference works. These treatment suggestions can only point the way. Your reward will be the smiles and appreciation of those who have been relieved of great discomfort.

Holistic relationships: interaction with other systems

Jerns Jernal writes in his article 'The field resonance approach in medicine' that the pineal gland, together with the pituitary and the hypothalamus, directs, via the hormones it produces, the activities of other glands. The pineal gland gives signals to the reproductive system which sets a child's birth in motion by producing a hormone that makes the womb contract and expel the baby. Also, the pineal gland is sensitive to ultra-violet radiation, that is, waves emitted by the sun. When there is no light, the pineal gland produces melatonin, which inhibits sexual activity and fertility. It is found that iron is essential for the production of seratonin which curbs melatonin production and stimulates sexual drive and fertility. Glandular chemistry requires metal ions which react to planetary vibration (e.g. lead to Saturn, iron to Mars, and silver to the moon.) This is one of the ways the glands react to the vibrations in the universe and correspond to various mental attitudes and stresses which are also part of the biochemistry of life.

The pineal gland plays a major role as a receiver and transformer of these universal vibratory signals and then sends messages so that the rest of the body can respond and adjust. No doubt, this process has a lot to do with the adaptive changes that take place over cycles of change in world history.

Another significant function is that the lactogenic hormone (prolactin) stimulates the mammary gland after birth and after placenta expulsion and together with the oxytocin from the posterior lobe stimulates the milk secretions.

The sex hormones produced by all three zones of the adrenal cortex influence the development and maintenance of secondary sex characteristics and increase the deposition of protein in muscles and the reduction of excretion of nitrogen in the male.

When there is hypersecretion of these hormones in adults, females develop male attributes and vice versa. Ovarian hormones, oestrogen and progesterone in response to pituitary secretions call gonadotrophins, set in motion the phases of the female menstrual cycle. The male testes secrete the male hormone testosterone, necessary for the development and function of the male reproductive organs, puberty changes in the male and the proper function of the seminiferous tubules. The testes are stimulated by the pituitary gland gonadotrophic hormones which stimulate the seminiferous tubules to produce spermatozoa and the interstitial cells of the testes to produce the testosterone hormone.

The thymus gland inhibits the sex glands while children are maturing, and the healthier the gland is, the more one's energy is available for non-sexual expressions of love and warmth. The adrenals accelerate the sex expression, and the thyroid and pituitary glands, also play a major role in sex expression.

Adrenals stimulate sexual expression, so whenever the adrenals are hypoactive due to exhaustion of the sympathetic response or high levels of toxin, the sex glands are weakened. Thyroid and pituitary exhaustion also weaken the sex drive.

The endocrine and circulatory systems
These systems are closely related as the hormones are secreted into the blood and carried all over the body.

Poor circulation affects the thyroid as it takes longer for hormones to reach areas of repair. Wherever a sodium ring (for instance) slows and inhibits circulation, these areas become starved not only of nourishment and cleansing, but also of the hormone crystals required for balancing and tuning the human organism.

There is also considerable influence of the adrenal hormones, adrenaline and noradrenaline on the circulatory system. This sympathetic stimulation to prepare for flight or fight causes a number of dilatory stimulations which increase blood supply, oxygen supply and blood pressure. The blood pressure is also raised by the antidiuretic hormone of the pitiutary posterior lobe when the blood vessels are contracted.

The reproductive and circulatory system

Mother's milk is actually blood without the red corpuscles. Obviously a conscientious health minded mother-to-be would appreciate cleansing procedures which would render the blood stream as clean as possible. As we have learned, this is largely dependent on bowel cleanliness and liver function. The foetus receives its nourishment from the maternal blood, via the circulation of foetal blood between the foetus and the placenta. The health and strength of the baby's growth and development depends on the nutrients and cleanliness of the mother's blood stream. Whenever anaemia hinders the quality of blood and the circulation of nutrients the reproductive system suffers.

The endocrine and respiratory systems

The thyroxine and triiodothyronine secretions affect the utilization of oxygen and increase oxygen consumption. The adrenal medulla secretions in response to sympathetic stimulation cause dilation of the bronchi, allowing a higher intake of air per breath.

The endocrine and digestive system

Pituitary secretions from the anterior lobe affect protein anabolism, absorption of calcium for the bowel and conversion of glycogen to glucose, all related to growth activity. The thyrotrophic hormone stimulates the thyroid's uptake of iodine. Thyroid activity influences the rate that digestion moves through the bowels, thus affecting the absorption of nutrient. Thyroxine and triiodothyronine influence carbohydrate absorption and metabolism. Hyperthyroidism causes loss of weight together with increase of appetite. Adrenal stimulation slows peristalsis and limits saliva flow so that energy is released for flight and fight. Secretions of the adrenal cortex, hydrocortisone and cortisone, regulate carbohydrate metabolism, the change of glycogen to glucose, and the utilization of carbohydrates derived from protein. Of course, the pancreas plays a vital role in digestion. Secretions from alpha cells act on the liver to break down its sugar store or increase sugar concentration in the blood. They also affect the breakdown and metabolism of fatty acids and the conversion of amino acids to glucose (protein metabolism). The beta cells secrete the protein insulin and influence the uptake of sugar.

The endocrine system and the lymphatic system

The thymus is the ambassador of the lymphatic system in the endocrine system. Before puberty it is a source of lymphocytes. It secretes thymosin hormone which enhances the development of 'T' lymphocytes, which secrete a substance that attacks the protein of certain tumour cells, foreign cells, microorganisms etc. This plays a significant and essential role in immunity and body defence. It is interesting that this gland, which functions better in a loving person, secretes the substances which attack and destroy invaders to the organism.

The endocrine system and the nervous system

The endocrine and nervous systems work together for harmonious communication and coordination of the internal environment, a condition of health and balance called homeostasis. Nervous system messages travel along the nerve pathways, but hormone secretions are chemical agent 'crystals' which pass directly into the blood stream and are carried to their destination. Thyroxine and triiodothyronine secretions from the thyroid influence nerve stability and proper nerve activity. Hyperthyroidism causes increased mental and physical activity which could be very wearing on the nervous system. The sympathetic system stimulates the adrenals to secrete hormones to prepare for flight or fight response.

The endocrine system and the muscular system

The muscular system is involved in the growth processes guided most directly by the thyroid. A hypothyroid condition stunts growth and the development of muscles and body tissues, while hyperthyroidism increases this activity, but often with a loss of weight. Also, the pituitary secretions from the anterior lobe affect the thyroid controlling growth and activity. The thyroxine and triiodothyronine hormones from the thyroid also affect the growth and maintenance of skin and hair. There is an effect in hypothyroidism which causes muscle spasms known as tetany, and in hyperthyroidism, weak muscles. Excess calcium due to malfunctioning parathyroids can also be deposited in tissues such as the arteries, lungs, etc. Adrenal stimulation causes 'goose flesh' and increased sweat gland activity in the skin. It also causes muscular sphincters in the anus and urethra to become inhibited. Whenever there are hypersecretions of hormones from the adrenal cortex, muscle wasting due to protein breakdown excesses, and muscular weakness due to potassium loss through kidneys takes place. The antidiuretic hormone from the pituitary posterior lobe contracts smooth muscles of intestines, gall bladder, urinary bladder and blood vessels. Skin pigmentation may be affected by secretions from the middle lobe of the pituitary.

Endocrine system and the skeletal system

The anterior lobe of the pituitary secretes growth hormones, one of which determines the growth of long bones, and the other absorption of calcium from the bowel which would affect the nutritional side of bone growth. The relationship of the parathyroids to the skeletal system is very close, as hypoparathyroidism causes usable calcium to be reduced in the blood (hypocalcaemia) and hyperparathyroidism causes the calcium level to be increased in the blood (hypercalcaemia). The hyperparathyroidism causes softening of bones, destruction of bone, and the development of fibrous cysts on the bones as the calcium is drawn out of the bones and is either deposited in arteries, lungs and other tissues, or secreted in the urine, often causing renal calculi. This condition should always be considered whenever the sodium ring or parathyroid markings are evident, as well as in cases of arthritis and rheumatism. Excessive bone growth of face, hands and feet is the result of hypersecretion of pituitary glands.

Endocrine system and the urinary system

The posterior lobe of the pituitary gland secretes an antidiuretic hormone which maintains the body's water balance, and adjusts osmotic pressure. The hypothalamus stimulates or inhibits this secretion and lack of this hormone results in large amounts of urine being excreted. Bladder function is inhibited by sympathetic stimulation of the adrenal gland. The adrenal cortex is involved with water metabolism via aldosterone (secretion stimulated by kidney angiotensin secretion) and controls excretion of potassium and reabsorption of sodium.

THE URINARY SYSTEM

Water is the sea in which all the cells of our body float, the ocean, the mother of all life. The nature of water is to seek the lowest place, and it falls until it is released from the body. Water becomes part of our body through eating, drinking and skin absorption. Water is released through the urine, exhaled during respiration and through the skin. The heat of our body fire releases water into gases. **How the urinary system works**

Both absorption and elimination of air and water take place on the skin's surface. We can live for a reasonably long time without food, a shorter time without drink, and only three minutes without air.

The urinary system is an eliminative channel for urea, toxins, metabolic by-products and unessential chemicals dissolved in water. It also plays an important role in maintaining electrical, chemical and concentration balances as well as working to preserve a constant acid-alkaline balance. Before elimination occurs, discriminatory processes monitor, then balance the blood. Only what is truly not needed is allowed to pass out, and this varies from person to person and moment to moment. What is passed out one day is retained the next, as the body constantly adjusts to maintain balance in a constantly changing input of water, foods, and environmental influences. When this process breaks down so that this discriminatory function is inaccurate, the body secretes what is needed and continues the progression towards illness at an ever increasing rate. This is where the value of auto-urine therapy is of paramount importance, because it replaces what is being lost so the body can work to return to balanced normal function.

Whenever the body is over-acidic, the urinary system suffers the most,

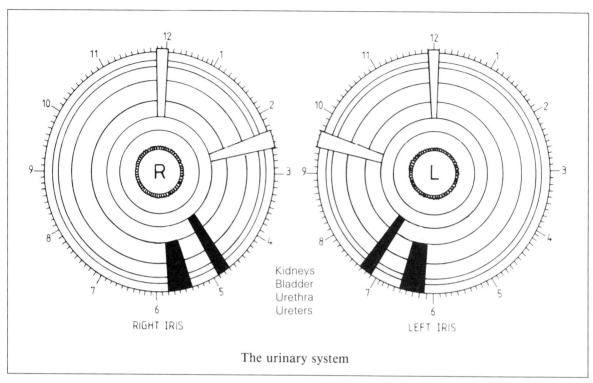

Kidneys
Bladder
Urethra
Ureters

RIGHT IRIS   LEFT IRIS

The urinary system

as it has to work overtime to try to eliminate and balance the acid alkaline in the blood. It is very important in such a condition to eat alkaline foods and to drink as much fluid as possible. Whenever other eliminative channels fail or work inefficiently it is also the kidneys which take on the extra burden. The acupuncturists refer to the kidney energy as the bottom line energy. The kidney meridian is one which runs up the centre of the body. When a person stands up straight they reflect strong kidney energy. According to their view of the body, the kidneys also store energy which is drawn on in different times. Kidney energy is the slowest to regenerate. Adrenal and kidneys are very close when we consider such subtle aspects of the urinary system.

The Japanese macrobiotic students consider excess yin to be a water disease, affecting kidney function. Homeopaths refer to the hydrogenoid constitution, where there is an excess of water. Here of course, the urinary and lymphatic systems would both be intensely involved in such an imbalance.

The urinary system in the iris

Kidneys

Inherent weaknesses are commonly recognized in iris analysis. Sometimes the lacunae are on one eye and sometimes on both. Look for the kidney medussa, an arc, usually white, which radiates in a curve from the adrenal by the ANW down on both sides of the kidney. European iridologists recognize this sign as an integrated dysfunction of the kidney/adrenals, together with inflammation.

White or pink/red vascularized *reflexive fibres* signify irritation. When they are combined with darker openings where the fibres separate this is a stronger indication of chronic trouble.

Radials from the anxiety area opposite the kidney adrenals stimulate the adrenal hormones which affect the kidneys when filtering blood. This shows the close relationship between the SNS and the adrenals.

Lymphatic tophi show as white inflammatory clouds in the outer zone, or as yellow to brown when toxins collect in the kidney area.

When *nerve rings* stop and start in the kidney zone, this indicates a relationship between the two areas of the iris. Often the other end of the nerve ring lies either in the lung, throat or medulla area, showing the relationship between these areas in the body as reflected on the iris map.

Bladder
Whenever kidneys show abnormal iris signs always check out the bladder area, and vice versa.

Kriege gives evidence for *radial* relationships between bladder signs and ear areas. This radial differs on the right iris (hereditary) and on the left (infection). When the ears open up as an eliminative channel, this shows a failure of the other eliminative channels and the blood purifying organs.

White *reflexive fibres* together with *lymphatic clouds* and wisps indicate acute inflammation, pain, excess mucus and catarrh.

Nerve rings will suggest pressure, cramps or irritations.

Dark colours in the bladder indicate hypofunction, muscular weaknesses and an overload of toxins.

Lacunae extending into the fifth zone warn of the possibility of cystic paralysis. Opening of fibres and other lacunae close to the ANW reveal connective tissue weakness and impaired circulation and elimination.

Uric acid diathesis constitutional type
Josef Deck identifies the iris type associated with hereditary or acquired susceptibility to weak urinary function, together with excess acidity. The blue eye will show a whitish grey colour, like large clouds or plates in the zones from the ANW to the ciliary edge. In brown eyes, this colour is more greyish brown. The tendency is towards rheumatic diseases, gout and the formation of stones.

Although this is a hereditary condition, it is worsened by incorrect lifestyle. Because of the tendency to retain and deposit uric acids, foods with excess acidity, stimulants, excess protein, high levels of meat eating, fats, cholesterol, etc. will increase the problem. Therapeutic indications include alkaline foods, stimulation of other eliminative channels and kidney function together with an increase in urine secretion.

Because Deck's work on the urinary system is highly developed we are including a copy of his iris chart which shows a different, perhaps more accurate map of the urinary system.

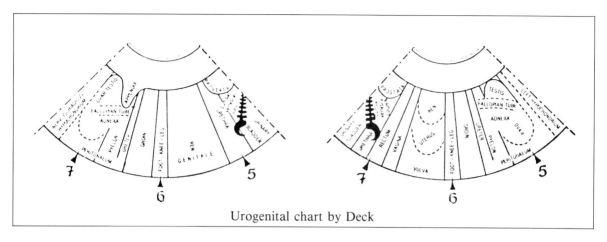

Urogenital chart by Deck

For treatment for the urinary system, please see Chapter 4, pages 133 to 135.

Holistic relationship: The urinary system and the nervous system
interaction with Emotions affect the nervous stimulation of the bladder via the
other systems sympathetic nervous system and the heart centre. The SNS relaxes the bladder and the PSNS contracts it. When we are nervous or anxious we pass water more often. Although there is a reflex action of pressure release of the bladder it can also be controlled by the will. The bladder is controlled by both the hypogastric plexus, sympathetic nerve fibres and pelvic nerves. In acupuncture the kidneys are said to control the nervous system – and the kidney energy rises up the central meridian.

The urinary system and the digestive system
As electrolytes are tissue salts such as sodium and potassium chloride, they are excreted to balance what is taken in food or drink. The composition of the urine depends on what is passing through the digestive system. This is also true especially of the ingestion of proteins (particularly meat and acidic foods) as this increases the amount of uric acid which needs to be excreted. It is also important how much fluid is taken in as the kidneys work to maintain water balance in the body. Imbalances of body chemistry together with other factors, cause the formation of renal calculi. Fluids are also taken up in the large colon, some of which will proceed via the blood stream to the kidneys to be eliminated. Constipation, and the retention and distribution of toxins in the pelvic area, will weaken the kidneys.

The urinary system and the circulatory system
Urine is closely related to the composition of blood, both in terms of concentration of salts and the acid alkaline balance in the blood. Blood is filtered through the kidney glomerulus, letting the plasma salts, glucose and small substances through. This glomerular filtrate passes along renal tubules, retaining or excreting varying amounts according to

the needs to maintain the balance of the blood. We can recognize and admire this selective discrimination. In astrology the sign of Libra describes this balancing process. It is important that an adequate blood supply reaches the kidneys at all times. Poor circulation and low blood pressure inhibits the proper function of the kidneys, and may cause renal failure. Left iris bladder/ear radials need to be correlated during interpretation with aortic signs, as circulation of blood would be a significant factor.

The urinary system and the lymphatic system

The urinary system contains lymphatic fluids throughout all its parts. Proper drainage of cell wastes and defence against infections is especially important in the pelvic area. As the pelvis often collects excess stagnant lymph fluids it is important to assess these factors in any analysis.

The urinary system and the endocrine system

The adrenals sit on top of the kidneys showing off the close relationship and intertwining function of these parts of the urinary and endocrine systems. The adrenals are our flight or fight centre, manifesting strength and staying power. They show the subtle aspect of how strength and power must have the foundation of balance and discrimination. When adrenal hormones are inadequate the kidneys excrete too much sodium and Addison's disease results.

The urinary system and the reproductive system

Often referred to as the *urogenital system.* In the male, both urine and sperm pass through the same organ – the penis. In the female the urine passes close by the vagina. Any unhealthy condition of either system closely affects the other.

The urinary system and the muscular system

The muscular system holds the pelvic organs in place and the condition of these tissues in terms of nutrition and adequate elimination influences the health of the organs themselves. Any prolapse from above will cause pressure and displacement of the urinary system, and perhaps impaired or painful function. The quality of the muscular tissue in the bladder, together with proper nerve supply, determines bladder balance and maintains body temperature.

The urinary system and the skeletal system

The skeletal system supports the pelvic cavity, giving a framework for the organs. Proper posture and position of the vertebrae affect nerve supply to the kidneys. Often when people complain of pain in the lumbar region it is actually kidney pain. Tense muscles caused by spinal displacement also influence the kidneys.

The urinary system and the respiratory system
The close relationship of lungs and kidneys comes out of their similar functions of blood purification, and the intake and exhalation of air. Kriege makes the point that there is no lung TB without kidney signs in the left iris. As they are both eliminative channels the function of one affects the function of the other.

THE MUSCULAR SYSTEM

The quickest way to understand the muscular system is to imagine it as the largest organ in the body. It is made up of billions of cells vibrant with dynamic life processes. It is a connecting system, holding everything in place and allowing movement. All the nerve and fluid pathways move through it, activating it, nourishing it and eliminating its toxins. The skin which is the interacting edge or body frontier, allows direct absorption from the outside environment as well as elimination from the pores. Movement itself takes place because of the close interaction of bones, muscles and nerves, in a most complex and sensitive way.

Posture and the wide range of movements, as well as digestive pulsations and the processes of body organs, all maintain life and produce heat.

The following description of the workings of the hand from *I Am Joe's Body* by J.D. Ratcliff, gives an indication of the complex workings of the muscular system. 'Structurally, we are the most intricate components of Joe's body. In no other part of the body is so much machinery packed into so small a space. ..... I have thousands of nerve endings per square inch, most heavily concentrated in my fingertips. Sensitivity here is extraordinary .... My tendons are the power trains, the connecting linkup between my many jointed bones and the remote muscles which move them (Joe can feel tendons in his forearm move when he flexes a finger). For binding material I have a maze of ligaments, plus fascia, which is a layer of connective tissue providing foundation material for nerves, blood vessels and other components. I don't have room for a big network of arteries and veins, but I do have a rich network of capillaries ....' This gives an excellent description of the complexity and diversity of the interrelated parts which make the muscular system so efficient in its ability for movement from the most strong to the most delicate, from quick to slow, from coordinated smooth action to rough jerky movements, etc.

It is good to remember the most important muscles, the diaphragm and the heart. Both these muscles begin working when we are born and never stop until we die. Both respond to internal rhythms, the heart beat and the pulse of the diaphragm marks the breathing pattern of the individual. We can only pause to admire the power and strength of these internal muscles and the vital role they play in our lives.

The muscular system in the iris   Heart, lower bowel, rectum, anus, bladder, all muscles, tendons and ligaments surrounding the spinal area and scapula, oesophagus, tongue,

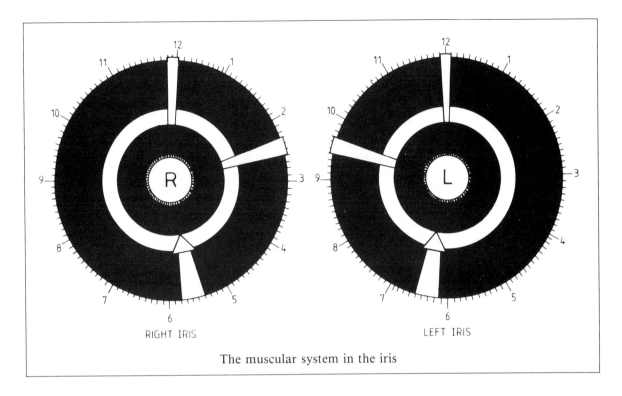

The muscular system in the iris

mouth, nose, facial muscles around the jaw, eye, neck, shoulder, chest muscles, arm, hand, diaphragm, abdominal wall, groin, the leg area, and vocal cords: all these can be seen in the iris.

Comb-like concentric lines within the scurf rim denote excessive perspiration, and the suppression of toxins as the lines move further inwards. Areas of distention indicate catarrhal encumbrance in corresponding organs. These lines are commonly found in the lung area where the suppression of catarrh is often caused by treatment of symptoms. Look for a bulging out on the iris at Left Iris 3 pm and Right Iris 9 pm. This can also occur in the larynx, pharynx and naso-pharynx areas. The brain zone is another major zone for the appearance of these lines which indicate passive congestion and encumbrances causing symptoms of dullness, lack of concentration, impaired memory, poor circulation in the scalp and tissues, dandruff and hair loss. When the spleen or liver areas are marked by these lines this would suggest the absorption of poisons by these organs has resulted in suppressed fevers, such as measles, chicken pox, scarlet fever and smallpox.

Markings in the scurf rim iris zone

Dark spots in cerebral area indicate suppressed scabies and hair lice as well as headaches and epilepsy.

Scurf rim domination of left or right irides can be the result of reposing on only one side during sleep where the constant pressure on one side inhibits both circulation and lymphatic drainage. This may also relate as to whether the congestion is more to the interior of the body (when it is medial) or to the exterior (when it is lateral on the irides).

Dark spots on generative organs denotes suppression of gonorrheal or leucorrheal discharges.

Dark spots on the anal area occur when this area is irritated by haemorrhoids, itching, fistulas and fissures. These iritations often have reflex disturbances the nervous system, because of the constant irritation and influence on the sympathetic nervous system.

Dark spots on the foot area indicate chronic perspiration, which is actually an imbalanced elimination which compensates for inactive kidneys. This can be a danger signal for impaired vital functions as suppression causes serious conditions, both physical and mental.

Hereditary lesions are dark spots surrounded by white borders when they appear in the scurf rim. Ask the patient about their mother's and father's illnesses, weaknesses and cause of death.

Deep dark scurf rims manifest in the irides of those who perspire profusely, due to chronic inflammation of the sweat glands caused by the retention of poisons, as excess perspiration produced in this manner is a secretion of local moisture by the sweat glands and is not effective as systemic drainage. Daily cold baths can also cause hyperactivity or over-irritation of the sweat glands.

Inherent weakness lesions indicate that the connective tissue and muscles are weak, lacking in recuperative power, and ability to absorb nutrient and eliminate wastes is hampered. When the lesion is coloured, this also adds to the interpretation, depending on whether it is white, yellow, brown or black.

White colours may appear in several different ways.
1. lymphatic congestion
2. acidic radiations from fermented bowels, and as a part of the uric acid diathesis lymphatic type which retains uric acid deposits in the tissues of the nose, ear, throat, vagina, etc.
3. exudative arcs showing acute eliminative processes (often via mucous membranes)
4. reflexive fibres suggesting pressure and irritation in the tissues
5. whitened nerve rings showing spasms and muscle contractions
6. sodium/calcium ring or hypercholesterol rings
7. transversals indicate a variety of conditions depending on their pattern:
   a. inverted V or rooftop transversal commonly found in the hip, leg zone and the pelvis and spine suggests inflammation due to arthritis.
   b. Crossed transversal (like an x or a y) accompanies pelvic inflammatory diseases, particularly in the pelvis, adrenal and abdominal areas of females.

c. Submerged transversals (they move in and out like weaving) indicate adhesions and scarring and the low grade infection and inflammatory process which causes them. This is common in women's irides.

8. Josef Deck seriously considers areas of the iris which 'brighten', where defects or pigmentation are surrounded by a lightened area, indicating inflammatory and destructive processes.

Yellow to brown colours indicate sluggish activity and deposits of incomplete enzyme activity.

Dark brown psora show inherited weakness and toxins which inhibit and block normal function.

Black is indicative of destructive processes in the advanced stages of chronic disease.

Contraction rings tell the story of the relationship of the nervous system to the muscular system, where irritative tension results in lasting contractive spasms, which inhibit the normal flow of fluids carrying nutrient and wastes.

Radii soleris reveal the pathways of toxic secretions into various areas of the body.

Treatment of the muscular system

The following principles should be observed:

1. Evaluate, balance, and restore the function of all the eliminative channels.
2. Provide adequate nourishment and the means of balancing body chemistry so that food is assimilated.
3. Support blood purifying organs such as the liver, and the respiratory and urinary systems.
4. Stimulate and strengthen the heart and the circulatory system to carry the nutrient to all the tissue cells.
5. Nourish, relax and relieve the nervous system.
6. Make sure the respiratory system is providing enough oxygen.

In addition, the following natural therapies are useful:

1. osteopathy and chiropractic
2. body work of all kinds: reflexology, massage, rolfing, connective tissue massage, Alexander technique, shiatsu, Esalen massage
3. aromatherapy and herbal baths
4. fomentations and poultices
5. exercise, stretching, activity of all kinds to keep life processes moving through the tissues
6. proper function of the skin
7. lymph drainage massage

The following herbal formulae can be tried:

1. Body building formula

2. Calcium formula
3. Seaweeds for minerals in balanced proportion. Alkaline formula
4. Multi-minerals/vitamins naturally formula

Skin diseases
It is important to mention here that skin diseases reflect the unhealthy condition of total body function, usually involving bowel toxins, inactive skin elimination, poor liver ability to purify the blood, inhibition of other eliminative channels, inadequate respiration, improper diet and living habits and reduced nerve function. When the skin becomes an eliminative channel, one approaches treatment as follows:

1. Analyse the irides so that your treatment can relieve the skin by reducing internal toxins.
2. Reduce intake of toxins, processed foods, mucus forming foods and wrong combinations of food.
3. Put the patient on a purification and regeneration regimen.
4. Treat the skin direcly via ointments, baths, poultices and fomentations.

The skin forms a triad with the respiratory system and the urinary system. The function of each affects very closely the functions of the other. Look at the skin zone in the iris, make your evaluation and then proceed with unified holistic treatment.

Holistic relationships: interaction with other systems

The muscular system and the circulatory system
These two systems are closely interlinked. The arteries, veins and capillaries pass through this system, providing nourishment and removing toxins. It is very important that the force and range of circulation is complete and that some areas are not deficient. The blood vessels in the skin area play an important and complex role, radiating heat on hot days to get rid of excess and holding heat in on cold days to retain body heat. The heart muscle provides the force for circulatory fluids to move throughout the body.

The muscular system and the respiratory system
As discussed in an earlier section, the waves of inspiration and expiration at the cellular level are essential to healthy tissue life which requires oxygen and the elimination of wastes. Muscles such as the diaphragm provides the lungs with the ability to inhale and exhale.

The muscular system and the digestive system
Muscles form a very important part of the digestive process, beginning with the opening of the mouth, chewing, swallowing, continuing the involuntary peristalsis of digestion as it moves through the gastro intestinal tract to the elimination at the anus by sphincter muscles. The

digestive system provides the nourishment to build and maintain the muscular system.

The muscular system and the urinary system
Bladder muscles govern the retention and elimination of urine. The urinary system helps to relieve the body of tissue wastes and uric acid wastes released by muscular activity.

The muscular system and the nervous system
The nervous system provides the stimuli to move the muscles. In *I Am Joe's Body* the author refers to an area of skin the size of a fingernail and about one eighth of an inch thick, as containing 12 feet of nerves! Thousands of messages to and from the brain are necessary for even the simplest of movements. Whether the nerve impulses come from the central nervous system or the autonomic nervous system, the activation of conscious and unconscious muscles is a miracle of engineering.

THE SKELETAL SYSTEM

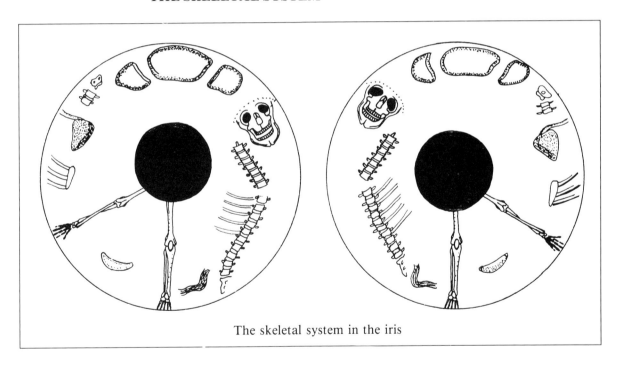

The skeletal system in the iris

Cranial bones
Facial bones – frontal bone, orbit, nasal bone, upper and lower jaw and teeth
Cervical vertebrae
Ear bones
Shoulder and clavicle bones
Scapula bones
Spine and ribs
Sternum and ribs

Hand and arm bones
True pelvis
Pelvic crests
Foot and leg bones

It is very easy to take the skeletal and muscular systems for granted, to be unconscious of the incredible microscopic world of metabolic activity existing in their living tissues. Here we have an opportunity to challenge our perspective of reality, to explore the inner world of microcosmic space, to imagine, magnify and visualize thc beauty and power of living tissue. Those fortunate enough to have seen the TV documentary of the inner world of the male and female reproductive processes have glimpsed some of the power and beauty of these usually invisible and mysterious internal processes.

The bones are the densest, hardest crystallization in the human body, yet within the hard framework are spaces which are very much alive and vibrant with life. The bones of a living person are living tissue, almost a forgotten world, sheltering processes like the manufacture of red blood cells and white lymphatic leucocytes in the red bone marrow, and the storage and release of calcium.

Blood vessels circulate supplies of food and oxygen to the cells inside the bone. The bone itself is a living tissue containing osteocytes which live in small spaces in the bone, connected to each other by canaliculi which lead to the large haversian canals which contain the capillaries. The canaliculi distribute food and oxygen via tissue fluid to the osteocytes.

The periosteum sheath which covers bone is a fibrous cellular vascular and highly sensitive life support, being a source of bone developing cells during growth and after fracture.

Bone is the hardest connective tissue in the body even though it still contains nearly 50 per cent water. Mineral and cellular matter make up the rest of the composition of bone. A proper balance of digestive and endocrine function is essential so that bone does not suffer from too much or too little nutrient. Adequate circulation to all parts is essential so that the nutrient can be drawn up into the bone.

Iris signs in the skeletal system
The most significant information about the skeletal system is found on the spine area. This is very important information for practitioners of osteopathy and chiropractic. Here analysis and interpretation can be made concerning balance of chemistry, weakness, inflammation, and the effect on the muscles and autonomic nervous system.

Also significant are the readings of the leg area and the pelvic bones. Remember the circular zone for bone markings, and that lesions or reflexive signs, or radials coming from the nerve wreath are an indication of nerve and bowel irritation, not bone markings. These ANW signs may indicate the effect to the nervous system through spinal damage or weakness.

White signs in bone areas indicate inflammation and pain, an acute condition, as well as more long term arthritis and rheumatism.

Darker signs in bone areas mean that the condition is more chronic.

Small black defect markings show intervertebral disc injuries together with small sclera vein markings pointing to that area.

Structural lesions means weakness, either inherited or caused by accident or stress.

Yellow to brown colours indicate the sluggish, toxic condition of metabolic processes in these areas.

Treatment of the skeletal system

Balancing any disease of the skeletal system requires consideration of nutrition and digestion, evaluation of the endocrine system (particularly the parathyroid control of calcium levels in the blood), and the strength of the circulatory system. These points would be considered after the evaluation of the eliminative channels and weakest organs and systems and a total plan of purification and regenerative treatment had been formed.

As the skeletal system is held in place by the muscular system, it is always essential to consider the play of mind and emotions which pull the muscles into patterns of tension which would offset correct posture and affect the skeletal system.

Equally important is how one walks and moves. Alexander technique provides a superb treatment designed to reconnect one's consciousness into a pattern of harmony together with strength and flexibility of muscles.

One's very life is reflected in the way one stands. The balanced position of the foundation pelvis is essential. Tai chi provides a marvellous exercise where you stand with your legs straight under your pelvis. First you become aware of your feet relaxed and sure on the ground, your body standing straight above them. Then you imagine that you are suspended along the spine by a string from the top of the head. A lovely soft relaxed posture results when you hold your neck, head and shoulders from this string, the rest of the body hanging from the head. All is in place, your nervous system is free, muscles are balanced and relaxed. The body is in equilibrium in its environment so that the flow of energies and fluids can take place. The miraculous life processes of the body can now work unhindered.

Whenever there are suspected spinal displacements it is essential that the patient be treated by an osteopath or chiropractor. The treatments described here together with these adjustments have produced amazing successes.

A patient referred to me suffering from dizziness and lightheadedness was told he may be suffering from Meniere's disease. The family was upset and the man visited several specialists both in England and Europe, feeling quite hopeless. When he was recommended to me for treatment the consultation revealed that the signs had occurred after minor neck injuries from family play and work. Iris examination revealed a small inherent weakness in the ear area and marks on the cervical vertebrae. Herbs, diet and four visits to the osteopath cleared all symptoms to the family's great relief.

Herbs
1. Body building formula
2. Alkaline formula for the high balanced mineral content
3. Comfrey (knitbone) to help rebuild spinal areas or heal fractures
4. Thyroid formula to help balance parathyroid function
5. Calcium formula to provide adequate nutrition. Calcium is also essential for pregnancy when the foetus bones are forming, and during nursing when the child's bones are growing and developing. As a person ages it is essential that the system does not get overburdened with excess inorganic calcium or suffer from lack of calcium. The balance of calcium/phosphorus is essential for proper growth and maintenance of the skeletal system. Vitamin D is also essential to promote the absorption of calcium, necessary for bone calcification.

Other treatments
1. Exercise
2. Osteopathy and chiropractic
3. Fomentations on the spine (see Jethro Kloss, *Back to Eden*)
4. Comfrey poultices on fractures or sprains
5. Slippery elm and lobelia poultices on congestion and inflammation

A really superb description of the bone organs and their important functions are in the chapter on the thighbone in *I Am Joe's Body* by J.D. Ratcliff, essential reading for anyone wanting to visualize body processes. To quote,

'Bones are *organs,* with a host of responsibilities beyond supporting Joe's body. We contain virtually all the body's mineral supply – 99% of his calcium and 88% of his phosphorus, for example, plus smaller amounts of copper, cobalt and other essential trace elements. As a high turnover warehouse we operate 24 hours a day, moving inventory in and out.

We also have a busy manufacturing division – our marrow. In a single minute, 180 million of Joe's red cells die of old age. Joe's spleen and his liver supply a few replacements but the vast bulk come from us. In the spongy interior of our marrow chambers we also produce most of the white blood cells that protect Joe from infection ...

My role in storing and releasing calcium is crucial. It is via the blood that I transact all of my business – I have, of course, my own surprisingly rich supply of blood vessels. I expose my mineral crystals to the current, plucking excess calcium from the blood or supplying it when there is a lack. The surface of crystal we bones expose to the bloodstream is vast; all flattened out, it would cover 100 acres of land!'

The skeletal system and the muscular system

The muscular system holds the skeletal system in place, both systems being large organs of microcosmic activity. A total of 400 muscles and 1000 ligaments support the spine. It is important to exercise, stretch and strengthen muscles, and keep one's posture upright so that muscles do not become weak. Environmental considerations such as chairs, beds, work, living habits etc. can cause problems which will affect the structural system through the muscles.

The posture reflects the mental and emotional attitudes of the individual. A straight, balanced spine relieves the nervous system of distress and allows muscles to hold and move the body in a relaxed way, without imbalances and tension.

There is a tendency in some areas of alternative medicine to regard the subtler energies as higher or superior. One must move from that prejudice to the holistic point of view where all parts contain the whole and all support and complete each other. The activity of the hardest densest bone matter is essential to the completion and polarity of the subtle energies. Health is balanced function of the whole. When we choose a part and concentrate on it to the detriment of the whole that attitude is not superior or higher. These subtle points of consciousness are essential to the evolution of a student of iridology. We are involved in a new way of perceiving life in the body, that is slowly transforming us. The holding on of prejudices or outdated limited views of consciousness will limit your effectiveness as an iridologist.

The skeletal and the nervous system

Here, the support of the skeletal system allows the free flow of nerve impulses when the spine is straight and balanced. Pain, inflammation, diminished nerve flow, all these symptoms and considerations are a result of misplaced vertebrae, and a spine out of alignment.

The skeletal system and the digestive system

The skeletal system is built out of the nutrient circulated in the blood stream. A full and complete diet is essential for proper bone development and maintenance in all stages of life. Correct alignment of vertebrae related to autonomic nerves which govern digestive functions is essential to the functions of the digestive organs. Calcium is also stored in the bones, to be released into the body when needed.

The skeletal system and the circulatory system

The skeletal system is dependent on the circulation of blood to receive the nutrient for its growth and development. Weak circulation, toxic blood, a labouring heart, all of these will limit the level and quality of blood exposed to the surfaces which absorb nutrient into the structural system. Exercise is also important here, as it plays its part in the movements of blood and lymphatic fluids throughout all parts of the body and into the capillaries. Here the structural system plays an active contributory role by its manufacture of red blood cells. The blood also transports calcium released by the bones when needed. It is stored in the bones until required.

The skeletal system and the respiratory system

The skeletal system is affected by respiration which is closely integrated with the circulatory system. The movement of oxygen and nutrient throughout the body and the exchange of wastes has been fully discussed in an earlier section. The skeletal system, while dependent on the other systems, contributes its support and nutritional balancing.

The skeletal system and the endocrine system

The parathyroids play a crucial role in monitoring blood calcium levels. The bone builders or bone destroyers absorb or release calcium from or to the blood stream as required. Whenever imbalances occur, whether too much or too little calcium in the bones or the blood, the parathyroids would be involved as well as other causes, such as improper diet, high mineral levels in food and water, and the contributing role of toxic and weak organs and systems. Endocrine secretions from the pituitary determine growth patterns and the length of the long bones.

The skeletal system and the lymphatic system

The lymphatic system provides the means of transporting wastes out of the structural system and the skeletal system produces a major part of the white lymphatic leucocytes, so necessary to fight infection. In this sense the bone marrow of the skeletal system is an essential part of the lymphatic system.

The skeletal system and the reproductive system

It is very important that proper nutrition be provided when the foetus is being formed, and after birth, during nursing, when the infant is dependent on the mother's milk provided by the mammary glands. There is a great interest now in preconception regimens which attempt to balance and build up a complete nutritional level to provide the essentials of human life from the earliest stages of conception.

The size and shape of the pelvic skeleton, and its flexibility, will also influence the birth processes. Difficult births are often the result of improperly formed bones during childhood years due to lack of or inadequate nutrition. The chain of body weakness can be broken as regards hereditary and generations, if the patient is willing to do the work of developing and maintaining healthy natural living. Children conceived and born after the parent's completed purification and regeneration programmes do not inherit their parent's weaknesses. The child's tissue integrity is at a higher level than the parents. It is important to know that how we live our lives will affect the lives of our children, their children, and so on.

The skeletal system and the urinary system
The urinary system is easily affected by lower back weakness and misalignment of vertebrae. Often people find it difficult to distinguish between back pain and kidney pain. Proper nerve supply allowed by the correct position of the spine is essential to urinary function.

Chapter 6

Putting it all together

THE TRUE PHYSICIAN

Almost anyone can study iridology, memorize the symbolic language, recognize the markings as they appear in the iris, and learn by rote what treatment should follow what sign. However, the sensitive practitioner will observe far more than the concrete facts. Each living iris will be a unique experience. He or she will not follow rules and regulations and try to make the individual iris fit set patterns. He or she will find the truth of each living iris even if it takes him or her to frontiers of uncharted territory. In many ways an iridologist is like a detective or an explorer who creates a synthesis of each person's iris print, who approaches each patient's eyes with reverence and awe for the miracle of life and how it manifests itself in the iris.

There is an intuitive, subjective element in iridology as there is in every branch of medicine. The true physician looks beyond objectively observable data and sees directly into the inner person. Paracelsus wrote, 'That which is perceptible to the senses may be seen by everybody who is not a physician; but a physician should be able to see things that not everybody can see. There are natural physicians and there are artificially made physicians. The former see things which the latter cannot see, but the others dispute the existence of such things because they cannot see them. They see the exterior of things, but the true physicians see the interior. The inner man is the substantial reality; while the outer one is only an apparition; and therefore the true physician sees the real man and the quack sees only an illusion.'

Said J.C. Burnett, 'I don't look where you look, I let my imaginations play about a case.' It was by such 'looking' and such play of his imagination that Burnett was able to see a nexus between the ringworm parasite and the bacillus of tuberculosis, which further led him to cure many cases of ringworm with Bacillinum or Tuberculinum, which in his day was not to be found in *Materia Medica* or *Repertory*.

William Blake was not a physician, but he was a Seer. He wrote, 'My business is not to argue and compare; my business is to create. I must create a system for myself, or else be the slave of some other man's.' 'Let him who has power to be his own not be the property of any other man' is Paracelsus' way of saying the same thing.

True physicians follow their own genius without being fettered by authority, be it Hippocrates, Hahnemann, Galen, Avicenna or Culpepper. Every physician must create his own system from his own experience and from the teachings of others. Other men's works provide the nutrient required to form the egg of mental concepts. Wisdom is hatched later out of experience. Those who can put their experiences into a shape that enables others to make them live again are true teachers who guide students to their own truth.

INTERPRETATION

If the interpretation is done in stages it is easier to come up with a balanced diagnosis which has evolved out of a combination of observation, intuition and analysis.

The first impression of an iris reveals a mandalic pattern. What stands out as the most important signs or patterns reveals significant predispositions. The iris has already manifested outstanding signs in selected areas.

During the iris reading the iridologist selects the main markings to record on the iris drawing. If diagnosing from slides the practitioner is also selecting, but the multitude of surrounding details still accompanies the main markings. The drawing is an excellent means to grasp the interpretation on return visits without having to re-diagnose the slides. If relying on slides, the iridologist should also look in the iris to confirm correct positions and note the effects of the camera flash because it may have created shadows which look like toxic dark areas.

Evaluation of the constitution is the first priority. This offers a short cut to understanding the causes of illness.

The evaluation of the eliminative channels is also of prime importance. Their clearing will accomplish over half the work to restore harmonious body function. Against the background of the constitution and the eliminative systems all other markings and their relationships are considered.

The symptom pattern only needs to be considered if any of the symptoms are extremely strong. It is best that the symptoms be eliminated by interior transformation of their causes. When exhaustion is deep, the patient needs tonic herbs, or sometimes local treatments for conditions such as ear infections may be applied. Asthma may require extra support. A skin disease may call for an ointment. These extra symptomatic aids accompany internal treatments.

The first level of treatment needs to include support for all the weak eliminative channels, combined with constitutionally weak systems and organs. This is usually enough to create miracles of healing and reversal of symptoms. Add any other extra treatment that is appropriate.

Follow-up treatment requires adjustment and variation. New symptoms may appear that require attention. All aspects of the iridology reading may not have been able to be treated at the first visit. Herbs and diet regimen will need variation and alternations. The

practitioner is like a symphony conductor working with all the body
organs and systems to create harmonious order.

RELATIONSHIPS

Once the essential language of iridology has been grasped and the ability
to select significant patterns and form them into the individual mandala
iris print has been achieved, the practitioner can absorb another
dimension, that of relationships.

One has to stand back and gain another perspective in order to
observe relationships. The eye has to travel from top to bottom, side to
side, eye to eye and across the iris to discover the relationship patterns
and their meanings.

There are several patterns which guide us to observe relationships.

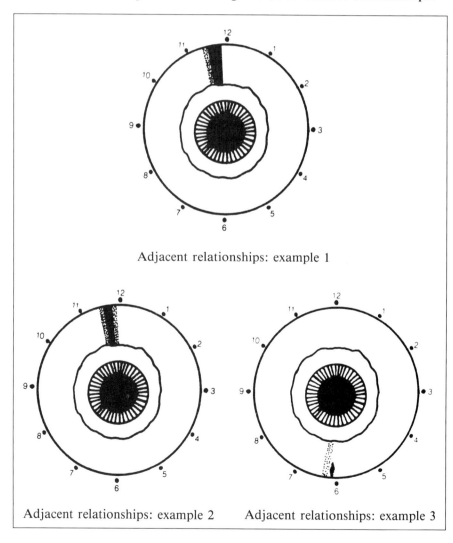

Adjacent relationships: example 1

Adjacent relationships: example 2   Adjacent relationships: example 3

Adjacent relationships
Iris areas affect the iris areas next to them. These are significant relationships to consider in iridology. Examples are:

1. Fear and worry spilling over from the anxiety brain area into either the sexuality area or the sensory motor area.
2. Perfectionism pressure spilling over and affecting the function of the five senses area or the listening learning speaking area.
3. Overacidity in the kidney area causing gout in the foot area.

The spillover may occur in different forms:

1. Lacunae may include two areas, so both zones are affected and affect each other.
2. Toxins may spread from a lacuna or radii soleris.
3. Reflexive fibres may include the adjacent zone.
4. Lymphatic tophi at the end of an organ, gland or body area may also include the adjacent area.

You can only learn this by observation. When you notice these relationships they have to be interpreted in terms of the patient, the symptoms and the total iris reading. It should add a catalytic spark which will increase the holistic understanding of the patient's case, or it may explain a confusing symptom pattern.

Body systems
As each body system is made up of many different parts, the more parts that appear with abnormal markings in the iris the higher the priority for treatment. Sometimes when you add up the signs one or two body systems have an outstanding number of markings displayed in the iris reading. This often explains confusing symptom patterns.

Observation of more than one body system shows interrelationships based on holistic anatomy and physiology as discussed in Chapter 5.

Circular relationships
Notice whether abnormal markings like psora, nerve rings, lesions or radii occur in the same circular zone. This will indicate a relationship between the body systems and parts of the zone as they function together during metabolic processes. (See diagram overleaf.)

Cross relationships
Crosses establish segmental relationships at the same time that radials are formed. Crosses divide the iris into a pattern defining body areas.

1. *Mind body equilibrium cross.* This pattern shows a narrowly spiritual attitude to life: a mind/body split and lack of balance. The few people who have manifested this pattern in my practice were

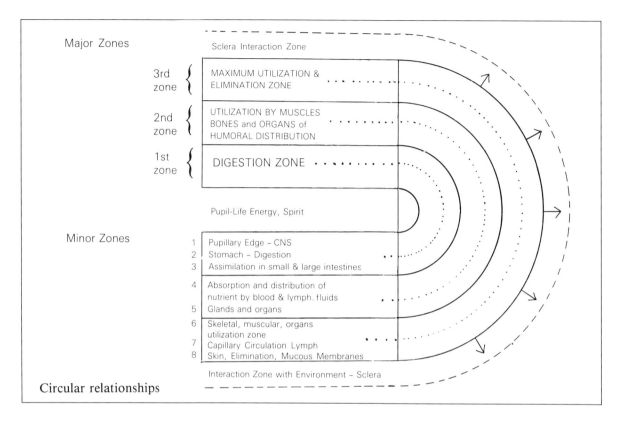

Major Zones

Sclera Interaction Zone

3rd zone { MAXIMUM UTILIZATION & ELIMINATION ZONE

2nd zone { UTILIZATION BY MUSCLES BONES and ORGANS of HUMORAL DISTRIBUTION

1st zone { DIGESTION ZONE

Pupil-Life Energy, Spirit

Minor Zones

1 Pupillary Edge – CNS
2 Stomach – Digestion
3 Assimilation in small & large intestines
4 Absorption and distribution of nutrient by blood & lymph. fluids
5 Glands and organs
6 Skeletal, muscular, organs utilization zone
7 Capillary Circulation Lymph
8 Skin, Elimination, Mucous Membranes

Interaction Zone with Environment – Sclera

Circular relationships

spiritual aspirants who denied themselves all the pleasures and support of the world. They usually succumbed to nervous disorders because of the intensity of their aspiration.

2. *Brain pelvis cross.* This pattern displays the higher and lower

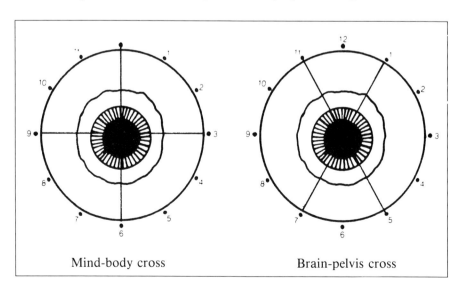

Mind-body cross   Brain-pelvis cross

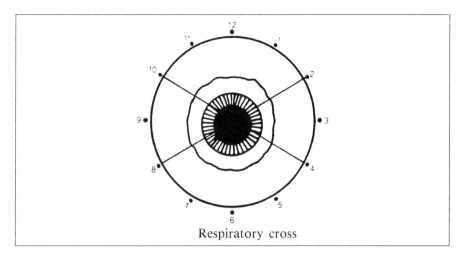

Respiratory cross

aspects of one's being and the struggle between the mind and the body. Observe the differences of texture, colour and abnormal markings in both segments. Their lives will reveal their choice, whether mind or body is allowed to dominate.

3. *Respiratory cross.* This pattern may be formed of radials, but you may also notice it when large lesions cover the respiratory area, which is confined within the shoulder/torso part of the body.

Lateral/medial relationship

Often nerve rings only appear on the lateral side of the iris, and this may be repeated in the other eye. Notice similarities. If nerve rings are medial, tension is deeper, more interior. If they are lateral it affects the outer body and possibly shoulder to groin muscles and neck tension. Posture may play its part also.

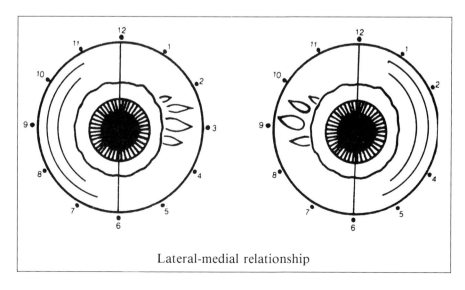

Lateral-medial relationship

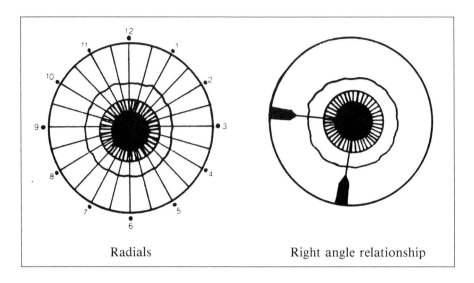

Radials   Right angle relationship

Radials relationships
These lines reveal polarity reflex and opposite relationships. Refer to the individual radial descriptions in Chapter 3.

Right angle relationships
Adrenal/kidney to thyroid. Here the thyroid influences the function of the adrenal response.

Right/left irides and pupil relationships
Observe any differences between rings on one iris or the other and write them down. Look for more nerve rings, radii, lacunae, etc., on one eye then the other, or for pupillary flattening, placement and size. Determine whether the person is right or left dominant by establishing an excess of markings and/or lacunae on either the right or left iris (Rayid). The right iris refers to the left brain and the left iris to the right brain as well as personality traits of masculine (right iris) and feminine (left iris).

Rings
Sometimes when you look in an iris two rings stand out. There are various combinations. These relationships tell us much about the systems which are breaking down or weakening and the cause of symptoms.

1. *White stomach halo and sodium ring.* Sodium/calcium imbalance. Digestive chemistry as a causative factor in sodium/calcium imbalance in the blood and the plaquing of the arterial walls which result in the hypercholesterol ring. Check out the thyroid, liver and heart as contributory factors.

2. *White ANW and lymph rosary.* Nerve and lymph hyperactivity and sensitivity. Here the individual is keyed for acute reaction. Check

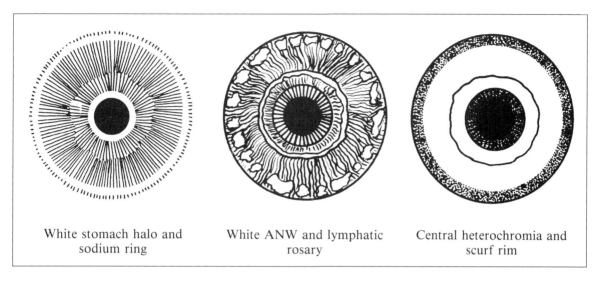

White stomach halo and sodium ring

White ANW and lymphatic rosary

Central heterochromia and scurf rim

out the condition of the adrenals and use nourishing herbs to strengthen the nervous system. As the physical body is purified the lymphatic system will be less reactive. Bach flower remedies will also be helpful.

3. *Central heterochromia and scurf rim.* Toxins in both the digestive system and the skin zone. Often the lymphatic zone may also be involved. Toxins have spread from the bowels overloading the lymph. Here two major eliminative channels are insufficient, toxins are collecting and creating a ground for disease to flourish. Increase the activity and effectiveness of all five eliminative channels to relieve this condition.

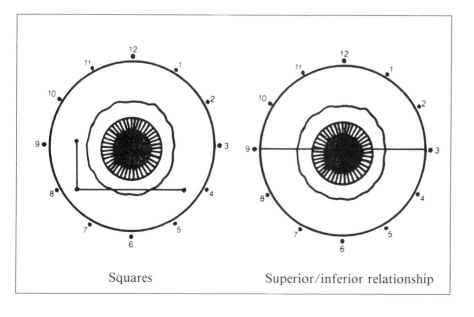

Squares

Superior/inferior relationship

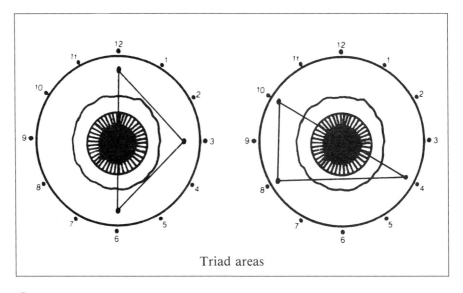

Triad areas

Squares
In chronic pancreas cases the disease sign appears in several areas, forming a square. European charts reveal these pancreas placements in more than one place in both irides. Whenever there are pancreas signs check out all areas. Squaring of the ANW indicates advanced chronic disease.

Superior/inferior
Often there are noticeable differences between the top of the iris and the bottom. Possibly there may be more toxins in the pelvis or more reflexive fibres in the brain area. Toxins and circulation may be weaker in either head or torso areas. Equalization of circulation and tissue and blood purification will help to restore the balance. Perhaps the head is too active and they never exercise. Many interesting possibilities come from observing this relationship.

Triad areas
A malfunctioning heart area influences the life force zone causing exhaustion, weak will and low energy, thus influencing lack of movement and use of the legs.

Liver/gall bladder distress leads to congestion and pain in the right shoulder and scapula areas. Gas pressure causes swelling and congestive lumps around the scapula.

THE ELEMENTS IN THE IRIS
If a patient manifests symptoms mostly in water signs, fire signs, air or earth signs it is worth considering astrology, polarity therapy or acupuncture based on the balancing of elements.

In the book by French iridologist Gilbert Jausas (*Traité pratique d'Iridologie Medicale*) astro-iridology is considered significant as he has reached correlations consistently of 70 per cent between the localization of iris signs and planetary positions on astrological charts.

Shock will produce certain vivid markings in the iris and these should be considered when seeking to integrate mind, body, and emotion with a patient. I have often seen large white markings in the heart area, or in the ANW just where the heart area lies. On asking certain delicate questions, it was revealed that a strong trauma or a great sensitivity affected their heart, either with palpitations, or emotional pains which prevented them from establishing close relationships. Any area of the ANW which breaks out of regular formation with white jagged areas reflects the overactivity of that area, and is usually an escape valve. If this is the brain area, note carefully any markings in the sector the ANW points to.

One can also look at the iris from the points of view of patient self help: what does this person need to work on? How best can they develop or complete themselves? For instance, one person needs to develop sensitivity to others, compassion, consideration, etc. and the next person more strength of will and perseverance. Besides these obvious indications, there are other more subtle ones. The person with a tight small pupil exercises too much self control and needs to learn how to respond to outside influences. Patients with excessive markings in the digestive organs should seek to clear their emotional life of its destructive influence on physical tissue. This approach will serve to present difficult information in a way that the patient will be able to accept. After the treatment is over, it is often good to suggest further therapies such as Alexander technique if there are problems with posture; Acupuncture; Gestalt, etc.

Looking at the constitution either from the European point of view, or as Dorothy Hall sees it in terms of personality, will also give strong indications about potential life attitudes to consider in any mental and emotional work. They are classed in effect as personality types, and especially in the European school the homeopathic type remedies can be useful in diminishing the effect of the constitution on body weaknesses.

This interesting area requires that we use our full potential to assess the messages that stream through the iris patterns into the life of the person we are looking into. We need to use both our long and short vision, to gain understanding, to examine both the close up details and stand back and catch the overall view patterns of the iris mandala. If we freeze ourselves we will miss out. We need to take different views, different perspectives and fresh viewpoints.

Some iridologists like to follow the same patterns of examination every time they look in the irides; for example, Dorothy Hall likes to look at the head areas first and then evaluate how the rest of the body reflects the patterns there. My personal preference is to see what stands out, and go from there. In some patients it may be the brain zone, in others the digestive system. Sometimes a patient will manifest only one major sign, like a brilliant white ANW or an orange lymph system. You will find that this will be the key to their personality. The white ANW will reflect a frustrated overactive nature, lost in doing and perfectionism and the orange lymph will indicate toxic accumulation, but also the congestion of conflict and unresolved emotions.

Above all, you will learn that we are what we eat, yes, but more so what we think and what we feel and how we live our daily lives. You will discover the keys to help each person unlock their understanding of themselves. Patients are lost in unrelated symptoms and a confusion of feelings and emotions. It is up to us to give a fresh vision of clarity and understanding that will give a sense of faith and trust in the body and help to stimulate the healing process. It is always a joy to see the happiness that comes over patients' faces when you explain why they have the symptoms they do, and why the body is doing what it is. It is a relief to know. There is nothing worse than not knowing and feeling at the mercy of unknown and unseen forces.

MIND BODY EMOTION RELATIONSHIPS IN THE IRIS

When you begin to perceive the whole life of the person in the iris you will know that you have reached a new level of professional expertise. Sometimes with one or more patients it will evade you, but with others the picture will be so clear that you will be astonished and amazed. Your patients will teach you many of these subtle mysteries, but here are a few examples to guide the way.

I was working with a patient who had been suffering from extreme grief for over two years. Her much beloved father had died suddenly and she was unable to accept this reality. Her mother, a most exquisite, proper and perfect lady, could not bear to see her daughter grieve in such a heartbroken way and forced her to suppress her feelings, with the result that she swelled up, and gained over a stone in weight within a few days. During the two years she had been to various practitioners seeking help, and had tried many diets. For the past year she had been the patient of a well known Auryvedic doctor who had helped her considerably, but the problems were complicated and chronic.

On analysis she revealed severe anxiety tetanic eyes, with heavy self-destructive radii soleris contained within dark nerve rings. She would complain, 'I cannot forgive my father for leaving me'. She made considerable progress in the treatment. I referred her to reflexology (which got her periods going again) and acupuncture to help stabilize her emotions. From time to time I would feel her contained anger, and once found myself hoping that I would never be the target of the anger. She had ended several therapeutic relationships in difficult and emotional circumstances and asked me to write a letter to help her bring a case against one doctor who had been treating her.

She invited me to her apartment because I was interested to purchase music she had collected and I wanted to hear it. I was astounded on entering to see a large collection of owls made of ceramic, metal or glass. They peeked from every shelf and covered every table, and she was very proud of them, telling how she had been collecting them for years.

On holiday in Crete I noticed lovely owl knick-knacks and bought a little bronze one for her, noticing for the first time that the eye markings on the little sculpture exactly matched the ones on my patient ... pure anxiety tetanic. There was more than met the eye in this similarity. Think of the owl: fluffy feathers, soft, with large round eyes (like my patient, an initial sweetness) then you notice the hard beak which swerves to swoop down on defenceless victims in the dead of night. Within a short time I was to experience most clearly that deep and powerful destructive force within her that the outer nerve rings struggled to control so that she could present the gentle, mannerly and sociable image outside that her mother demanded of her. I should never have gained such a deep understanding of the anxiety tetanic type without knowing the patient in her own home. It was an unusual exception. I was fortunate to have learned such a valuable lesson.

Another example came in the case of an attractive, sincere, troubled young man. He was in the music world, and lived with a girlfriend. When I looked in his iris I noticed that the brain areas for anxiety and sexuality on the right iris were filled with brilliant white radials.

'Do you have any worries in your sex life'? I asked him.

With surprise, he answered immediately, 'Yes! How did you know'?

I showed him the chart and asked whether he would like to share his problems. He said he would, after explaining that he had never talked to anyone else about it before. It turned out that he had been seduced by an older cousin who had come to stay when he was in his early teens. They had to share a bed as there was no other place to stay. He felt guilty about it, but he also admitted that he enjoyed the pleasure. Although he had never again experienced sexual relations with a man, he said that he struggled with this in his mind and that he felt attracted to certain men and wondered about it all the time. He had a very permanent and loving relationship with his girlfriend, and would never sleep with other women because he did not want to hurt her or their good relationship. He admitted feeling attracted to other women as well.

The problem here was not one of mental illness, but sheer overactivity of thought he could not resolve. I helped him to understand his feelings and questions were normal, and the Bach flower remedies eased the mental strain so he could rise above the worries. The white iris markings in the brain area calmed down as well.

The very first eyes that I looked in several years ago reflected a poignant picture of that individual. He was a young man in his mid twenties, who had remained celibate all his life due to devotion to a spiritual path and a strong sense of discipline. He also was a recluse, limiting everything in his existence to the bare minimum - possessions, relationships and food, going out as little as possible, except in connection with his spiritual group. His eyes revealed a strong constitution and were very clean and clear blue eyes. The only strong markings were a cross on either eye. Both the 12–6 and the 9–3 radials were evident on both eyes. I was so astounded that this Christ-like person should have crosses in his eyes. If you read about these two radials, showing the mind body spilt with the horizontal line and the grounding on the earth with the vertical line you can understand how those eyes reflected the total life of that person.

As I have mentioned before, differences in markings on the left and right irides reveal much about the person, especially concerning male and female energies, both in the life of the person and their relation to parents and spouses. Individuals who exhibit lack of trust and unusual fear which inhibits receptivity will manifest deep strong left sided nerve rings, usually started at the groin. Unusually aggressive, overactive or successful dynamic people may exhibit excessive nerve rings on the right side. There are so many interesting permutations on this theme which you only get to understand by talking to the person, and asking the right questions.

Another key is to consider the five elements and how they manifest themselves in the reading. The list below shows how the elements are related to various organs and areas of the body, based on the astrological signs.

Aries - eyes and head   Taurus - neck   Gemini - arms, shoulder
Cancer - breast   Leo - solar plexus   Virgo - abdomen   Libra - kidneys   Scorpio - genitals   Sagittarius - thighs   Capricorn - knees   Aquarius - ankles   Pisces - feet.

It is also interesting to look at the iris by the elements themselves:
Earth: Bones, faeces, calcifications, teeth

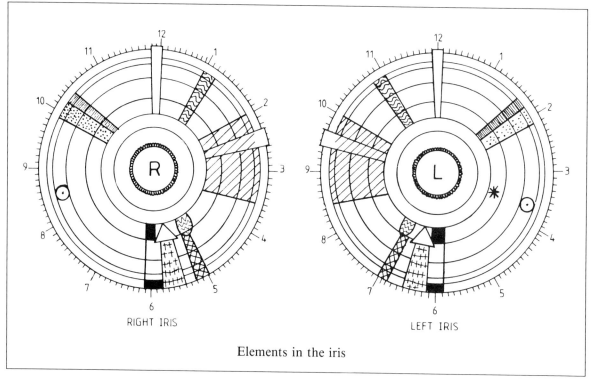

Elements in the iris

Water: Urine, lymph, mother's milk, secretions, saliva etc. (fluids)

Fire: Digestion: stomach, intestines, bowels, liver, gall bladder, pancreas, duodenum (warmth)
Circulation: Heart, blood

Air: Breathing processes, nerve system of communication

IRIDOLOGY CHART FOR EMOTIONS

RIGHT EYE – *Male Principle. Relationships with men and one's male energy.*

12:00	AGGRESSION OR EXPRESSION, Creativity, I am. Suppressed vitality, frustration, determination to succeed or always acting and doing.	Life force
12:30	WHO AM I? Proving for self and/or others.	Perfectionism pressure
1:00	Clarity of thought affected by emotion.	Intelligence
2:00	Determination OR frustration, grin and bear it.	Jaw
2:00	Expression through voice OR suppression.	Throat
2:30	Rhythm of life (hyper- or hypoactive).	Thyroid
4:00	Strong convictions. Strength.	Spine
5:00	Lack of trust. Fear. Lack of normal sexuality.	Vagina
5:30	Balance, ability to make decisions, knowing.	Kidneys
6:00	Grounded, stand on own feet, responsible (Knees for stubbornness) OR flexibility.	Legs, feet
6:30	Stress.	Appendix
7:30	Suppressed sexuality OR over sexuality.	Testes, ovary
7:20	Valve of expression/repression of emotions.	Diaphragm
7:30	Bitter gall, anger, jealousy, resentment, hate.	Liver/gall bladder

8:00	Don't handle giving and receiving well. Difficulty reaching out to others needs and wants. Feeding one's self (denying OR overindulging)	Arms, hands
8:30	Difficulty with giving and receiving nourishment. Nurturing inhibited or expressed.	Breast
10:00	Responsibility for self and others. Shoulders bent over in fear and protection	Shoulders
11:00	Basic physical functions affected by emotions.	Medulla
11:30	Lost in fantasies, dreams, hallucinations.	Mental sexuality

LEFT EYE – *Female principle. Relationships with women and one's female energy.*
Lack of confidence. Fear overrules doing.

12:00	Lack of motivation. Apathy.	Life force
12:15	Comfortable or uncomfortable in relation to environment and social background.	Sensory motor
12:30	Fear of being in the moment, or accepting reality.	Anxiety
2:30	Either loving warmth OR depression and fear. Generosity OR life is not worth living.	Heart
4:30	Cannot think clearly or concentrate. Longing for sun and warmth.	Spleen
6:45	Fear. Won't let go or eliminate. Holding on.	Anus
7:15	Acute reactions to emotional stress (Bedwetting in children; cystitis).	Bladder
11:15	Invasion of psyche. Spirit weak. Lack of will.	Pineal
11:30	Lack of connection to higher forces and their guidance. Unable to govern life from higher centre. Unable to have children.	Pituitary

Chapter 7

Case Histories

BARBARA

Barbara came for a consultation because she had experienced a very dramatic physical breakdown and was not recovering. Stress had built up in her personal life because she could not make a decision about whether to marry her steady live-in boyfriend or to follow through with a strong romantic attachment to a colleague at work. She felt she was coping, but in January when she went for a check up her vaginal smear was abnormal and in March she had laser therapy. She experienced this as a deep shock which she could not get over. In May she had a physical breakdown where her body shook severely. She fainted every one half to one hour, had severe diarrhoea, low energy and was extremely thirsty no matter how much she drank. She also suffered from bad headaches, had no appetite and lost a stone in weight. A visit to a neurologist only resulted in tranquillizers and hypnotherapy brought no relief. The attacks would come most often after a meal. She would become very

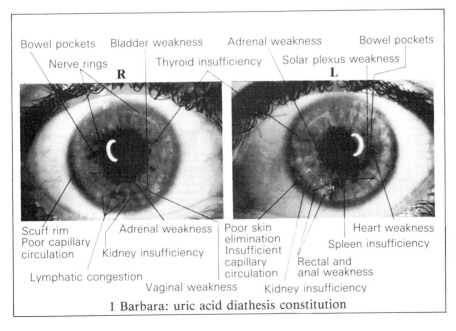

Bowel pockets Bladder weakness Adrenal weakness Bowel pockets
Nerve rings **R** Thyroid insufficiency Solar plexus weakness **L**

Scurf rim Adrenal weakness Poor skin elimination Heart weakness
Poor capillary circulation Kidney insufficiency Insufficient capillary circulation Spleen insufficiency
Lymphatic congestion Rectal and anal weakness
Vaginal weakness Kidney insufficiency

1 Barbara: uric acid diathesis constitution

hot, dizzy and shake all over, suffering from exhaustion, and extreme sensitivity. Her hair had started to thin on top. Arthritis was beginning to appear in her fingers. Backaches in the sacrum and kidney areas were becoming daily events as well as aches and pains in the front and back passage. She looked very weak and depleted, her hair was limp and dull and she had a poor complexion.

When she came to me for an iridology consultation, I diagnosed weakness and imbalances in the following areas: thyroid glands; liver; gall bladder; left kidney; adrenals; rectum and anal passage; adrenal glands; bowels; lymphatic system.

I prescribed the bowel, lymph, kidney, adrenal and liver formulae. Her Bach flower remedy contained Star of Bethlehem to relieve the shock of the operation, Agrimony to bring to the surface her relationship problems, Walnut for protection from the extreme sensitivity, Mimulus for anxiety and Centaury to strengthen her will.

Three weeks later she reported that her bowels were more active, her appendix area softening and becoming less sore, there were no headaches and both the arthritis and the pains in the front and back passage were relieved. Her energy was better and on the fasting day on Sunday she slept in until 1 pm. Her complexion was clearing. On this visit she received bowel, heart, circulation, chronic, thyroid formulae as well as lady's slipper for the nervous system. The Bach flower remedy was repeated.

On the next visit three weeks later she said she felt quite well although she was breathless at times and had odd twinges and palpitations in her chest. Her hands and feet still felt cold. The bowel movements continue to improve. Headaches occurred only fleetingly and the aches and pains in the front and back passage are fewer. Both the hair and the lower eyelashes are growing. Herbs prescribed were kidney/bladder, adrenal, heart, nerve, bowel, circulation, exhaustion formulae and chaparral herb to aid purification.

A month later she reported further improvements. Her strength had returned and even though she could handle her job again she got a new job to avoid long hours travelling. The relationship problem came to the surface and we talked through the options of her attractions to both men. The Bach flower remedy contained Scleranthus to help her make a decision. The diarrhoea vanished and her fingers were rarely stiff. All panic feelings were gone. Periods had been easy. I prescribed the same herbs as on the last visit except for the addition of the heavy metal formula for deep purification.

On the next visit about three months later, she came in absolutely radiant and looking happy and beautiful. It was extraordinary. I couldn't help enquiring as to what had happened after I complimented her. She decided to have a love affair with the man she was attracted to at work and said it was one of the best things she had ever done. 'I was such a wimp, before,' she commented, 'always afraid to go for what I wanted.' After several weeks she realized that she did not want to marry this man, and slowly the romance ebbed and now they are just friends.

She decided to marry her boyfriend and they are planning to have a child. She has cleared all the conflicts and stresses out of her life. This is a case that clearly shows the emotional base that led to stress and eventual physical and emotional breakdown. The conflict at the root of her life was destroying her. The herbal treatment strengthened and cleared the physical weakness while the counselling together with the Bach flower remedies helped her to find her way through her problems.

LINDA

When Linda came for consultation she was suffering from severe stomach pains in the left spleenic area. She had been to the doctor many times and had gone twice to the hospital for X-rays and internal examinations, but they could not find anything. They advised a telescopic exploratory but did not want to do this because of the risk of the general anaesthetic. She also suffered intensely from indigestion with pains higher up on the left side. Aches at the top of the spine and the upper arm together with headaches, a poor memory and depression gave her quite a strong condition of ill health.

Because she was a publican and spent most of the day around food and drink she did not eat regular meals, only snacks. It was clear immediately that poor eating habits and nutritional deficiency were main causes of her condition. She also took excessive doses of aspirin for the headaches.

Her iridology consultation revealed a large bowel pocket in the spleenic area where she suffered pain; stomach acidity; hyperactive autonomic nervous system (the nerves affect digestion); congested and inactive lymphatic system.

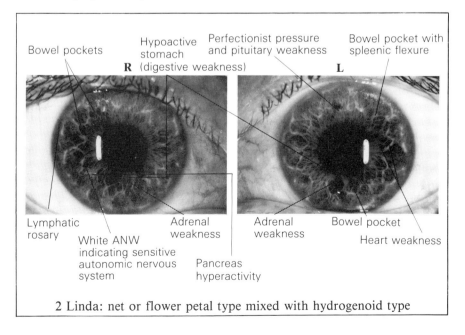

2 Linda: net or flower petal type mixed with hydrogenoid type

On the first visit she was given bowel, lymph, stomach acidity herbal formulae and wild yam root for indigestion and flatulence. She was also asked to drink waterbalance tea twice daily, and to take slippery elm with soya milk and honey regularly through the day to provide nutrition and to soothe the stomach wall. The castor oil pack was prescribed to help eliminate bowel toxins and to reduce pain in the spleenic flexure. Bach flower remedies were also prescribed: Mustard for depression, Hornbeam to relieve tiredness and boredom with her daily routine, Agrimony to help her express her inner feelings and Crab Apple to encourage cleansing and for her distress about her condition. Holly was also given to reduce her irritable anger with her work at the pub.

Three weeks later when I asked her how she was she replied, 'Very well'. Although she still had the pain on the left side she felt better in herself. She did not need the castor oil pack. Digestion was better, in fact she was following the diet plan I had given her and cut out meat, fats and bread. The headaches were better and she had only had one immediately after taking chocolate. The same herbs were repeated.

A month later she again announced that she was doing very well. She was now pain free, and had had only two headaches. She used the castor oil packs. The aches in her arms were much less. When prescribing her herbs I added the liver/gall bladder, alkaline and the kidney formulae and continued with the bowel, stomach acidity and wild yam root. She is now drinking meadowsweet and wood betony tea for her digestion.

She now monitors her own orders of herbs, taking them as needed and continues to make special efforts to eat and drink properly. This is a case which could have resulted in major surgery. Iridology guided cleansing and rejuvenating treatments and provided the direction for a change in life habits.

SIMON

When Simon attended his first consultation he complained of severe exhaustion, weakness, very poor circulation (his fingers were blue and purple), intense sensitivity, insomnia and a very delicate digestion. He looked so thin, delicate and fragile, he seemed hardly alive. I asked him how he could continue working and he explained that was all that he could do: work, eat and sleep. He had no energy for anything else, still lived with his parents at 50 years old, and had no relationships with anyone other than his mother and father. He explained that he had trained for years to be a concert pianist but his nerves were so bad that he could not play properly at recitals. Eventually he had to give up his career and the only job he could get was a telephone operator. This had a disastrous effect on him and he became very depressed and hopeless, and eventually gave up playing the piano altogether.

The iridology consultation revealed a weak digestive system, a depleted nervous system, a deficient circulation, an ineffective lymphatic system, and finally a weak kidney/bladder system.

Three years previous Simon had suffered from Bell's palsy and had lost the function of the left side of his face. For a long time he could not

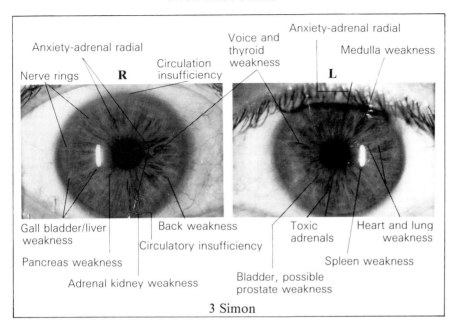

Anxiety-adrenal radial

Voice and thyroid weakness

Anxiety-adrenal radial

Medulla weakness

Anxiety-adrenal radial

Circulation insufficiency

Nerve rings

R

L

Gall bladder/liver weakness

Back weakness

Toxic adrenals

Heart and lung weakness

Circulatory insufficiency

Pancreas weakness

Spleen weakness

Adrenal kidney weakness

Bladder, possible prostate weakness

3 Simon

close his left eye and the left cheek had dropped. It was still very stiff and the left foot and left eye were very weak. He suffered from cold, blue hands and feet and constant chilblains, even in summer.

The Bach flower remedies given were Star of Bethlehem to relieve past shock and sorrow for his failed pianist career and his comfortless life, Crab Apple for present symptoms, Water Violet because he is such a solitary person, Wild Oat to help him find out what to do in his present life to make it more fulfilling, and Mimulus for anxiety. Herbal formulae included nerve tonic, circulation, lymphatic, kidney/bladder and bowel tonic.

He could only eat the simplest raw foods, most of which were cleansing. He was not able to digest any building, strengthening or heating foods. He was completely right brain or yin with his diet. Everything he did was actually increasing his problems.

On his second visit he announced that the constipation was improved and that he was feeling much better. Now he could eat a little at tea time and still sleep all right. He was pleased that the nervous system felt stronger. The colour of his hands and feet were better and his circulation had improved. His hands were less clammy and he was calmer and more relaxed. He felt there had been a positive improvement and seemed more hopeful. He continued on the raw diet but added avocados blended with juices at lunch – his first protein in a long time. I prescribed bowel, circulation, chronic purifier and two nerve formulae as well as the waterbalance tea. When making up his Bach flower remedy, I used the same remedies except Crab Apple was exchanged for Walnut to give him added protection at work.

On the next visit he felt he had progressed further and was feeling stronger. He was able to stay up two hours later, going to bed at 7 o'clock instead of 5 o'clock. He rose at 4 o'clock instead of 5 o'clock (it was summer) and worked in the garden before going to work. Just being able to do this gave him much happiness. He was not suffering from insomnia at all now but he still felt very depleted and tired after work. At this visit I gave him the exhaustion, adrenal, alkaline, bowel, multi mineral, and nerve formulae as well as wild yam root and gentian to aid his digestion.

In September he was again improved and announced happily that he was not so weary and exhausted anymore. He now went to bed at half past seven and still rose early. He was coping well at work. He was now able to eat steamed vegetables and oats which had been soaked overnight. He said that he felt as if he was now a part of the world. He had gained half a stone, was more positive and would like to live a more spiritual life. He was investigating various paths of meditation. It seemed that a meaningful direction had opened to him at last, and one which did not require physical energy. During this period he also had four metamorphic technique treatments which he felt were very beneficial. I repeated the same herbs again.

In November he said he was feeling well and certainly he looked happier and stronger. He is now enjoying reading books on spiritual paths and meditation. He says that he is much happier and not so worried. He meditates before sleep and does not need to take herbs for sleep, only the nerve tonic during the day. He does not feel that he suffers from stress any more and is able to enjoy his life now. Although he still suffers from minor problems and has to live very carefully his improvement is substantial.

From time to time Simon comes for assessment and herbs, although he takes a minimal dose now, often ordering what he needs on his own. He lives a normal life and pursues his interests. It is rewarding to see how the nutritive aspects of herbal medicine are able to strengthen a case of weakness, sensitivity and emotional despair. The downward spiral of hopelessness is now an upward spiral with a new goal of the spiritual life before him.

SANDY

Sandy was thirty-five and a head teacher. When she came for iridology analysis, she was extremely tense, her fingernails were covered with white marks, her abdomen was bloated and she suffered from wind and digestive discomfort, and she had aches and pains in her knees, wrists and lower back. She was obsessively tidy, and needed to know where everything was. When tired or upset, she got rid of any stress by cleaning and organizing everything; she spent her vacations organizing her teaching material so that everything would be perfect for the start of term. Her hair was kept very short, almost shaved; she could not bear it to grow.

She had been raised as her mother's favourite child and helper in a very strict Catholic household. Her mother was obsessively tidy and everything has to be just so. When she fell in love and had a relationship

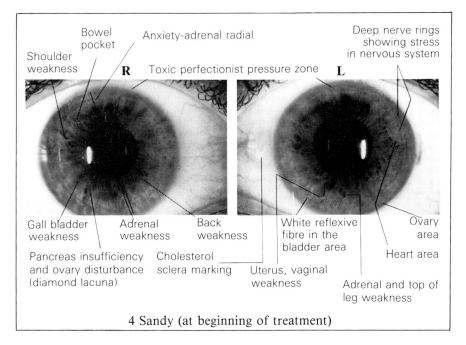

Shoulder
weakness

Bowel
pocket

Anxiety-adrenal radial

R   Toxic perfectionist pressure zone   **L**

Deep nerve rings
showing stress
in nervous system

Gall bladder
weakness

Adrenal
weakness

Back
weakness

White reflexive
fibre in the
bladder area

Ovary
area

Pancreas insufficiency
and ovary disturbance
(diamond lacuna)

Cholesterol
sclera marking

Uterus, vaginal
weakness

Heart area

Adrenal and top of
leg weakness

4 Sandy (at beginning of treatment)

her mother refused to see her and speak to her. This resulted in a complete break from all her family, except for very rare contact with her brother, over most of her adult life. Although she eventually married, she separated from her husband but never divorced because she could not bear to see him.

This case demonstrates a complete inability to deal with emotional situations, with relief being found by ordering and dominating the material world even though the internal world is a contained volcano of emotional pain. Considerable energy is required to contain these unresolved conflicts which shows in the deep strong nerve rings in the iris.

She realized she needed help and that she would be in trouble if some changes were not made. When the iris interpretation was given and the physical and psychological markings explained she immediately turned her strong intelligence and obsessive tendencies to doing the treatment fully, and she achieved the results. At about the six month mark she received a letter from both her husband and her father requesting communication and hopeful resolution. The opportunity appeared because she was ready to resolve the situation.

As the marking in the perfectionist pressure zone diminished she relaxed more in life and felt the need to clear accounts and tie up loose ends. New job opportunities came her way. She began using her holidays to relax and enjoy herself. She is very conscious of her obsessive tendencies now and works to adjust them. She has let her hair grow for the first time in years and looks feminine and attractive. She attracted a loving and very affectionate boyfriend and she bloomed with happiness.

Treatment was based on intensive purification by the use of herbs, special diets, juice fasting and supportive treatments such as skin scrubbing, enemas, and daily jogging. She was an ideal patient and cooperated fully in the healing process.

BETH

Elizabeth came for iridology analysis and natural treatment because conventional medicine and surgery had not solved her problems. She was suffering from severe abdominal pains, periodic nausea and general lethargy. She has already had five abdominal operations including an appendectomy, laparotomy, hysterectomy and two further laparotomies. Although there were some problems with adopted children she had a very happy marriage. The abdominal troubles were ruining her life. Preceding the hysterectomy she had had several miscarriages and persistent pain with her periods, which came irregularly every three or four months. When she was fourteen years old she had a dream that she would never have a baby and this had been a source of worry all her life. After her first operation the tissues stuck together and became the cause for further operations. Her state of fear was intense. She was convinced that if she had another operation, she would die. All the time she was telling me about herself she was holding her stomach and shaking with fear.

I felt she needed immediate treatment so I applied comfrey and slippery elm poultices to her abdomen to soothe the abdominal distress and taught her how to apply them daily at home. When I gave her a foot reflexology treatment, the bottom of her feet were extremely tender. Her Bach flower remedies included Star of Bethlehem to relieve the shock of her operations, Pine for the guilt of not being able to have

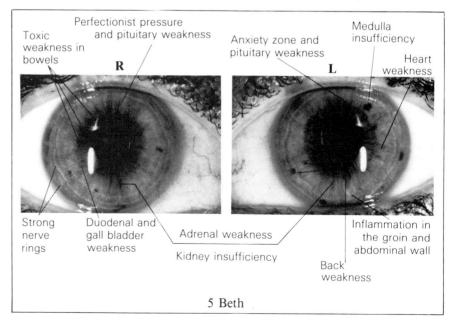

5 Beth

children, Agrimony to bring her in touch with her deeper feelings and Mimulus to ease the worry about her condition. I gave her bowel cleansing herbs, kidney tea, serenitea for the nervous system, as well as several tissue salts. She was also advised to take regular supplements of kelp and lecithin and keep to a strict purifying diet. The poultices were to be done daily. (This was many years ago and I had not developed my present system of herbal formulae, which is slightly different).

Two weeks later on her return she looked and felt much better. I repeated the reflexology treatment and after an abdominal massage applied a lobelia poultice to the abdomen. I taught her how to do catnip enemas which she would administer three times a week. She also agreed to do lobelia emetics daily for a week to cleanse the stomach.

Three weeks later she was pain free. The bowels were clean and the packs had softened the tense rigid tissues. She had also lost nearly seven pounds. She continued to take care of herself, watch her diet and administer treatments as necessary. When she came some time later to ask for help it was because she had returned to former dietary habits. She now knew that she would have to adopt a simple vegetarian diet for the rest of her life. Her efforts at establishing a new lifestyle were so successful that she became a lecturer and teacher of vegetarian cookery and years later took iridology and herbal medicine diplomas. She is now a successful practitioner guiding others to health and well-being and is a living testimony to the success of the methods.

Herbal Formulae, Teas and Tinctures, Oils and Ointments

NUTRITIONAL HERBS AND TREATMENTS

All the herbs described herein are non-toxic and non-habit-forming. It is recommended that patients take the herbs under the guidance of a qualified iridologist and herbalist. Students and practitioners are welcome to use the formulae in their work.

Special instructions

1 All herbs are combined in equal parts except where otherwise stated in brackets. For example, (2) means two parts, and (0.5) means one half part.
2 Because herbal formulae are combined with other formulae in this system of medicine, I have limited the amount of carrier and dispersing herbs such as ginger, cayenne, cloves, black pepper, etc. so that patient does not become overloaded with stimulating, hot herbs. If the practitioner uses the formulae separately it might be wise to add a stimulant such as cayenne to ensure that the formula is dispersed throughout the system, whenever a carrier herb is not part of the formula.

Adrenal formula

In these days of stress, nervous tension, anxiety and hyperactivity, the adrenal glands take a beating whenever we run on our nerves. This formula provides the nutrient to strengthen, support and rebuild these endocrine glands which deal with the input from the outer environment and the signals of the sympathetic nervous system which stimulate the response required to deal with the situation. A balancing formula to restore normal function to either hypoactive adrenals contributing to systemic exhaustion or hyperactive adrenals at the mercy of a sympathetic dominant nervous system in continuous sensitive response to outside stimuli.

Borage, Mullein, Lobelia, Ginseng, Gotu Kola, Hawthorn Berries, Cayenne, Parsley Root.

Alkaline formula

'From the ocean cometh all life.' The seaweeds which constitute this formula contain almost the full range of basic nutrients that are required by the human body and when they are given to the patient the body selects what it needs. A valuable source of all the trace elements, this formula is effective whenever the iris or symptoms indicate an imbalance of chemistry or a lack of some essential mineral or trace element. This formula will help to balance acid/alkaline and normalize body chemistry. We use this as an effective part of arthritis and rheumatism treatment, for nutritional imbalance and as an aid in tablet making, where its hygroscopic properties help to form a cohesive mixture.

Irish Moss, Kelp, Iceland Moss, Bladderwrack.

Allergy formula

Whenever the immune system is overburdened, the body reacts to aggravating stimulis with acute reactions such as hayfever, rashes or other allergies and weak eliminative systems will create an uncomfortable exudation of mucus. Although it is essential to nourish and balance the systems and organs and adjust diet and living habits, the force of the discomfort can be alleviated with this formula. There is no subsitute for treating the cause of the distress, so unless the body system is cleared and returned to balanced function, a true cure would not take place. For best effectiveness, use this formula as a part of the foundation level of treatment, the restoration of the active normal function of the eliminative channels, together with the regeneration of any weak or unbalanced body systems and organs and essential guidance in diet and living habits.

Black Pepper, Burdock Root, Cinnamon, Elecampane, Ephaedra, Ginger Root, Licorice Root, Marshmallow Root.

Anaemia formula

This formula provides strength and power to a sluggish system and helps to restore an adequate supply of iron, so necessary for body metabolism and energy. Especially valuable to pregnant and nursing mothers, this formula provides assimilable iron which does not cause any side effects such as constipation. The formula contains all the additional ingredients to utilize the iron in the system.

Barberry, Comfrey Root, Sarsaparilla, Sassafras, Cayenne, Quassia Root, Yellow Dock Root, Lobelia(0.5).

Antibiotics naturally formula

Whenever acute distress requires strong activation of the lymphatic immune defence system, this formula provides an alternative to synthetic antibiotics, if used in combination with naturopathic first aid techniques and an understanding of the body cleansing required to relieve obstructions to faulty elimination. It is essential that the bowels are cleansed, and stomach juices neutralized and purified with peppermint and thyme tea. Strong mustard baths and steaming under quilts will produce copious skin elimination to relieve a burdened system. Other complementary treatments are also recommended depending on the symptoms, whether there is fever, sore throats, pain, cough, nausea, inflammation, swelling, etc. It is important to consult your practitioner or refer to excellent reference works.

This formula will have a hard time working against morbid accumulations, but if the system is cleansed and the patient is flushing out the system with herb teas, lemon water, juices and enemas, there is an excellent chance of overcoming the problem in a natural way. The dosage can be increased considerably during acute crisis, taking tablets or capsules more often and in increasing quantities. Once when dental surgery pierced through the root of my tooth and caused a severe infection, my pendulum indicated half hour doses of 24 tablets of my combined formulae. I was taking nearly 125-150 tablets a day for a period of four days. My dentist was amazed when the infection was completely cleared up without any abcess. I received the additional benefit of a complete inner-clean at the same time, so instead of feeling depleted by an acute illness I was actually rejuvenated and restored. These are the benefits of living with nature's natural pharmacy. Every health problem becomes a challenge which leaves one with greater understanding.

This formula can be effectively combined with a Sore Throat Syrup, hot water, honey, apple cider vinegar, garlic, ginger and cayenne pepper, slowly simmered and then drunk regularly after gargling in the throat. Proportions may be adjusted to suit individual tastes. The combining neutralizes the strong flavours and the result should be a thoroughly delectable soothing and healing drink which helps restore the mucous membranes to normal function, and ease soreness. Any of the following: cinnamon, lemon juice, sassafras, sarsaparilla, cloves, mullein, licorice root, aniseed, fennel and peppermint may also be added for the personal touch.

Golden Seal, Burdock, Lobelia, Mullein, Poke Root, Chaparral, Cayenne, Echinacea(1.5), Cloves(0.5), Thyme(0.5).

Anti-inflammatory formula

Inflammation means congestion of fluids, irritation, and therefore pain. This formula was designed to work with constitutional treatment, the arthritis formula, the alkaline formula as well as the clearing of the eliminative systems and systemic balancing to reduce the level of discomfort for sufferers of such diseases as arthritis and rheumatism. Containing such herbs as white willow bark, the original source of the aspirin, the formula seeks to reduce inflammation without providing the side effects of stronger synthetic drugs. While the process may take longer and must also be coordinated with diet reform, the results are longer lasting and the patient also learns to adjust living so that the progress of the condition is inhibited while the herbal nutrients seek to restore and balance function.

White Willow Bark, Prickly Ash, Yarrow, Poke Root, Elderflower, Black Cohosh, Nettle, Sarsaparilla, Guiacus.

Anti weight and water formula

This powerful herbal combination seeks to reduce adipose tissue and eliminate excess water without depleting the system. Once the foundation level of treatment has been achieved and the eliminative channels are working efficiently, this formula will support the restoration to normal body weight by increasing the activity of essential body systems that have become sluggish or overburdened, with the overall effect that weight loss, once achieved, is maintained, because of the restoration of normal body function.

Burdock Root, Bladderwrack(3), Fennel Seeds, Echinacea, Parsley Root, Spirulina.

Arthritis formula

As a complement to systemic treatment, cleansing and diet reform, this formula helps to relieve the discomfort of arthritis and rheumatism. Working to purify the blood, lymph and tissues and reduce inflammation, this herbal combination helps an overburdened system to recover equilibrium of function.

This formula can also be used as a tea 3 times a day, or every 2 hours (half a cup) when discomfort is acute.

Mountain Grape(2), Parsley Root(2), Sassafras, Prickly Ash, Black Cohosh, Ginger.

Asthma formula

The treatment of asthma is an intricate challenge to the most qualified and experienced practitioner, involving cleansing, balancing and activation of the eliminative functions, as well as sensitive counselling for mental and emotional causes and the introduction of living habits which will lessen mucus formation and support the herbal formulae. The addition of this formula to systemic treatment steps up the success rate admirably, as it encourages the thinning, loosening and expellation of excess mucus from the lungs. This formula can be taken as a tea (4 cups or more per day) depending on need or in combination with other herbs in capsules or tablets. It is also useful in combination with the respiratory and alkaline formulae. Add antibiotics naturally formulae if there is evidence of infection.

Slippery Elm, Comfrey Root, Marshmallow Root, Licorice Root, Elecampane(2).

Blood circulation A

The herbs which make up this formula combine together to increase the range and power of circulation, especially to those areas of the body which have been deficient, usually the extremities and the capillary circulation. This equalization of the circulation restores normal blood pressure, whether it had been high or low. It is especially important to use this formula to carry herbs to deficient areas if there is any doubt that the force of circulation is weak or sluggish. Herbal nutrients travel through the blood and the lymph fluids, so it is essential that all areas of the body receive adequate and regular supplies of blood. Saffron tea and a large amount of garlic in the diet will complement this formula.

Bayberry, Cayenne, Ginger, Ginseng, Golden Seal, Hawthorn Berries.

Blood circulation B

This complementary formula provides an alternative to blood circulation A so that long term treatment of circulatory disorders do not have to rely on continued use of one formula. Concentrating more on relieving cerebral insufficiency, this formula restores adequate blood flow to the brain areas, relieving tiredness, poor memory, senility and negative mental states. It is important that it be combined with herbal formulae to discharge morbid accumulations or obstructions in other body areas, organs and systems, and to consider heart and liver functions. Every part of the body relies on every other part. When one part of the body is not performing adequately all the other parts suffer. Poor circulation also affects body temperature and the inadequate nourishment of various organs and tissues. It is essential that it be restored if the individual is to regain normal health.

St John's Wort, Bayberry, Cloves, Prickly Ash, Cayenne, Sage.

Blood purifying

Alterative blood purifying herbs help to relieve the blood stream from morbid accumulations which have settled there because of living habits, insufficient liver function, and the inadequate function of the lymph, bowels, skin and respiratory systems. Whenever the eliminative channels are not functioning properly, toxins accumulate in the blood and tissues.

Echinacea, Oregon Grape Root, Poke Root, Red Clover Blossoms, Sarsaparilla, Sassafras, Yellow Dock Root.

Body building formula

Wherever superior nutrition is needed to provide the raw materials to rebuild damaged and weak bone, muscles and tissue, this formula will provide the means for regeneration. Take internally and apply as poultices directly on areas of need (over wounds, damaged vertebrae, broken bones, sprains etc.) This is especially important because if a damaged area does not need to draw nutrient to it through the blood and lymph, causing congestion, swelling and inflammation in the process, the healing proceeds much more quickly. As the poultice nutrient is drawn in through the skin into the lymph and circulation of the damaged area, it provides all that is needed without depleting any other body area or causing excess fluids to be drawn to the damaged areas.

Comfrey Root, Comfrey Leaves, Irish Moss, Marshmallow Root, Mullein, Plantain, White Oak Bark.

Bowel tonic A

Bowel cleansing and rejuvenation is required by almost every human being. The cleaner the colon, the purer the blood stream and lymph, and the better the nutrient is distributed throughout the body because the walls of the colon allow the absorption of nutrient into the blood and lymph. A clean colon gives an uplift physically, mentally and emotionally. One feels lighter, cleaner and clearer, and the brain functions better.

This formula normalizes bowel function, whether the problem is constipation or diarrhoea. In fact, diarrhoea is considered the worst kind of constipation. Visualize a colon wall that is coated with toxic mucus lining. The lymph and blood are not able to draw off the fluid containing the nutrient so the faeces are more liquid than they should be. When the walls of the colon are clean, the liquid can be absorbed in a normal way.

So many symptoms find their source in colon toxins. So many chronic diseases owe their early development to toxins in various parts of the bowels. If you alter the foundation level of the causes of ill health, the whole pyramid shifts and the way to healing opens. Nutrient becomes available to the body, blood and lymph are cleaner, and as the burden on the eliminative channels becomes less, the whole being rejoices. 'Cleanliness is next to godliness', the old saying goes. This is proven every day whenever patients use this formula.

It is important to realize that this formula accomplishes a very individual result and therefore the dosage must be monitored and adjusted according to response. In chronic cases of constipation individuals have taken up to 45 capsules per day for up to three weeks before the body releases its accumulated faecal matter. This initial release can be aided by the use of the Castor Oil Pack – see Appendix II. Also, if diarrhoea is persistent, use mullein tea to relieve the symptoms.

The aim of this formula is to restore normal bowel function, not to create a dependence, like most laxatives. Because its ingredients work simultaneously on normalizing bowel function, toning colon muscles, restoring peristalsis, clearing out bowel pockets and diverticuli, healing raw or inflamed areas and relaxing areas of tension, it is an overall formula which will ultimately leave the patient without the need to continue the formula. In some cases, the use of this formula may need to extend to nine months, but often bowel function is restored and the colon cleansed in approximately six months. Long-term use of this formula requires that after seven weeks thyme should be substituted for golden seal due to the astringent properties of this herb. Its use can be recontinued after a further seven weeks if desired. Of course, the iris reading is an excellent monitor of this cleansing process.

Each individual needs to understand that the bowels should eliminate as often as the person eats meals in a day. Usually three good movements a day will ensure that the faecal matter is not retained in the bowel for more than 24 hours, so that fermentation and absorption of faecal toxins is minimal.

As a complement, occasional discriminate use of enemas or colonics will prove invaluable.

Cascara Sagrada, Ginger Root, Golden Seal (or Thyme), Slippery Elm, Turkey Rhubarb, Wahoo(0.25), Culver's Root(0.25).

Bowel tonic B

This herbal combination developed out of a need for a formula which would work as well as bowel tonic A, stimulate peristalsis by activating the liver, and not rely on the continued use of golden seal, which is contraindicated during pregnancy and should not be taken over long periods of time due to its astringent qualities. Happily, this formula, which has been well tested by all our school and clinic staff, combines all the positive aspects of bowel tonic A along with a gentle stimulation of natural peristalsis. Dosage is to be adjusted according to response, and can be alternated with bowel tonic A.

Mandrake Root, Ginger, Licorice Root, Wild Yam Root, Alfalfa

Burdock

Burdock is added whenever boils, psoriasis, eczema, itch and other skin diseases present strong symptoms. Its strongly purifying influence also increases urine flow, stimulates the lymphatic system and reduced fatty tissue.

Calcium formula

A superior intake of calcium is valuable for many conditions, including pregnancy, nursing, muscular cramps, hair and nail weakness and with imbalances of body chemistry leading to weak bones, calcification of the joints etc. It is also a help to teething babies, because irritability and discomfort are relieved when their body has enough calcium to form their teeth without drawing calcium from other areas of their body, thus causing congestion and pressure on nerves, with resultant pain.

Horsetail(6), Oatstraw(4), Lobelia, Marshmallow Root(2), Kelp, Parsley Root.

Cayenne pepper or capsicum herb

This stimulant herb has many valuable uses. As a dietary supplement it increases the circulatory power and provides the means to reach sluggish areas where the blood is having difficulty. One of its main uses is as an antiseptic. It is also an essential part of any home herbal first aid kit because of its ability to stem the flow of bleeding. It is even used in childbirth to stop haemorrhages. If there is heart trouble, even heart attacks, spoonfuls of cayenne will help relieve the condition. It is worthwhile reading in depth about the many uses of this excellent herb. It is an essential part of many herbal formulae. The book *Back to Eden* by Jethro Kloss contains a number of pages devoted to the use of this excellent herb and Dr John Christopher found the herb so effective that he devoted an entire book to it: *Capsicum.*

Chaparral herb

A North American Indian Herb, this desert plant is one of our greatest and strongest purifiers. Whenever it rains in the western desert, the fragrance of this plant is released and the very air carries its healing aroma and energy. It is especially useful for arthritic and cancerous conditions, while also providing healing to the urinary system and the lower bowel. It can also be used individually in cleansing programmes. However, if this herb is used over a long period of time it will cleanse too drastically, and the patient may feel minor distress from an accumulation of mucus in the alimentary tract in the stomach and throat areas. It is best used in strong doses over a short period of time (for example 6 capsules 3 times a day for 3 weeks). Chaparral baths are an excellent way of absorbing the nutrient of this powerful purifier directly into the body through the skin.

Chickweed

Once, two days after I had seen a new patient who suffered from severe eczema, I received a telephone call at 6.30 in the morning to hear that she was in an acute crisis. She was hysterical, screaming that she had had these crises before and had to be hospitalized, but did not want to go to the hospital again. I said: 'Come right over and we'll see what we can do', then I rushed to my herbal books and looked up herbs for 'itching' and decided to try chickweed. By the time she arrived, I had a chickweed bath waiting, and this sobbing, burning, itching woman, quickly climbed into it. Within seconds the heat and the painful itch were relieved. She soaked for a couple of hours and I sent her away with a large bag of chickweed. For the next few days, she either sat in a chickweed bath, or was wrapped in cloths soaked in chickweed infusion as she weathered out the crisis. To complement the treatment, she fasted on juices and herbs. She has never had a repeat of this terrible crisis and over the next few months, the condition was cleared by systemic treatment and restoration of the nervous system, which proved to be the cause of the irritation. She eventually had to change her job at a mental home.

Use chickweed internally as tea and externally to relieve itching and help eliminate the acids which cause the itching.

Chronic purifier formula

Dr Shook created this formula to provide a deep level of blood, tissue and lymph purification in chronic disease, dyscrasia, syphilis and cancer. Use after the eliminative channels are activated and working efficiently.

Mimosa Gum (3), Echinacea, Blue Flag(3), Comfrey Root, Irish Moss, Cloves.

Colitis formula

This formula, together with the bowel tonic and nerve formulae will work together to unravel the complicated causes of this illness. It is also important to counsel, offer Bach flower remedies to assist the changes in mental and emotional attitudes, and to ensure that the eliminative channels are all working efficiently.

Barberry, Golden Seal, White Oak Bark, Myrrh(0.25), Slippery Elm, Aniseed.

Colds and flu formula

There are few common ailments as uncomfortable as acute cold or flu symptoms. This formula, together with antibiotics naturally formula, mustard baths, and fasting on herb teas, will relieve the system and ensure a quick response without the suppression of toxins which result from the use of drugs. Working with the body's acute responses to eliminate accumulated toxins, these herbal aids and associated treatments will support nature, speed recovery and leave the patient stronger and fitter without laying the ground for the development of chronic disease. Hot ginger, yarrow or ephaedra tea are highly recommended when anyone is suffering from colds or flu. Also use the Sore Throat Syrup given under the antibiotics naturally formula.

Elderflower and peppermint tea taken copiously day and night.

Ear treatment

The combination of the antiseptic qualities of the garlic oil and the ability of mullein to reach the lymph glands around the ear provide an all-around ear treatment which relieves pain, swelling and infection, and also improves the chances of restoring hearing quality.

Instructions: Drop 4–6 drops of each oil into the ear every night for six days, plugging with damp cotton wool. Syringe with a mixture of apple cider vinegar/water (10ml each) on the seventh day. Then repeat this seven day cycle until the condition is relieved.

Echinacea

This lymphatic herb has a strong specific action for stimulating leucocyte action. Therefore, its powers for clearing up infection, pus and foul discharges can be well used both internally and externally wherever tissue decay threatens or healing repair is slow. Can be added to poultices wherever there is infection and taken internally to stimulate the auto-immune system. Combine with herbal formulae for the eliminative channels and systemic treatment.

Enema mix

This formula evolved out of discussions with Margaret Strauss, granddaughter of Dr Gerson, the founder of the Gerson Therapy for Cancer and severe chronic diseases. After I confided in her my appreciation of his treatments, I told her about the problems related to adapting it for use with completely vegetarian patients. We then discussed possible solutions. She felt clear that if her grandfather had lived longer, he would have found substitutions for the liver and thyroid extracts as well as adopting other methods which are not so strong and stimulating as the coffee enemas. This herbal mix is an excellent substitute for coffee enemas with the added advantage of the superior nutrition being readily available for direct healing of the walls of the colon, as well as for absorption into the blood and the lymph to be transported throughout the body. After taking this enema one is truly aware of strength and nourishment, and the liver is stimulated to dump bile. The system is relieved, and the pain and discomfort of the healing crises is reduced.

Red Clover, Red Raspberry, Burdock, Yellow Dock.

Exhaustion formulae

Although exhaustion has many possible causes – mental, emotional and physical – the treatment of this condition usually requires high levels of minerals and vitamins, together with herbs to aid the digestion and assimilation of the nutrient. It is important to calm the digestive system if there have been emotional or mental upsets. This formula, when it is combined with systemic treatment which is guided by iridology, produces excellent recuperative energy to bring a person back to their normal energy level. The Bach flower remedies and flower essences are a great help here also.

Gentian Root, Gotu Kola, Chondrus Crispus, Cetraria, Cloves, Alfalfa, Calumba Root.

Eye wash formula

This eye wash has been successfully used by herbalists for many years in treatment of cataract, glaucoma, eye weakness and infection. This combination of herbs stimulates the circulation to the eye, relieves congestion, feeds the eye and provides healing herbs to cure any infection. Although there is some mild stinging when you first start using the eye wash, this soon passes and the eyes feel bright, refreshed and strengthened. Use $\frac{1}{8}$ tsp of the herb to $\frac{1}{2}$ cup water.

Pour boiling water over the powder and allow to steep until warm and strain well through a fine cloth or coffee filter. Then, using an eye cup, open and close each eye under the infusion for at least 1 minute. Do this once, twice or three times a day as needed, and continue until the condition is improved. If your eyes are particularly sensitive, dilute the strained infusion further.

Eyebright, Golden Seal.

Female reproductive formula

This herbal combination strengthens, tones, regulates and heals the reproductive organs. Whatever the problem or symptoms, this formula provides the nutrient to support regeneration and harmonizing of this body system. It is essential, however, that the eliminative channels be fully cleansed and activated and that systemic weakness be supported if long term benefit is to be realized. While working at deeper levels, the formula relieves cramps, menstrual flooding and pain, and prepares the reproductive system for healthy childbearing. It is excellent to combine this formula with the women's period pain formula.

Blue Cohosh, Licorice, Motherwort, Parsley Root, Red Raspberry, Squaw Vine, True Unicorn Root.

Fenugreek

The highest vegetable source of vitamin D, fenugreek provides the basis for an excellent skin rejuvenation programme. Whenever the iris shows that the skin is not eliminating properly, the person does not perspire, or the skin is dry and scaly, put the patient on a programme of 6–8 cups of fenugreek tea a day. Use 1 level teaspoon of powder per cup or simmer the seeds very gently for 15 minutes. This concentrated use will stimulate perspiration. Often patients need to bathe more often as the skin will eliminate acids and toxins during the early stages of the treatment. After bathing rub the skin with a mixture of almond and wheat germ oil, and scrub the skin twice daily with a natural bristle brush.

Fungus formula

Although many cases of thrush clear up with systemic and vaginal ovule treatment, some stubborn cases resist. Also, with other patients, fungal infections on fingers or elsewhere prove resistant. There is so much written about Candida Albicans and I wanted to create a herbal formula which would form a powerful part of a total approach to clearing the system while relieving the irritating symptoms at the same time. The results have been excellent when supported as a part of the full programme as determined by iris diagnosis. Use internally and externally as a poultice, bath or douche.

For best results, do not mix with herbs or formulae containing seaweeds as iodine neutralizes the action of the formula.

Thyme, Poke Root, Myrrh, Clivers, Cayenne, Meadowsweet.

Gall bladder cleanse formula (Frank Roberts)

This formula completes the cleanse detailed in *Herbs of Grace*. It should be taken for at least six weeks after the cleanse to reduce inflammation and strengthen and heal the gall bladder.

Black Root, Euonymous, Kava, Marshmallow Root(2).

Gentian root

This herb is added to eliminative and systemic treatment when absorption of nutrient, digestive weakness and exhaustion are a major problem. A strengthening and revitalizing tonic, gentian tones the liver and makes an effective digestive tonic.

Hairwash formula

Whenever hair has become weak or brittle or is falling out, use this formula to complement systemic treatment. It is essential that the circulation formula together with purifying herbs also be used. One must consider the absorption and assimilation of nutrient and whether it is reaching the head area.

Make a herbal tea of sage, yarrow and yellow dock, a strong brew of 3 tablespoons per cup of water. While this is steeping, wash your hair. Massage the tea into it, and leave it on all day.

Make a mixture of castor oil, wheatgerm oil, and olive oil and massage into the head before bed. Steam with hot towels and then wrap in a dry towel. Wash the hair well in the morning and then massage in the herb tea for the day.

During this time do inversion postures or slant board exercises, drink sage tea, take one or both of the blood circulation formulae, and take high doses of vitamin E. Continue this treatment for a full seven-week cycle, and repeat at regular intervals for best results.

Sage, Yarrow, Yellow Dock.

Heart tonic

A normalizing heart formula needs to take into consideration blood pressure, water retention, heart rate, whether there are deposits in the blood vessels, the force of the heart contraction, peripheral circulation and the influence of the nervous system. This tonic for the heart provides a wide range of nutrient to balance, strengthen and nourish, and often needs to be combined with either of the two circulation formulae.

Hawthorn Berries(6), Motherwort(3), Ginseng(3), Ginger Root(2), Comfrey Root (2), Lily of the Valley(3), Broom(2), Dandelion(2), Scullcap(2), Lime Blossom(2), Bugleweed(2).

Heavy metal purifier

After a certain level of eliminative function and systemic balance has been achieved, the practitioner decides when this formula can be applied to release a deeper level of cleansing. However, it is essential that all the eliminative channels are working well or the patient will experience headaches, nausea and weakness.

Often, the urinary system is put to the test so it is essential that this formula be combined with the kidney/bladder formula, taken as usual between meals with a glass of water or herb tea. Daily Epsom Salts baths will increase the elimination from the skin.

This formula will slowly reduce the shape and size of psora markings. Take it over a three week period, rest three weeks, then it can be taken again. The heavy metal formula reaches deep into the tissues where toxins have collected in weak areas. It is best to choose a time when the body can easily handle the purification. If the treatment is guided properly, the patients should feel neither discomfort or weakness, and purification should proceed easily.

Yellow Dock, Bugleweed, Lobelia, Chaparral, Uva Ursi.

Hormone balance formula

The herbs in this formula contain natural hormones, offered within complex plant chemistry, so that the patient, whether male or female, will be provided with the required range of nutrients. Their body will select what is needed to balance their system. Use confidently during pregnancy, puberty or menopause, or whenever the endocrine function needs tuning.

Black Cohosh, Sarsaparilla, Ginseng, Holy Thistle, Licorice Root, False Unicorn, Squaw Vine, Chasteberry.

Hydrangea root

Use a strong decoction of hydrangea root to dissolve calcarious kidney stones. Take at least 4–6 cups daily for seven weeks while following a purification diet and systemic internal herbal treatment guided by an iridologist.

Ileocaecal valve formula

This formula is an excellent aid to regulate ileocaecal imbalances, whether overfunctioning or underfunctioning. The Touch for Health or Applied Kinesiology practitioners do wonderful work to adjust this valve and to teach people about its influence on the digestive system. If you have this problem, this formula will help to normalize the function of the valve. However, it is also essential to treat the nervous system and the mental and emotional attitudes associated with the condition.

Ginger(0.5), Quassia, Bistort, Bayberry Root Bark, Angelica Root.

Infection formula

Acute infections require special herbal treatment, high doses closer together, for shorter periods of time, to stimulate the lymphatic system to deal with the invasion. Keep this formula in your first aid kit and administer doses every half hour, 4–8 capsules. Reduce to 2 capsules for children under 12 years, and to 1 capsule for children under 7, and $\frac{1}{2}$ capsule for children under 2 years of age. Useful for colds, flu, fever, infected wounds, bronchitis, treatment of burns, etc. It is best to have the guidance of a doctor in any serious condition, and certainly if natural medicines are to be used, it is essential that the bowels and stomach are clean and clear, and that any tendency to fever is supported by hot mustard baths, followed by steaming and perspiring under quilts, and regular intake of red raspberry, catnip and peppermint teas.

Echinacea(2), Garlic, Golden Seal, Lobelia, Mullein, Plantain.

Intestinal infection formula

Whether this formula is used as a part of bowel cleansing treatment or because of infections in tropical climates, it will help to eliminate harmful microbial parasites and infections in bowel pockets and diverticuli. Although its influence will be strong enough to encourage elimination of various types of intestinal worms, if there is a severe manifestation it is necessary to consult a practitioner. Also eat large amounts of pumpkin seeds daily until condition is cleared.

Gentian, Burdock, Wormwood(2), Sage, Fennel, Cloves, Mullein, Myrrh, Thyme, Quassia.

Kidney/bladder formula

This formula combines several actions to cleanse, heal and balance urine flow, to dissolve sediment and to tone and strengthen the function of the entire urinary tract. Kidney problems are not always directly due to kidney weakness. They also suffer because of the lack of support from other eliminative channels, or because of improper drinking habits. Within the framework of systemic and eliminative channel treatment, this will bring the function of the urinary tract to a healthy balanced level.

Buchu, Clivers, Gravel Root, Juniper Berries, Marshmallow Root, Parsley Root, Uva Ursi.

Lady's slipper

One of my favorite herbs, lady's slipper breaks the action of stress and strain, gives an excellent sleep and relieves emotional sensitivity so that you can make a fresh start in the morning. It produces a most relaxed state which is a complete relief to any nervous system wound up by work, family or personal crises. It is an excellent aid for jet travel, allowing total relaxation and releasing anxious tension so that you arrive feeling fresh and rested. For the constitutional types who proceed to illness through the nervous system, this is a prime remedy because when balance is restored by complete rest and a good sleep, the nervous system is not allowed to influence the rest of the body towards disease.

Dosage: From 3-12 capsules, depending on the person and the circumstances, before bed.

Lady's slipper/valerian

This combination reduces the expense of pure lady's slipper, and it is also more suitable for those who run on nerves during the day, who are restless and unable to sit down or stop doing things. Divide into 3 daily doses. This formula prepares the body to withdraw from tranquillizers, relaxants, and it can also be used before sleep to ensure a good night rest.

Lady's Slipper, Valerian

Liver/gall bladder formula

The digestive chemical factory needs the full support of the liver-gall bladder function to secrete alkaline fluids into the duodenum to balance the acid secretions from the pancreas. There, together, they act on the food which comes from the stomach. This formula begins its good work in the stomach and proceeds to influence the digestive process of the liver as it deals with the metabolism of carbohydrates, proteins, fats and the storage and metabolism of vitamins. A healthy liver means clean blood and a good digestion. It is an essential part of good body function.

Barberry Bark(3), Wild Yam Root, Cramp Bark, Fennel, Catnip, Peppermint, Dandelion(2), Meadowsweet(2), Wahoo, Black Root.

Lymphatic formula

Whenever the lymph system needs rejuvenation, whether due to constitutional deficiency (indicated by a lymphatic rosary in the iris), the body's inability to deal with the high levels of catarrh formed by incorrect diet, high levels of toxins in the body, or invasion of viruses or germs, this formula will strengthen and activate the leucocytes, support the glands as they purify the lymph and stimulate balanced elimination. It is also important to consider the level of toxins and the functioning of the other eliminative channels and blood purifying organs such as the liver and the kidneys. It is helpful to use this formula in alternation with chronic purifier formula.

Echinacea, Lobelia, Mullein, Poke Root, Burdock, Cayenne, Chaparral.

Mucus congestion formula

This natural antihistamine will relieve the irritating sinus and nasal problems associated with colds, flu and hayfever. It makes your acute eliminations more comfortable.

Black Pepper, Aniseed, Ginger Root.

Mullein

Diarrhoea can be a severe problem during bowel illness and bowel rejuvenation programmes. It is essential to use a combination of treatments, to reduce the diarrhoea as quickly as possible because it is so uncomfortable and debilitating. The mullein tea, on its own or mixed with soya milk, will reduce diarrhoea. In stubborn cases, put the patient on a diet of stewed apples with very high amounts of cinnamon, baked potatoes and slippery elm tea. Use astringents (either infused or as rectal injections) such as red raspberry, witch hazel or bayberry.

Multi-minerals/vitamins naturally

A balanced herbal alternative to mineral and vitamin supplements! So many patients and students have requested a formula like this over the years. Although all our fresh, potent, unprocessed herbal nutrients are richly endowed with vitamins and minerals, this formula contains the full range made available in one formula (at a great saving when you compare what you would have to pay for processed packaged vitamin/mineral supplements). It also contains easily assimilable vegetarian alkaline protein and amino acids. Adjust dose according to need. Two teaspoons replace a meal and help to take away hunger pangs when dieting or on cleansing fasts.

Alfalfa, Alkaline Formula(4), Anaemia Formula, Calcium Formula(2), Spirulina, Rose Hips.

Nerve rejuvenator

This formula restores the nervous system, encourages deep rejuvenating sleep (take about 6–8 capsules before sleep) and rebuilds the system after nervous breakdown.

Gotu Kola(4), Valerian(2), Kava Kava, Irish Moss, Lady's Slipper.

Nerve tonic

Rebuilding the nervous system requires regular intake of nervine herbs which provide the nutrient for central, autonomic and peripheral nervous systems, as well as the nutrient to rebuild nerve sheaths. It is especially effective to combine this formula with the calcium formula, the sweet sleep formula or the thyroid formula, if there are problems with hyperactivity or insomnia.

Catnip, Gotu Kola(2), Lady's Slipper, Lobelia, Scullcap, Valerian.

Nerve vitalizer

This formula strengthens the nervous system during and after trauma or shock.

Prickly Ash Bark(4), Irish Moss, Bayberry Bark

Pain relief formula

Whether pain is from acute injuries, headaches, burns, or from chronic diseases like arthritis and rheumatism, this formula will soothe, diminish the discomfort, and encourage sleep. The dose can be adjusted from 3 times a day with meals, to every 15 minutes, $\frac{1}{2}$ hour, or every hour as needed. Works best in combination with professionally guided treatment to relieve the cause of the pain.

White Willow Bark, Jamaican Dogwood, Valerian, Cramp Bark.

Pancreas formula

The herbs in this formula contain natural insulin which help to lower blood sugar levels and strengthen and feed this gland. Use of this formula must be a part of a systemic program of treatment. Hypoglycaemia will also be relieved by this formula, especially if several cups of licorice tea are also drunk throughout the day. Diet regimen must also be maintained as recommended by your doctor or practitioner.

Elecampane(2), Golden Seal, Uva Ursi, Wahoo(2), Licorice Root, Mullein, Nettles, Allspice, Juniper Berries.

Pre-natal formula

The expectant mother should drink several cups of this tea during the last six weeks of pregnancy to aid the elasticity of the birth canal, and strengthen the reproductive organs for easier delivery. It is also good for the pregnant woman to take regular doses of the calcium formula and the anaemia formula throughout the entire pregnancy and when nursing. These are purely nutritive herbs and will not upset the mother or the baby. Adjust dose according to need. Also drink red raspberry tea all through pregnancy. Blue Cohosh Root decoction or tincture may be taken regularly from the early stages of labour to the birth to ease and relax the birth canal and minimize pain.

Holy Thistle, Red Raspberry, Squaw Vine, True Unicorn.

Prolapse formula

There are many factors which contribute to a prolapsed condition. After the iridology reading pinpoints the cause, and whether it is related to weak connective tissue, pressure from other organs, bowel toxins or nutritional deficiency, treatment by internal herbal treatment can be supported by specific feeding of the pelvic area by means of ovules and douches.

Black Cohosh, Witch Hazel, White Oak Bark (2), Lobelia, Yellow Dock, Marshmallow Root.

Prostate formula

Combine this formula with the bowel tonic and the lymph formula. Take over a period of eight weeks to strengthen this gland. Use in conjunction with the ovule for prostate conditions.

Echinacea, Saw Palmetto, Gravel Root, Parsley Root, Golden Seal (2), Marshmallow Root, Cayenne.

Psyllium seeds

Soak 1 teaspoon seeds in $\frac{1}{2}$ cup of warm water. Add juice to taste. This mucilaginous mixture sweeps the bowel walls clean and provides bulk to ease constipation. Take concurrently with the bowel or liver/bowel tonic combination.

Respiratory formula

This formula supports the respiratory system when it is actively eliminating, infected or chronically weak from conditions like asthma and bronchitis. It is best when combined with the asthma formula, as well as systemic treatment for activating and cleansing the eliminative channels and purifying and regenerating the body systems and organs.

Comfrey, Elecampane, Elderflowers, Mullein (2), Licorice, Lobelia.

Skin problems formula

Although chronic skin problems are deep seated and involve the blood purifying organs, toxic eliminative channels and the defence systems of the skin itself, this deeply purifying formula will work well to eliminate morbid conditions from the blood which cause the skin to suffer the consequences. Diet considerations are essential to healing skin problems, and sufferers are advised to consult trained practitioners.

Blue Flag, Burdock Root, Burdock Seeds, Cayenne, Echinacea, Poke Root, Red Clover.

Slippery elm

Whenever a sensitive digestive system reacts against foods or herbal formulae, slippery elm forms the perfect carrier to reduce discomfort.

Make a warm drink by mixing the slippery elm powder with warm soya milk or water, and add a dash of honey, cinnamon, lemon, etc., to taste. As well as soothing and protecting the intestinal wall, and easing digestion, this herbal nutrient is highly nutritious food, containing abundant calcium.

   This fine mucilaginous herb is also used with poultices and the vaginal ovule.

Smoking mix

This formula seems to reduce the need for nicotine, alter taste cravings so that the desire for smoking is reduced, and relieve pain in the resiratory system. I have known many patients who have completely stopped smoking after using this mix. Roll into a handmade herbal 'cigarette'. Excellent for relieving respiratory pain in chronic lung diseases. The lobelia relaxes the chest and disperses congestion while the other herbs soothe and comfort. Lobelia poultices are an excellent complement to this treatment.

Coltsfoot, Mullein, Yerba Santa, Lobelia.

Spirulina

This powerful energy nutrient algae from Mexico contains almost every mineral and vitamin, a high amount of B vitamins and assimilable alkaline protein. Whenever there is weakness, exhaustion or strong cravings and hunger, this nutrient will help to balance the digestion. It is an excellent supplement to take during fasts, juice cleanses and the purifying diets necessary for cleansing the body of accumulated toxins and acids.

Stomach acid/alkaline balancing formula

Imbalances of body chemistry often begin in the stomach. Whenever the stomach is too acid, or too alkaline, this formula will provide the wide range of nutrients to normalize the stomach environment. It is also useful to add this formula to other formulae if the patient has a sensitive digestion, as it will help to soothe and heal the stomach and ease other herbs into the system.

Dandelion Root, Slippery Elm, Calamus, Meadowsweet, Irish Moss, Iceland Moss.

Sweet sleep formula

Restful sleep depends to a large extent on the ability of our parasympathetic nervous system to relax and release us from the stress and strain of daily activities. These herbs combine to relax, mildly sedate, and encourage a sweet restful sleep that leaves one rested, yet alert in the morning. During times of stress or intense activity, this formula can also be taken at regular intervals with meals.

Passion Flower, Lady's Slipper, Scullcap, Hops, Broom, Lime Tree Flowers.

Swollen glands formula
Internally, and as a fomentation on the outside, this formula works to relieve congestion and reduce swelling and discomfort. Use with the lymphatic formula and antibiotics naturally for best results. Leave the fomentation on all night and day if necessary, 6 days a week.
Lobelia, Mullein(2), Parsley Root or Leaves, Plantain.

Tableting mix
For use with tableting rollers and cutters, or for hand-rolled tablets, reducing sticking and finishing the tablets with a pleasant tasting nutritive powder.
Alkaline Formula(2), Slippery Elm, Cinnamon.

Thyroid balancing formula
Whether the thyroid is underactive or overactive, the entire body is put out of balance if this master gland does not receive the nutrient required for balanced activity. Use this formula together with the nerve and sweet sleep formulae if the thyroid is overactive and with the exhaustion and multi-mineral/vitamin formulae if the thyroid is underactive.
Parsley Leaves, Kelp(2), Irish Moss, Iceland Moss, Nettles, Bladderwrack and Bugleweed.

Vaginal ovule or prostate treatment (see also page 238)
The vaginal ovule is an internal poultice which is used to transform the internal environment of the vagina, to offer superior healing agents and nutrition and to draw out poisons. Although the deeper cause may be inherited, or the result of mental, emotional and living influences together with systemic interaction, much can be gained by using the ovule locally to relieve irritation, itching and sores. The ovule will also influence deeper conditions such as cysts, tumours, inflammation, sores and cervical dysplasia, providing healing exactly where it is needed.

The herbs are absorbed into the mucous membranes and spread via the capillary circulation and lymph into the pelvis. When the ovule is balanced by herbal nutrients taken internally, the influences meet, contributing to total healing. We must visualize the pelvis as an internal environment where everything touches everything else, where toxins or healing are spread through the lymph and circulation from the bowel and where emotional tensions in the solar plexus inhibit peristalsis and the movement of blood and lymph carrying nutrient and cleansing the area. If healing is to take place, the pelvis must be restored to harmonious function within the total ecology of the whole person.
Squaw Vine, Echinacea, Comfrey Root, Marshmallow Root, Chickweed, Golden Seal Root.

Wild yam root
Whenever flatulence, gas, wind, spasms, colic or stomach discomfort

contribute strong symptoms of discomfort, this herb is added to the patient's total prescription. It is also excellent for uterine cramps, and can be taken in addition to the women's period pains formula, or throughout pregnancy as a tonic and to prevent miscarriage.

Women's period pains formula
If cramps and pain disturb the menstrual cycle use this formula just before the period is due and during the days of discomfort. Because the effect is accumulative, the need for it should lessen from month to month, especially if the causes are being dealt with by systemic treatment. Chamomile tea will also help to relive cramps if taken at the first sign that the period is due, and continued until the pain disappears.

Blue Cohosh, Cramp Bark(2), Lemon Balm, Ginger, Turmeric, Valerian.

Yellow dock root
We offer yellow dock separately because it is a part of the vaginal ovule treatment, where it is used as a vaginal douche. Its very high iron content attracts oxygen, increasing cellular metabolism and restoring health to the mucous membranes. Although it is a part of the anaemia formula which is also taken during pregnancy, yellow dock tea is an excellent way to take assimilable iron into the system. A valuable blood-purifying herb and a lymphatic stimulant. Yellow dock contributes positive influence whenever it is used.

Teas Teas are prepared by pouring one cup of boiling water over two teaspoonfuls of herb. Steep for at least five minutes. Top it up again with more herbs and more boiling water later on in the day.

a) Serenitea

If you would like to go into low gear before sleep, try one or two cups of this tea before retiring. Because it is a strong but pleasant tasting tea, milk and honey improve the flavour. This is also a useful tea to have on hand to weather crises or emotional upsets.

Catnip, Vervain, Mistletoe, Peppermint, Wood Betony(3), Valerian(0.5), Scullcap(0.5), Hops (0.5).

b) Waterbalance

This mildly diuretic tea beneficially influences the entire urinary tract and helps regulate the elimination of water. When acute conditions such as cystitis occur, drink a cup every half an hour until the symptoms are relieved.

Couchgrass, Parsley Leaves, Clivers, Buchu, Uva Ursi, Chickweed.

c) Digestea	This delightful tea improves the digestive chemistry, balances the acid/alkaline secretions in the stomach, improves digestion and increases the assimilation of nutrient. Take a cup or two, one half hour before or after eating, or for afternoon tea. *Meadowsweet, Wood Betony, Peppermint, Hibiscus, Lemon Grass, Rose Hips, Fennel.*
d) Chickweed	Neutralizes and eliminates acidity.
e) Oat Straw	A high source of silica and calcium, also useful for water cure baths and for footbaths.
f) Red Raspberry	High in iron, which attracts oxygen and increases metabolic activity, overcoming sluggishness.
g) Red Clover	An excellent blood purifier.
h) Sage	The ancient Chinese longevity tea, which stimulates cerebral circulation and increases brain activity.

Tinctures

a) Catnip/Fennel	To relieve colic, wind and discomfort in the digestion.
b) Wild Lettuce/Valerian	To calm and relax the nervous system, especially when sleep or digestion are disturbed.
c) Nervine	*Black Cohosh, Lady's Slipper, Scullcap, Lobelia, Blue Vervain.* Rubbed on the back of the neck under the skull, this tincture feeds the nerve centres and reduces hyperactivity. Take internally as well to calm the nervous system.
d) Echinacea	To assist the lymphatic defence system during acute infections or illnesses.
e) Antispasmodic	*Gotu Kola, Mistletoe, Lady's Slipper, Lobelia, Scullcap, Passion Flower.* For shocks, cramps, spasms, hysteria, epilepsy, asthma.
f) Saw Palmetto	A specific for mammary glands. Use to complement treatment for breast lumps, swollen breasts etc.
g) Lobelia	By prescription only for use as an emetic and to relieve asthma. Rub over congested areas to relieve pain, spasms and swelling.

h) Myrrh Superb addition to your dental regimen. After brushing your teeth put 3 drops on a clean toothbrush and rub into your gums. Good for sores, spots and herpes.

i) Wild Yam For colic, cramp, flatulence, bloating and wind.

j) Euphrasia Excellent eye wash to brighten and strengthen eyes.

k) Elderflower Highest herbal source of potassium. Use to complement treatment for excess acidity, fibroids and nutritional imbalance. Helps to maintain a youthful supple skin.

For adults, the tincture dose is 6–12 drops in a half cup of water 3–4 times daily.

Oils & ointments

a) Chickweed Relieves heat, itching, rashes.

b) Balm of Gilead Soothes and heals eczema, psoriasis.

c) Comfrey To aid cell growth, repair of cuts, wounds, fractures. Provides regenerative nutrient directly where it is needed.

d) Garlic Oil Useful for warts, spots, infected wounds. Apply directly on areas 2–3 times per day.

e) Mullein Oil 2–3 drops in the ear relieve earache, suppuration and inflammation of the ear. Can also be applied externally on sprains, bruises, sores, joints and for skin diseases.

Administering herbs to children

When children cannot swallow tablets or capsules, then tinctures are an excellent alternative. The powders can also be mixed with cinnamon and ground carob and/or mixed with dates, cream cheese or honey. If you offer herb teas to infants, they will accept the taste and be willing to take it during the rest of their childhood. I have had many young patients over the years and enjoy taking them into our herbal pharmacy, explaining how their own special medicine is made up and requesting their cooperation. They love to see their iris drawings and learn what they can do to feel better. Always, remember to congratulate them for their efforts when they are well. We are setting habits for a lifetime, so it is a wonderful opportunity to share a positive experience that will bring them back to natural methods when they are older.

Tinctures can be administered according to age, 3–4 times per day as required, or more often in acute conditions. Size, weight and sensitivity of the child are also a consideration for individual doses. The general doses are:

Up to 2 years of age: 2 drops in a quarter cup of water, 1–2 times per day. Sip as required.

From 2 years to 7:   4 drops in a half cup of water, 1–3 times per day.

Between 7 and 12 years: Use 6–8 drops in a cup of water depending on size, 1–4 times per day.

The full adult dose is: 6–12 drops in a half cup of water 3–4 times daily.

Appendix II

Enemas

Such is the current emphasis on external appearance that usually the mere mention of the word enema invokes expressions of repulsion or embarrassment. The yogis of old who maintained equilibrium between inner and outer cleanliness in a detached manner always included enema techniques in their way of life. Their ancient texts, as well as the Essene Gospel, include information on methods of internal bowel cleansing. Originally, it is said, birds were observed to draw water into their beaks, insert their beaks into their rectum and then expel the water. Man then followed this example.

In modern times, the science of iridology helps to prove the relation of the colon to reflex disease, toxins and symptoms. Essentially, the colon is a hub: each segment of the bowel with its intricate multitudinous connections of circulation, lymph and nerves connect to specific reflex areas throughout the entire body. If one area of the colon is toxic, spastic or inflamed, the symptoms are not only found in the bowel itself, but also in the reflex area.

Also, in allopathic medicine – in surgery and autopsy – the poisonous toxic conditions that exist inside the bowel, which pollute the body via the blood stream, can be viewed at first hand. The colon is supposed to serve as a reservoir from which the blood absorbs nutrients to circulate throughout the entire system. But when the colon is toxic, or impacted with faecal matter, poisons are distributed instead. Also the person is not satisfied by food, feels hungry and eats much more than he needs, because the nutrients are not absorbed and circulated.

In Dr Bernard Jensen's excellent book *Tissue Cleansing Through Bowel Management,* photographs clearly show the black toxic material which is eliminated during thorough bowel cleansing.

Often when a patient is asked if they are constipated, they immediately say, 'No'. On further discussion it is found that this may mean from one motion every day up to one every three days. This is considered normal by them. Does it follow that if you take in food three times or more a day, that you should eliminate only once a day or less? Children with relaxed healthy systems usually have about three movements per day. If you let food sit for three days, it deteriorates. Imagine how much more putrefactive it becomes if it stays in the bowel for three days. Gas is manufactured and pressure causes further problems as the colon develops swellings and pockets which hold further deposits of toxic waste. Poisons from these toxic areas are carried throughout the entire system, causing toxaemia.

Almost every person needs bowel cleansing, and once the bowels are brought to clean normal activity, a regular maintenance programme is advised. Just as a house requires spring cleaning and a car needs regular tune-ups, the bowel needs maintenance cleansing, so that toxic wastes do not build up.

Although complete bowel cleansing and maintenance requires herbs, diet, massage and often packs and poultices, enemas are a significant and useful aid which serve an important function in any bowel program. The various kinds of enemas and their suggested use are listed below.

You will require the following:

How to take an enema

1. A gravity flow enema bucket or bag, and
2. Two pints of enema fluid (various types listed below).

You will find your enema a simple and pleasant experience if you organize yourself well, set aside a relaxed half hour and provide yourself with something to do when you are retaining the enema (such as radio, book, tapes, etc.)

Many people like to take their enema while they are soaking in a warm bath. Others prefer to do it on a rug on the floor, so they can go up into the Yoga shoulder stand or the plough posture. Others choose the use of a slant-board or TIP-U-UP, allowing gravity to aid retention. The main suggestion is for each person to find out what they like and then make it a dutiful function of health care. It helps to have a hook in a convenient place from which to hang the enema bag or bucket.

When you have everything together, lie down on your back, or on your right side, and press the lubricated tip of the enema tube into the rectum until it is firmly in place, using a little soap, vaseline or oil for lubrication. Release the tube lock and let the liquid begin to flow into the rectum. It is best to have the liquid at room temperature, as hot water will of course be uncomfortable and cold water is harder to retain. You can control the flow of the liquid with the tube lock if it begins to get uncomfortable. If the water hits a block of impacted faeces, you can stop the flow, massage the area, turn or go up into the shoulder stand until you feel ready to inject more. Ideally, you should be able to inject and retain for at least ten minutes, an entire quart of enema fluid. Sometimes the urge to release cannot be ignored and it is wise to let it go and begin all over again. As the bowel condition improves, it will be easier and easier to accept and retain all the liquid with a minimum of discomfort.

As you want the liquid to flow up the descending colon, across the transverse, and down the ascending colon, it is helpful to change positions and massage the area. Often when a strong urge to release comes, it usually lasts only for a minute or so, and if you breathe quickly, and/or turn your feet in circles at the ankle in both directions you can ride the storm and will find that the crisis passes. Remember – the more you need the positivity and help of the enema, the more your bowels will try to reject the enema fluid prematurely. Each time you do an enema, try to hold it longer than the time before. Stay lying on the right side or in the inverted posture.

It is clearly necessary to recognize that once people experience the release of symptoms by the use of enemas, they may be tempted to overuse them, rather than master overeating or stricter aspects of habit change and body purification. Overuse of enemas can result in weakening of bowel tone, so it is important to realize when enemas should and should not be used.

The most important use of enemas is the service they add to any body purification program. Whenever any form of fasting or dietary regimen releases toxins into the blood and lymph, the enema is most effective in carrying away toxins out of the body. It is also a necessary part of any program dedicated to deep bowel cleansing. However, once the goal is achieved, the enema is used only on a maintenance basis, sometimes once a week and sometimes once a month, or whenever signs of impending colds or flu or digestive problems make themselves known. If the need for enemas is too often, the person should seek professional guidance, so that they do not weaken the system by overusing the enemas, also avoiding the cause of the congestion or problem.

Plain water enemas
A warm water enema will effectively cleanse the rectum and release toxins which may be causing headaches and flatulence. Its effects are superficial, but can be relied on whenever any of the other enema fluids are not readily available. Wash the colon clean with a plain water enema before you insert retention enemas.

Herbal enemas
Make a strong infusion of herbal teas or a decoction of roots and barks, strain and cool. Use two tablespoons of herb per pint of water. This may be made up in advance, but used preferably within 24 hours, though certain herbs keep up to 72 hours. However, once souring or scum appears, throw it away. It should be kept in a glass container in a fridge or cool place. Make herbal infusions or decoctions in stainless steel or enamelled pots only.

Catnip enema	Mildly nervine, calming, soothing, relaxing. Effectively brings down fevers. Excellent for use with children.
Chamomile enema	Excellent for recuperative periods after illness or a healing crisis.
Detoxifying	Make a decoction of yellow dock and burdock roots, then add red clover and red raspberry

	infusions. Stimulates the liver to dump bile, thereby relieving stress and pain in a healing crisis.
Slippery elm	Mucilagenous, soothing, softening and nourishing enema. Excellent to give if the patient is having trouble eating or retaining food, as the bowel absorbs the nutrient.
Sage	Warming, purifying
Garlic injection	Profoundly purifying, an excellent aid in the treatment of worms. Liquidize four cloves in 1 pint warm water and strain.
Astringent	Witch hazel, bayberry, or white oak bark, used to help stop diaorrhea and dysentery.
Flaxseed enema	Relieves inflammation, pain and bleeding (more effective if you add two teaspoons of liquid chlorophyll). Also aids healing process.
Wheatgrass implant	Inject pure chlorophyll juice of wheatgrass which restores positivity to bowel and blood stream. Excellent for chronic diseases. Can be mixed 1:1 with rejuvelac (water from soaking wheat). Wash colon clean first with a plain water enema.

Coffee enemas

The coffee enema is widely publicized these days as a part of cancer therapy and chronic care naturopathy. It is excellent to relieve healing crisis pain and discomfort, to stimulate the liver to dump bile by absorption of the coffee into the haemorrhoidal veins and the portal vein, and to encourage deep cleansing of the colon by stimulating peristaltic activity.

It is a regular part of the Gerson Therapy regimen and the Kelly cancer programme. The coffee enema is prepared by putting three tablespoons of drip ground coffee into one quart of distilled water which has just been brought to the boil. Continue on the boil for three minutes and then simmer on very low heat for 20 minutes. Cool. Strain and inject while at body temperature. Retain 10–15 mintues. This can be done every morning when on a detoxification programme or fast, and every hour during an acute healing crisis. The bowels continue to operate independently even when taking the coffee enema regularly and start functioning easily on their own after the coffee enema is discontinued. The coffee enema is recommended after a lymph massage to cleanse the colon of the lymph which has drained into the bowel, but not before sleep as it is too stimulating. A herbal substitute for the coffee enema is: red clover, yellow dock root, burdock and red raspberry.

Spirulina enema

The use of spirulina plankton enemas together with fasting and purification programmes is an excellent way to cleanse the colon and purify the blood stream as quickly as possible. Spirulina has the unique advantage of supplying strength and power through the absorption of the plankton into the bowel wall, as well as cleansing at the same time by softening the impacted faecal matter and stimulating peristalsis. Direct nutrition absorbed by the colon provides proteins and essential amino acids, laying a balanced foundation for easy purification, since hunger and weakness are prevented by the spirulina intake. The spirulina enema may be made as follows: Heat one blender full of distilled water to body temperature. Mix two teaspoons spirulina powder with half a cup of cold water till you make a smooth paste. Add two teaspoons glycerine (obtainable from the chemists) and stir together. Add this loose paste to a blender half full of the warm distilled water, and mix at slow speed. You can also use a whisk. Add the remaining distilled water slowly, to fill the blender. Fill the enema bag right away and use quickly.

This method will wash out the lower and upper bowel and encourage a complete peristaltic downward action. The plankton is also absorbed into the bowel wall, helping to soften, loosen and dilute the bowel contents. Inject the mixture a little at a time while lying on the right side. Move back and forth from left to right side, and massage the bowel area. If you feel that retention is impossible, then eject, and start the process over again. With practice the bowel becomes accustomed and eventually you will be able to retain a full enema of two quarts for five to ten minutes, while massaging the abdomen. Use of the shoulder stand will help the spirulina to reach the whole of the intestinal tract. The glycerine helps to emulsify the mixture, soften the impacted faeces and lubricate the walls of the colon. Take the enema the first night of any fast and for the next two nights. While you continue the fast, take one every other day and after the fast take once a month on a regular basis for effective bowel maintenance. Spirulina powder is better than grinding up tablets, as it is without additives.

Enema equipment   There are a number of different types of enema kit available, the commonest being described here:

The *Enema/Douche Bucket* is a non-brittle, white plastic, 1.2 litre (2 pint) capacity, 4.25 inch diameter by 6.5 inches high, bucket with gravity feed pvc tube, enema and douche nozzles, and tap. It has a hole on one flattened side to allow it to be hung on a wall-mounted hook and is easily cleaned from oils and strong herbs.

The *Enema/Douche Bag* is a strong, collapsible, 2 litre capacity, plastic bag with reinforced top for mounting on a wall hook. It is easily cleaned inside. Packing into a small size, this enema kit is useful both for the home and when travelling, and comes complete with enema and douche nozzles and tap.

The *Enema/Douche Bag* is of the hot water bottle variety, with tube, clip, enema and douche nozzles, and a stopper for normal hot water bottle use. Useful for travelling as well as at home, but you can't get your hand inside it for cleaning. It is fine for warm water or well-strained herbal enemas.

There is also another variety, sometimes called a *Higginson's Syringe,* which is simply a squeezable rubber bulb with a nozzle. They are useful for some applications, such as implants, but generally they don't hold enough fluid for a decent enema.

A useful addition for implanting the enema fluid higher up in the colon is a soft, flexible, 14 inch *Rectal Implant Tube,* with two laterally positioned end holes (rather than a single one in the end that gets blocked up). It fits all the enema kits, slipping over the standard rectal nozzle, also making insertion smoother and easier.

Appendix III

Castor oil packs

Castor oil packs assist the enemas, because the absorption of the castor oil via the skin into the lymph system softens, relaxes, nourishes and balances the sympathetic and parasympathetic nervous systems when it is absorbed into the lacteals in the small intestine. It also disperses congestion and tension, and slowly helps to release the blockages in the bowel pockets. Dr Christopher also comments, 'castor oil helps to get rid of hardened mucus in the body, which may appear as cysts, tumors, or polyps.' Many patients resist this treatment because they fear it will be messy. When they finally do it and are rewarded by the results, they always wish they had done it earlier.

Directions:
1. Place a cotton tea towel over a plastic bin bag.
2. Soak the cotton cloth in castor oil.
3. Cover with second moist cotton cloth to provide heat.
4. Cover these two layers with plastic. Lift the cotton cloths off the bottom plastic bag and place over the abdomen, the cotton soaked in oil next to the skin.
5. Place a heating pad over this or use a hot water bottle (not so easy to manage). Don't fill hot water bottles too full or they are too heavy.
6. Cover the entire lot with a thick towel which wraps around the body to hold everything in place. Secure by ties or pins.
7. Enjoy this soothing and relaxing pack for one and a half hours, three days in a row. Place the two layers of cotton and top layer of plastic back on the first layer of plastic, roll it up and put it away.
8. For the next three days massage the entire area with olive oil.
9. Rest on the seventh day, then repeat the entire procedure again.

Make sure you have organized yourself well to enjoy your castor oil pack. You can choose reading, writing, resting, meditating, T.V., conversation or even go to sleep. When I am tired, I let myself go to sleep and vaguely remember waking up, taking it off onto the plastic beside my bed and then going back to sleep. The relaxation of the solar plexus and abdominal emotional brain is very soothing and especially valuable to the kind of constipation caused by muscular tension.

One of the happy results of a clean colon is a more stable emotional life. It is said among natural healers that the constipated person is an irritable, impatient one. If we could only realize consciously the importance of internal hygiene on general health, well-being and appearance, we would balance all our efforts for external appearance with internal cleanliness. It is certainly an essential aspect of any body cleansing programme, whether for preventive or curative treatment. Once it is accepted into your life and has a place along with other beauty and health routines, you will be able to apply it when needed for beneficial results. Many people have a resistance towards accepting enemas and we hope this information will help you to overcome that. Your life will be the better for this knowledge.

Appendix IV

Cold abdominal pack

This is a simple but effective home treatment.

Take two cloths, one of 100 per cent cotton wool, the other 100 per cent strong cotton, both 18 inches by 60 inches.

Wet the cotton cloth in cold water and wrap quickly around your body twice, covering the torso from the groin to the bottom of the ribs. This will feel cold and uncomfortable for just a moment but as soon as you wrap the 100 per cent wool around you twice it will already feel like body temperature. Tie the pack in place with a string which wraps around from top to bottom, a body stocking which holds it in place, or pins.

Generally the best time to apply the pack is in the evening at least two hours after eating. It is only necessary to wear it for an hour and a half, but if you fall asleep with it on it can be removed when you wake up. It is fine to walk around, sit up or lie down: whatever is best for you.

The cold abdominal pack increases circulation, activates metabolic functions, reduces inflammation and calms the nervous system. It produces a feeling of well-being and relief if pain or congestion is a problem in either digestive, reproductive or urinary organs.

Although it seems a simple treatment its effects are powerful. Don't underestimate the cold abdominal pack because its influence on internal organs and systems is most beneficial. It is especially helpful because it increases circulation to the kidneys.

Appendix V

Healing diets

One of the prime goals of treatment is to eliminate toxins, acids and mucus from the body organs and tissues. It is essential that diet be adjusted so that they are not being put back in the body as fast as they are being eliminated.

Eliminate	Substitute
Salt	Savoury herbs, cayenne pepper, freshly ground pepper, ground dandelion greens and seaweeds, soya sauce, olive oil (cold pressed).
Tea, coffee, alcohol	Herbal teas, dandelion and grain coffees, mulled juices with spices, miso drink, fresh juices. Coffee and tea contain high levels of tannin and neutralize iron. It is *essential* to eliminate the drinking of tea or coffee around the time you take herbal supplements, at least one hour before and one hour after.
Meat, fish, fowl and eggs	Purifying diets must eliminate these proteins. See list of high nutrition foods for acceptable proteins. The energy required for digestion should be minimized so that it can be used for healing.
Dairy products (butter, cheese, yoghurt, cottage cheese, milk)	Highly mucus-forming. A small amount of goat's milk products can be used or soya cheese.
Flour and flour products	When heated or baked, they are mucus-forming. Use chick-pea flour or rice.
Processed and preserved	Use fresh products only, without chemical additives and preservatives. Organically grown produce is best.

One of the best approaches to the transition phase of diet is to go through your cupboards and pack away all of the above products which are to be eliminated.

When that is done, make up a shopping list which lists all of the foods you can eat. If you decide to increase all that is good for you it will make it easier to eliminate other foods from your diet. The foods you need to increase are fresh fruit and vegetables. If a high proportion of these exist in your diet, you will not feel so hungry for other things. However it is also important not to overdo fruit, so that the sugar levels in the blood do not go out of balance.

Spirulina   If hunger and cravings for sweet, sour or salty foods are a problem, bowel cleansing combined with a regular intake of spirulina will make adequate nutrition available. Often when the cleansing current is strongest, we want to support regeneration. Whereas other proteins will stop the purification, spirulina balances purification with regeneration so that both continue at a more comfortable level. One to 3 tsps of spirulina per meal will provide adequate protein, but the addition of the alkaline and multi-mineral and vitamin formulae offers the complete range of nutrients.

Capsicum or cayenne pepper   A safe pure stimulant, antiseptic and toning agent which helps the system to throw off disease and establish equilibrium. Start with $\frac{1}{4}$ tsp. in yoghurt or tomato juice and take three times daily. Continue increasing the dose until you are taking 1 full tsp. three times daily. Although this herb is very hot and strong the first few times you take it, and it is best to drink it down quickly and follow it with a chaser, you soon get used to it and begin to enjoy its powerful energizing effect.

Honey and apple cider vinegar   Mix 1 tsp. honey and 1 tbsp. apple cider in $\frac{1}{4}-\frac{1}{2}$ cup of warm water three times a day to soothe, balance and alkalinize the digestion. The high potassium and antiseptic qualities of this drink have proved themselves over centuries of folk medicine.

Kelp   High mineral supplement and thyroid nutrient; 6–12 tablets daily.

Alfalfa   Herbal multi-vitamin, bowel cleanser and stimulant. Take 2–4 tablets per meal. The roots of the alfalfa plant go deep into the earth where they are able to pick up valuable trace elements. These tablets also have a gently softening and laxative effect in the bowels.

Wheat germ oil   1 tbsp. of fresh oil will provide vitamin E and other nutrients to assist the healing process. Take in juice or on salads.

Powder a mixture of sunflower, sesame and pumpkin seeds, and sprinkle over salads and vegetables for their high nutritive content. (See food value list.)

Three seeds

Add seaweeds to soups and salads, for their high mineral nutrition. Macrobiotic books are an excellent guide to the use of seaweeds. Wash, tear and mix with salads raw. Add to soups in the last few minutes.

Seaweeds

Soybean miso provides strengthening soup stocks and beverage bases. Miso vegetable soups for breakfast provide power, energy and warmth, offering a balancing alternative to fruit or cereal breakfasts.

Miso

Soybean curd provides alkaline, easily digestible protein. Boil lightly in soya sauce, add fresh cut peppers, herbs, tomatoes, etc. and eat as a savoury or cut, dice and add to soups, stews and nut loaves for top nutrition.

Tofu

Whenever alkalinizing is needed, take this broth daily for one meal. Soak 2 cups bran and 1 cup oatmeal overnight in 1.5 quarts water. Stir, then strain through a sieve in the morning. Add potatoes, carrots, onions, celery and parsley, then simmer gently in the bran-oatmeal water. Mash up vegetables and strain again if you wish. Season as desired with herbs, cayenne and spices.

Potassium broth

An excellent milk substitute for children and adults. Very tasty. Blanch 1 cup almonds and slip off skins. Liquify together with 1 quart water, $\frac{1}{2}$ tsp. honey and 1 tbsp. safflower oil. Strain the pulp if you wish for use in baked goods or desserts.

Almond milk

If your brain is active with mental work, you would do well to add this to your daily diet. High in phosphorus, it is known as brain food. Daily use of lecithin also helps to reduce cholesterol levels in the blood.

Lecithin

It is important not to be too strict or to deny yourself foods you love or crave unless you are in a life and death chronic disease programme. The tension and emotional imbalance caused by suppression of all desires and enjoyments, collects and causes one to react, eventually resulting in bingeing or giving up one's attempts altogether.

Food provides physical energy which goes downward through digestion, etheric energy which rises upwards through the palate to the central nervous system, emotional satisfaction, and delight to the

Comfort foods

senses, the eyes, nose, taste and touch. To deny any aspect of this range
of nourishment is asking for trouble.

Over the years so many patients (especially women) have said to me:
'When I'm upset, I head for bread and butter... or toast and jam.'
Inability to express emotions or to complete an encounter activates liver
distress which is calmed by chewing, the smell of the toast and the
warm, soft, sweet comfort of carbohydrates. For others, the comfort is
attained by chocolate, alcohol, or coffee and often we see the food that
is craved the most is actually causing further imbalances.

This craving is a very real need and while some patients find the will
and strength to stop indulging completely, others have a struggle.
Strong cravings can be reduced by the use of spirulina: 6 capsules or a
teaspoon mixed with juice. Acupuncture may be needed to restore
balance to the digestive system. Sometimes, also, our jaw is tight
because of emotions and shock, and the patient simply needs to chew.
Sunflower seeds or pumpkin seeds are excellent for this purpose.

The herbal treatment eases the craving by providing superior nutrient
for specific areas of need. This balances the body and cravings diminish.
Diets should not be made so rigid and strict that it causes other
imbalances or reactions. Because the herbal nutrients are so effective,
we can ease up on strict diets, especially in the early stages of treatment.

The elimination of harmful foods should be a comfortable natural
process which happens gradually. As strength and balance are created
from within, it gets easier and easier to maintain a purifying or
wholesome diet. Slowly, the enjoyment for vital, wholesome foods
returns and cravings for stimulants or synthetic tastes diminish or cease
altogether.

If you have been drinking 20 cups of coffee a day and need to stop,
the answer is not to say no and suffer. How can we approach this
problem in a positive light?

First, drinking other things leaves less space for drinking coffee. If the
patient is drinking 4 cups a day of herbal tea, that means 4 cups less of
coffee. The apple cider vinegar and honey drink eliminates another cup.
They can't drink at the time the herbs are taken, and so the
transformation begins. As energy builds from within, the need for
stimulation lessens and soon patients find they enjoy the coffee less and
less and are soon satisfied by beverages like Barleycup, grain coffee,
miso cup and dandelion coffee.

While excessive cravings reflect imbalances within, enjoyment of
occasional treats is a joy which should not be forbidden. The breaking
of an addiction to coffee, tea, chocolate or alcohol for instance will
release the cause which can then be explored, adjusted and transformed
as a part of the healing process.

It is wrong to assume that correct eating will not be enjoyable and
satisfying. Your tastes will rejoice in vital fresh simpler foods which will
leave you with a feeling of well-being, and when you want to enjoy a
food for the pure pleasure of it, your body will be able to handle it. You
will be in control, no longer at the mercy of blind cravings or habits

which are potentially destructive to your good health.

When you follow this diet, you will gradually adjust to your normal weight, receive more vitality and satisfaction from food, cleanse the system and save considerably on your food budget. Do not be concerned because this diet omits meat and dairy proteins. Remember that cows, horses, elephants and even gorillas eat only plants, grains, nuts and seeds.

Purification diet

On waking: Bach flower remedy. Herbal tea or other beverage.

Breakfast:
1. Liver flush – see section below.
2. Herbal formulae and supplements listed above, immediately before a breakfast of low-cooked whole grain cereal, fruit or miso soup.
3. Fill a thermos flask with $\frac{1}{3}$ whole grain cereal and then fill with boiling water. Shake a few times and allow it to sit overnight. By morning the grains should be soft. Add a little oil or fresh butter and honey. Organic grains are best. Low heat preserves full nutrition and the cereal is still a live food.

Mid-morning: Herb teas, fresh juice, Bach flower remedy.

Lunch: Tossed salad of mixed vegetables, leafy greens, fresh cut herbs together with an oil and apple cider vinegar dressing, with a dash of lemon. Grate fresh black pepper. Use garlic. Add 8–10 blanched almonds and seaweeds. Sprinkle the salad with the seed powder and lecithin, and take with your regular herbal medicines and supplements.

If you wish to make lunch your main meal of the day (this is preferred), you may add steamed or baked vegetables, potassium broth, soups or baked potatoes, sweet potatoes or yams. Top potatoes with a tasty mixture of soya sauce, olive oil and cayenne pepper.

Afternoon: Bach flower remedy.
Drink fresh juices during the afternoon (choose several and alternate them): carrot, grape, apple or vegetable mixtures. If bottled juices are necessary, be sure and choose brands which are sugarless and free of preservatives.

Evening meals: If the lunch was light, take the heavier meal at night, but if the lunch was heavy, take a simple light fruit salad with seeds, nuts, goat's yoghurt, honey and soaked, dried fruit. If you need to reduce sugar levels, take miso soup instead.

Evening & before bed: Juices. Warmed beverages. Fruit. Bach flower remedy.

Energy snacks   If the metabolism is very active and food moves quickly through the digestive system, or the expenditure of energy is considerable, often loss of weight or hunger occurs on the purifying or health building diets. Also, large or tall men, or men active over long hours and in physical work, require more food to sustain them. When this occurs under treatment, it is important to take regular snacks during the day to provide the needed nourishment. The following suggestions will fill out the diet programme.

a)   Fruit, seed, nut mixes. Keep a bag of raisins, currants, dates, nuts and seeds nearby for regular snacks, or when hunger strikes.

b)   Add extra herbal supplements of the multi-vitamin/mineral formula. Take it with juice and an apple 3–4 times a day.

c)   Miso soup or miso cup exerts a potent balancing and nourishing effect which reduces the need for sweets or stimulants which might give an immediate boost but which will leave you depleted and tired.

If the individual metabolism is hyperactive, through nervous or glandular imbalance, it may be necessary to add extra herbs to soothe, calm and slow down body functions. Also, formulae such as the exhaustion formula or gentian root will increase the body's ability to absorb nutrient. Longitudinal ridges on the nails indicate diminshed ability to absorb nutrient and will also reflect improvements in digestion.

Liver cleanse on a purifying diet: Cold pressed olive oil with lemon is a cleanser for the liver. Cooked and fried oils are harmful.

Daily breakfast: mix 3-4 tbsp. pure, cold pressed almond, olive or sesame seed oil, 6-8 tbsp. (twice the amount) of fresh squeezed lemon juice, fresh ginger juice may be added to taste. Liquify with 3-6 cloves of garlic. Drink and follow with herbal tea containing: licorice, anise, fennel, fenugreek (simmered) and add peppermint and violet leaves.

If constipated: add more licorice root and fresh garlic.

If diarrhoea: no licorice, ginger or liver flush but substitute cinnamon bark in the tea and use ground cinnamon with baked apples and dates, raisins or cinnamon cooked with rice or barley.

Also chew citrus seeds, keeping in the mouth for at least 15 minutes to gain the benefit of enzymes, vitamins and minerals. The bitter essence is helpful to the liver and also helps to relieve the garlic odour, along with parsley or whole cloves.

NO FOOD TO BE TAKEN WITH THIS MORNING CLEANSE!

Liver cleanse (when eating proteins)
Take 1–3 tbsp. of pure, cold-pressed almond or olive oil mixed with 3
times the amount of fresh lime or lemon juice – stir and drink. Then
take 2 cupfuls of HOT water with the juice of half to a whole lime or
lemon juice to each cupful. ALTERNATIVE: Take 1 glass (8 oz) fresh
orange, grapefruit, pineapple or pomegranate juice with the 1–3 tbsp. oil
added in and followed by 2 cupfuls of HOT lemon water as above.
**Also helps to relieve constipation. This health-building liver flush
may be followed by fresh fruit with a few almonds and raisins about 14
minutes after the liver flush. Heavier breakfast: may be taken 1 hour or
more after the liver flush.

Millet ($\frac{3}{4}$ cup) and Fenugreek ($\frac{1}{4}$ cup) steamed porridge with $\frac{1}{2}$ cup of
juice containing fresh pressed ginger juice and soaking water in which
raisins, dates and/or figs were soaked overnight.

Exercise

All patients MUST exercise. Whether you choose vigorous walking,
jogging, aerobics, home bouncers or gym workouts, it is essential to
stimulate circulation, exercise muscles, stretch, tone and get your
lymphatic system working.

Breathing

Deep breathing is essential to bring in life giving oxygen and to eliminate
poisonous gases and toxins. If you have difficulty in breathing fully
twice a day for 5 minutes, take up yoga classes and/or gentle aerobic
workouts.

Vital circuitry

Walk barefoot for at least 15 minutes per day. If the weather permits,
walk outside on the grass to ground your electrical force and release
stagnant energy. Regular use of cotton or natural fibre socks and
comfortable natural fibre shoes (open sandals when weather permits)
will also allow your feet to relax. Walk barefoot around your home
whenever possible. Disciplines such as Tai Chi develop sensitive foot
movements which bring your feet back to life and benefit your whole
being.

Natural fibres

The use of synthetic fabric builds up static electricity around the body
and inhibits skin function. Wear cotton, silk, linen and wool fibres, and
make sure your bedding is 100 per cent cotton. Quilts must be feathers
and down, not synthetic fillers. Your health is more important than easy
laundry care.

Mental and spiritual attitudes

Think positively. Know you can be healthy. Be grateful for this opportunity for healing. Be willing to let go of your toxins and the mental and emotional patterns that created them and, like the phoenix bird, let yourself be renewed. Find your growing edge and concentrate on that. Your old outer layers will die away and leave room for your real self to emerge. Imagine you are at the centre of an expanding flower and feel the beauty of that growth.

Purification diet

The purification diet will eliminate toxic lymph, mucus, catarrh and excess acids. It will help to normalize your weight and prepare the body for regeneration. The diet provides the highest nutritive and vibratory foods to rebuild vital parts of the body and eliminates static electricity, frustrations and confusions. Most patients say they feel very well on this diet, but sometimes the first day is rough. If hunger is a problem, add spirulina. This diet raises the cell regeneration level above the cell destruction level and expels negativity. The coffee enema or its herbal substitute will also relieve cleansing headaches, aches and pains, especially if taken first thing in the morning. Make sure the bowels are active.

1. On rising in the morning, drink a large glass of prune juice. If you make it yourself use 2 glasses of water and about 10 prunes, and liquidize it in the morning. This draws toxins from every part of the body to be eliminated through the bowels.

2. Every day take 2 tablespoons of cold-pressed olive oil to lubricate the liver and bile ducts. Small amounts in juice during the day will provide the required dose.

3. Choose one juice for each three day period. The cleanse can be repeated several times, by alternating a different juice for the next three day period. It is wise to alternate between fruit and vegetable juices so that balance is maintained between cleansing and regeneration.

4. In the morning make 2 quarts of fresh juice, or use the best bought juice from glass containers containing no sugar or preservatives. Mix this with 2 quarts of distilled water or the best low mineral content spring water available in glass bottles.

5. $\frac{1}{2}$ hour after the prune juice, drink an 8 ounce glass of the juice/water mixture. Every $\frac{1}{2}$ hour, drink a glass throughout the day. If hungry, eat fruit or vegetable of your chosen juice in the evening. If, for example, you are on apple juice, eat an apple in the evening.

6. Herbal preparations are to be taken regularly during the day. If you are not on an herbal programme at the moment, take the bowel formula as an essential part of the programme.

7. Whether you decide to come off the cleanse after 1 or more cycles of 3 days, it is essential to break the cleanse properly. Start with a

fruit salad for breakfast. You may add honey and finely grated blanched almonds on top. Drink 1 or 2 glasses of fruit or vegetable juice in the morning. For lunch, eat another fruit salad and drink vegetable juice during the afternoon. For the evening meal, take a full vegetable salad with the dressing outlined in the purification diet.

8. When conditions are ideal and you are in the right state of mind, it is always beneficial to fast 1-3 days on water at the end of the juice cleanse. However, when breaking the water fast, have one day of juice cleanse before breaking the fast with fruit and vegetable salads and juices. DO NOT eat any heavy foods immediately, but add these to your diet gradually. Use a morning enema each day of the water fast.

Results: Toxicity within the lymph system will have been eliminated and replaced by the alkaline nutrition of juices.

Most patients say that they experience an increase in energy, and a feeling of light well-being. Friends tell them their eyes are shining and that their skin glows. A cleanse should not be a suffering experience when you adjust any reactions by rest, coffee, enemas, aromatherapy, baths, exercise, breathing, release of emotions, or meditation; the overall experience should be one of uplift and rejuvenation. If it isn't, seek guidance and adjustment by herbal formulae. Fasts can always be complemented by massage, reflexology, acupuncture, etc., to make the maximum use out of the cleansing experience.

Acid-alkaline foods

Science has divided foods, like chemicals, into two classes: alkaline-forming, or practically safe foods, and acid-forming, or somewhat dangerous ones. If you eat over 80 per cent alkaline foods, thus preserving the normal alkalinity of the blood, you need not think about diets. This is the key to all balancing of foods. Because some items are acid-forming is not any reason to exclude them entirely – but use them judiciously and in the correct balance, so they will yield the greatest good.

Rest and sleep are alkalizers. So are exercise, fresh air, pleasure, laughter, good conversation, enjoyment – especially love! Acidifiers are worry, fear, anger, gossip, hatred, envy, selfishness and greed, so try to cleanse these out of your system as well.

Alkaline foods (80% of diet)

Fruits	Cantaloupe	Grapes	Raisins
Apples	Carob, pod	Mangoes	LEMONS &
Apricots	only	Melons (all)	LIMES***
Avocadoes	Cherries	Olives (fresh)	*Vegetables*
Bananas	Currants	Papayas	Asparagus,
(ripe)	Dates	Peaches	ripe
Berries (all)	Figs	Pears	Aubergine

Alkaline foods (cont.)

Beans -
  green,
  lima, string,
  sprouts
Beets and
  tops
Broccoli

Cabbage (red
  & white)
Carrots
Celery
Cauliflower
Chard
Chicory
Chives
Cowslip
Cucumber

Dandelion
  greens
Dill
Dock, green

Dulse,
  seaweed
Endive
Garlic
Kale
Lettuces
Mushrooms
  (most)
Parsnips
Peppers
  (green &
  red)
Potatoes, all
Pumpkin
Radish
Swede
Sorrel
Soybeans
Spinach

Spring greens
Squash

Turnips and
  tops
Watercress

Dairy
  Products
Acidophilus
Buttermilk
Milk (raw)
Whey
Goatsmilk
  yoghurt

Flesh foods
None

Cereals
Millet

Corn, green
  (1st 24
  hours)

Miscellaneous
Agar-agar
Alfalfa
  products
Coffee
  substitutes
Ginger, dried
Honey
Kelp
Tisanes –
  mint,
  clover,
  alfalfa,
  mate, sage
Apple cider
  vinegar

Nuts
Almonds
Chestnuts,
  roasted
Coconut,
  fresh

Acid foods

Fruits
Citrus fruits
All preserves,
  jellies,
  canned,
  sugared,
  glazed
  fruits
Bananas,
  green
Cranberries
Plums
Prunes and
  juice
Olives
  (pickles)

Vegetables
Asparagus
  tips
Beans, all
  dried

Brussel sprouts
Chickpeas
Lentils
Onions
Peanuts
Rhubarb
Tomatoes
Dairy
  products
Butter
Cheese, all
Cottage
  cheese
Cream, ice
  cream
Custards
  (ices)
Milk (boiled,
  cooked,
  dried,
  pasteurized,
  canned)

Flesh foods
All meat,
  fowl, fish
Beef tea
All fish,
  shellfish
Gelatin
Gravies
Cereals
All flour
  products
Buckwheat
Barley
Breads, all
  kinds
Cakes
Corn,
  cornmeal,
  flakes
Crackers, all
  biscuits
Doughnuts

Dumplings
Macaroni,
  spaghetti
Noodles
Oatmeal
Pies and
  pastry
Rice
Rye-Crisp

Nuts
All nuts
  (more so if
  roasted)
Coconut,
  dried
Peanuts

Miscellaneous
All alcohol
Candy
Cocoa
Chocolate

Acid foods (cont.)

Coca-Cola	Eggs, esp.	Preservatives	Overwork
Coffee	the whites	Cornflour	Worry
Condiments	Ginger,	Soda Water	Tension
Dressings	preserve	Tobacco	Anger
Sauces	Jams, Jellies	Vinegar	Jealousy
Drugs, e.g.	Flavourings		Resentment
aspirin	Marmalades	Lack of Sleep	

Neutral   **Remedy (for acidity)

Oils: olive,	Lemon juice	Oranges
corn	with 1 tsp.	Calcium
Cotton seed,	cider	Nat. Phos.
soy,	vinegar	Tissue Salt
sesame,	Add hot	
etc.	water &	
Fat	honey.	

***(page 323) Citrus fruits are acidic, yet because of their high calcium content, they produce an alkaline effect during the digestive process. Some patients experience citrus fruits as acid, and others as alkaline.

High source of nutrition in herbs and food

	Herbs	*Food*
Bromine	bladderwrack	watermelon, celery, melons
Calcium	comfrey, marestail, oatstraw, marshmallow, licorice, red clover, hawthorn berries	sesame seeds, seaweeds, kale, turnip, almonds, soybeans
Chlorine	kelp	tomato, celery, lettuce, spinach, cabbage, kale, parsnip
Copper	ephaedra (desert herb)	peach, turnip
Iodine	black walnut, irish moss, bladderwrack, iceland moss, kelp, dulse	turnip
Iron	red raspberry, yellow dock, kelp, dandelion, gentian	dulse, wheat & rice bran wheat germ, pumpkin, squash & sesame seeds
Manganese	comfrey, cramp bark, uva ursi, gravel root, oat straw	apple, peach, rye, turnip
Magnesium	valerian, kelp, dandelion	wheat bran & germ, almonds, cashews

Potassium	kelp, dulse, irish moss	soybean, banana, cayenne pepper beans, peas
Silica	marestail, oatstraw	lettuce, parsnip, asparagus, dandelion, greens
Sodium	kelp, seaweeds, marigold, bladderwrack, irish moss	olives, cayenne pepper, dulse
Sulphur	garlic, kelp, black cohosh, dandelion	onion, watercress
Phosphorus	kelp	rice & wheat bran, wheat germ, pumpkin & squash seeds, sunflower seeds, sesame seeds, brazil nuts
Zinc	red raspberry, eyebright, alfalfa, uva ursi, slippery elm, hydrangea, cramp bark, echinacea, yellow dock	apricot, peach
Vitamin A	alfalfa, oatstraw	carrots, mustard greens, asparagus, cayenne pepper, dandelion greens, dock, sorrel, kale, spinach, cress, sweet potatoes, parsley, apple, garlic, ginger, papaya, rye
Vitamin B1 Thiamine	oatstraw, red clover, alfalfa	rice bran, wheat germ, sunflower seed, sesame seed, apple, garlic, ginger, papaya, turnip, rye
Vitamin B2 Riboflavin	alfalfa, oatstraw, red clover	hot red pepper, almond, wheat germ, millet, apple, garlic, ginger, rye
Vitamin B3	alfalfa, red clover	apple, garlic, ginger, onion, papaya, parsley, rye, turnip, watercress, wheat
Vitamin B5 Pantothenic Acid	barberry	rye, turnip, garlic, papaya, parsley

Choline	dandelion	parsley, turnip
B12	alfalfa, comfrey, red clover	rye, sprouted seeds, legumes
B17		apricot, peach seeds

Brewer's yeast and other yeast cultures contain all B vitamins, as do spirulina, and molasses.

Vitamin C	alfalfa, barberry, hawthorn berry, marigold, rosehips	oranges, apple, watercress, garlic, onion, turnip, cayenne, sweet red pepper, blackcurrants, parsley, walnuts, lemons
Vitamin D	alfalfa, fenugreek seeds	apple, watercress
Vitamin E	alfalfa, flaxseed, marigold, peppermint, rosehips	apple, parsley, rye, wheatgerm oil, watercress, wheat, soybean oil
Vitamin F & FF	red clover, evening primrose, borage	garlic
Vitamin K	alfalfa, oatstraw	apricot, garlic
Vitamin P Rutin	oatstraw	buckwheat
Niacin	kelp	rice & wheat bran, hot dry pepper, wild rice, sesame & sunflower seeds
Protein	spirulina	almond, pumpkin & squash seeds, wheat germ, dulse, beans, lentils, peas, sunflower seeds, soybean curd (tofu), avocado, millet, brewer's yeast

Highest alkaline foods are cantaloupe, avocado, melons, chinese cabbage, coconut, olives, blackcurrants, lettuce, watercress, chicory, carrots.

Vocabulary

Vocabulary abbreviations: Certain abbreviations are used throughout the book and on iris charts

AO	Aorta	P	Pineal
ANS	Autonomic nervous system	Pit	Pituitary gland
		PP	Peyer's patches
ANW	Autonomic nerve wreath	PT	Parathyroid
		PNS	Parasympathetic nervous system
CNS	Central nervous system		
CO2	Carbon dioxide	SNS	Sympathetic nervous system
HCl	Hydrochloric acid		
IOC	Ileocaecal valve		
MES	Mesentery		

A

Vocabulary

Aberrant fibres – white reflexive fibres which change direction, can become vascularized if long term

Absorption ring – alternative term for pupillary ruff or margin

Acid stomach – shows in iris as hyperactive white stomach halo indicating excess HCl acid

Acquired condition – not inherent, but the result of living, diet, environment and accidents

Acute – a condition arising suddenly and manifesting intense severity, usually accompanied by pain and inflammation, but lasting only a short time

Adhesions – abnormal union of structures or parts (sticking together of muscles and tissues)

Adjacent zone – spillover from iris area next to an area in the iris, especially valid in brain areas; e.g. anxiety zone or inherent mental zone affect sex impulse zone; or acids from kidney area relate to gout in leg and foot

Alimentary canal – gastro-intestinal tract

Anaemia of the extremities – lack of circulation in head, hands, feet

Anaemia ring – bluish haze outside ciliary edge (on the sclera) due to lack of circulation, low oxygen and iron

Analysis – the division of the physical whole into its constituent parts to examine or determine the condition and relationship of the whole

Anisocoria – pupils are different sizes in right and left eye of a person

Animation life centre – central 12 o'clock brain radial related to vitality and will (according to Dr Jensen) or Life force zone

Anterior – descriptive term for at or near the front

Anterior border or margin – first layer of iris, composed of two layers which are:

1) anterior fibroblastic layer   2) posterior pigmented layer

Anxiety-tetanic type – a brown eye classification of a type of person prone to neuromuscular disturbances, showing nerve rings in the iris

Arcus senilis – cerebral anaemia called 'pannus' by opthalmologist; (iris indication) white arc across top of iris

Ascending colon – area of large intestine which rises on the right side of the body from the ileo-caecal valve to the hepatic flexure

Asparagus shaped lacuna or lesion – organ sufficiency; danger sign; indicates predisposition to cancer

Assimilation ring – alternative term for pupillary ruff or margin

Ataxia – lack of muscular co-ordination

Autogenous – self generated or self-produced pigmentation (melanin & lipofuscin)

Autointoxication – alternative term for toxaemia (poisoned by own wastes)

Autonomic nerve wreath – separates ciliary zone from pupillary zone; indicates the shape of the bowels (large and small intestines)

B

Ballooned bowel – constipation and backup of faeces together with weak muscle tone causes bowel wall to stretch out; iris indication – dilation of part of the autonomic nerve wreath

Basal metabolism – the amount of energy required by an individual in the resting state for such functions as breathing and circulation of blood

Bowel pockets – formed by gas pressure or backup of faeces, cause the bowel to form pockets which hold putrefactive bowel matter, which is not eliminated in daily movements

Brain flair – Dr Jensen's term for each of the separate brain area sectors

Breaks in autonomic nerve wreath – crypts or radii soleris break through ANW, indicating diminished function of the ANS; is considered a serious sign

Bridge trabeculae – medical term for white healing lines or calcium luteum lines

Brushfield spots – medical term for lymphatic rosary

Butterfly lesion – large lesion flanked by two smaller ones or one small lesion flanked by two larger ones

C

Calcium luteum – white healing lines or trabaculae

Canthus – the inner or outer corner of the angle of the eye, formed by the natural junction of the eyelids

Cardiac renal syndrome – inherent weakness in both heart and adrenal kidney zones (the ratio of intensity of light falling on the surface)

Cardiac rings – alternative name for nerve rings; heart trouble people are constant worriers thus they always have nerve rings

Cataract – the partial or total opacity of the crystalline lens of the eye. An opaque area covering part of the eye

Catarrh – inflammation of a mucous membrane with increased production of mucus

Catarrhal encumbrance – accumulation of catarrh due to excess acids and breakdown of eliminative channels which inhibits function of that area

Central heterachromia – pupillary zone consisting of stomach and bowel areas is darkened (can be either yellow, rust, brown or black) while the rest of the eye is the true colour. Indicates toxins

Cerebellum – one of the major divisions of the vertebrate brain, situated above the medulla oblongata and beneath the cerebrum

Cerebrum – the anterior portion of the brain of vertebrates, consisting of two lateral hemispheres joined by a thick band of fibres. The dominant part of the brain in man associated with intellectual function, emotion and personality

Cervicals – neck vertebrae

Cholesterol ring – alternative term for sodium or mineral ring

Choroid – part of iris: the brownish vascular membrane of the eyeball between the sclera and the retina

Chromatophores – heavily pigmented cells in the anterior limiting iris layer; tightly packed in brown eyes; thin or nonexistent in blue irises

Chronic – long standing complaint; shows as dark sign in iris

Chrysanthemum type – abdominal reservoir type; inherently weak digestive circle where the lacunae make circles around the ANW, like a flower

Circulus arteriosus iridis minor – arterial ring arising from ciliary blood vessels, called ANW in iridology

Closed lesions – cut off from circulation and eliminative functions, indicates serious disorder, and not much hope of recovery without very deep cleansing. A completed disease process in the chronic stage

Clustered lesions – many lesions together

Colitis – inflammation of the colon

Collarette – medical term for minor vascular circle/iris frill/ANW

Colon – term for large intestine (ascending, transverse, descending or sigmoid)

Congenital – condition existing from birth, not necessarily hereditary

Constitution – physical make-up and structure; person's state of health; disposition of mind and temperament; inherent structural pattern shown in the iris by the weave or knit of the iris fibres

Contraction furrows – alternative name for nerve or cramp rings

Cornea – transparent continuation of the sclera which covers the frontal portion of the eye

Corununcle – fatty ball, nasal medial, in corner of eye; attracts plaquing deposits

Cramp rings – alternative name for nerve or contraction rings

Crisis – either a healing crisis (which is an acute state of elimination which leads to healing and health), or a disease crisis (which is a progression towards chronic and degenerative conditions). The iridologist can distinguish between the two because in the healing crisis most or all of the eliminative channels are white, and are the result of the reversal process

Cross fibres – white healing lines

Crypts – deep lesions or lacunae in rhombic form indicated organ insufficiency, possible cysts, necrosis; often break through ANW

D

Daisy petal eye – alternative term for chrysanthemum type, inherent weakness lacunae circle the pupillary zone like flower petals

Defects – small lesions or lacunae in any of the following shapes (lancet, dots, tear-like rips, cuts, streaks) signifying loss of substance. Often in stomach area or skin zone or inside other larger lesions

Degenerative stage – tissue breakdown has reached final stages of degeneration and toxic non-function; shows in iris as black mark

Depolarization lines or radials – relationship of opposite parts of the iris to one another; draw a line right through the iris and pupil to opposite side; these lines indicate relationships of function

Descending colon – part of large colon on left side of body leading down from the splenic flexure to the sigmoid colon

Diamond-shaped lacunae – indicate weakness, organ insufficiencies

Dilator papillae – muscle which dilates pupil

Diverticula, diverticulum – any sac or pouch formed by herniation of the wall of tubular organ or part, especially the intestines, which collect faeces, forming a putrefactive breeding ground for parasites and bacteria

Divided lesion – organ insufficiency, weakness

Drug spots – alternative name for psoric spots or mineral spots; pigmentation indicating accumulation of chemicals or by-products of faulty metabolism. Various colours: yellow, rust, brown, black

E

Echo lesion – remainder of past lesion damage now showing as parting or separation of fibres

Ego pressure brain sector or Perfectionist pressure zone – one's concept of oneself which motivates behaviour, attitude towards goals

Eliminative channels – five main channels for elimination of toxic waste from the body are lungs, bowels, kidneys, skin and lymph

Ellipse – pupil deformation where the pupils shifted on angle

Embryotoxon – baby born with arcus senilis condition

Emunctories – relating to a bodily organ or duct having an excretory function

Encapsulated lesion – alternative term for closed lesion

Encumbrances – that which hinders or impedes upon another or makes proper function difficult. To fill with superfluous or useless matter

Endothelial – first anterior layer of iris

Endogeneous – developing or originating within an organism or part of an organism (either the haemoglobin group, or the autogeneous group)

Epithelial pigment – layer of iris containing pigment

Equilibrium – balance created by a stable condition in which forces cancel one another

Etiology – study of the causes of disease; philosophy of causation

Exogenous – developing or originating outside an organism (heavy metal compounds or mineral compounds producing pigmentation in the iris)

Exudate arcs – white radial fibres indicating irritation in the acute eliminatory phase; most often in areas experiencing painful symptoms

F

Ferrum chromatosis – alternative term for iron pigmentation and deposits

Fibre density – alternative term for texture, showing inherent constitution

Field weakness – open lesion indicating weakness, prognosis for improvement is excellent as the area is open to circulation and elimination

Fish hooks – psychosomatic irritations; e.g. ulcerated nervous stomach

Flaccid – term for weakness, as in weak muscle tone

Flocculations – woolly cloud-like masses in the iris (e.g. lymphatic tophi)

Fuch's crypts – medical term for inherent weakness, closed lesions

G

Ganglion – any encapsulated collection of nerve-cell bodies, usually located outside the brain spinal cord

Gastric mucosa – iris stomach zone

General Adaption Syndrome – (GAS) by Selye 1976: defines the importance of inflammation as a defensive three phase response. 1. alarm; pain and inflammation. 2. resistance; symptom-free. 3. exhaustion; collapse and degeneration. This corresponds to pathways of disease, acute to degenerative stages of disease

Genotypes – genetic irreversible signs

Glaucoma – a disease of the eye in which increased pressure within the eyeball causes damage to the optic disc and impaired vision, sometimes progressing to blindness

H

Haemosiderin – iron containing pigment, red to dark brown; by-product of destruction of large quantities of red blood corpuscles

Halo – term used to describe stomach ring when its in acute white stage

Healing crisis – according to Hering's Law of Cure, when the body reaches a level of positive health, it will throw off disease. Identified in the iris as all or most of the eliminative channels become white

Hepatic flexure – part of large intestine near liver where the ascending colon curves into the transverse colon

Hepatotrophic – dark brown pathological polychromia signs; drug and mineral signs

Hering's Law of Cure – healing proceeds from within out, from the top down, in reverse order and from vital organs to less vital organs

Heterochromia – 'different colour'. In the iris – a sector or zone of the eye displaying a different colour than the true eye colour

Heterostasis – body defence; opposite of homeostasis

Histology – the microscopic study of the structure of a tissue or organ

Holistic – describes a philosophy or attitude of perceiving the body and life as an ecological system in harmonious integration with mind, emotions and spirit as well as the outer environment, nature and social structure

Homeostasis – (Gr.) state of equilibrium which living systems maintain when in normal health; subject to natural laws; deviation results in disease

Honeycomb lacuna – honeycomb shaped; indicating disturbance of local cell metabolism as a result of insufficient tissue nutrition

Hyperacid stomach – acute condition, excess HCl; white stomach ring in the iris

Hyperacidity – over acidic acute condition; shows as white in the iris

Hypercholesterosis – alternative name for sodium ring

Hyperpigmentation – alternative term for psora or drug spots

Hypoacidity – lack of acid and diminished function in weak and chronic conditions

I

Iatrogenic – diseases caused or worsened by medical treatment

Inferior – descriptive term (opposite of superior) indicating the bottom of the iris

Inflammation – the reaction of living tissue to injury or infection characterized by heat, redness, swelling and pain

Inherent strengths – constitution as indicated by density of iris fibre texture showing positive factors

Inherent weaknesses – weakness in fibre structure shown as lacunae

Inorganic – that which does not live or grow; cannot be assimilated into or become part of the tissues of human beings

Interaction zone – zone outside ciliary edge, on the sclera which indicate type of interaction between person and environment

Intrafocal signs – lesion or cavity signs within the lesion

Irides – relating to iris of the eye; plural of iris

Iridology – study of the tissues of the body through study of the iris of the eye

Iridoscopy – European term for iridology

Iris – the coloured muscular diaphragm that surrounds and controls the size of the pupil

Iris density – alternative term for iris texture or constitution

Iris frill – ANW

Iris root – outer edge of iris; ciliary edge

Iris zone – division of the iris on a chart into specific circular area

Ischaemia – an inadequate supply of blood to an organ or part, as from an obstructed blood flow

J

Jellyfish lesion – jellyfish shaped lacuna indicating organ insufficiency

K

Kidney medussa – a 'U'-shaped arch with the bottom of the arch on the ANW with the tips pointing towards the ciliary edge; indicates weakness. Sometimes also seen in lung areas

L

Lacunae – inherent weaknesses or lesions in a variety of shapes, types and sizes showing weakened function and organ insufficiency. Latin meaning is 'hole or pit'

Lance lacunae – lance or spear-shaped lacunae, indicating weakness and insufficiency

Landmarks – significant iris markings (like kidney or heart) that form the basic pattern of an analysis; selected iris markings which stand out clearly when you look at the iris

Lateral – descriptive term for the side of the iris closest to the temple, the outside of the head (opposite of medial)

Lattice structure – neuron net inside a lacuna signifying nervous blemishes due to nutritional disturbances and lack of alkalinity

Law of Cure – See Hering's Law of Cure

Leaf lacuna – leaf-shaped lacuna, often seen in thoracic area and in lung or heart weakness

Lesion conglomerate – can consist of a double lesion, honeycomb, butterfly or a giant lesion

Lesions – alternative term for lacunae (see above)

Lipid fat deposits – show upon sclera indicating congestion and wrong diet

Lymphatic rosary – string of white to yellow or brown clouds forming a pattern in the lymph zone, indicating excess collection of mucus

Lymphatic type – blue eye iris type with a tendency to lymphatic congestion and weakness; possibly born with lymphatic rosary; difficulty digesting dairy or mucus forming foods

Lypofuscin – pigmentation deposits ranging from light yellow to dark brown; considered the wear-and-tear pigment of old age

M

Mechanical signs – iris signs showing structural defects or organ displacement (like prolapse) causing pressure on organs

Medial – descriptive term for the side of the iris closest to the nose; opposite of lateral

Medulla – brain area on top of spine stem which controls automatic body functions especially respiratory ones

Melanin – pigmentation originating in melanocytes subject to hormone control which migrates within the body, especially to areas of inflammation. If found on the anterior surface of the eye it means serious metabolic disturbances, and pre-cancerous conditions

Melanocytes – special dendron cells which derive from the embryonic nerve crest where melanin originates

Mesentery – the double layer of peritoneum that is attached to the back wall of the abdominal cavity and supports most of the small intestine

Metabolism – the sum total of the chemical processes that occur in living organisms resulting in growth, production of energy and elimination of waste material

Miasm – (Greek) 'defilement.' Inherited taints from ancestral disease

Mineral ring – alternative term for sodium or cholesterol ring

Minor arterial circle – alternative term for ANW

Miosis – abnormal pupil contraction

Mucus – slimy protective secretion of the mucous membranes, consisting mainly of mucin

Mydriasis – abnormal dilation of the pupil

N

Naturopathy – system of treatment which recognizes the vital curative force within nature and within man, and seeks to support and strengthen that force by natural treatment and by removing obstacles to the proper function of that force

Necrosis – the death of body cells, usually within a localized area, as from an interruption of blood supply to that organ or part

Nerve rings – contractions in iris tissue indicating stress, irritation and tension

Nerve wreath – alternative term for ANW

Neurasthenic ring – pupillary, pigment border, ruff or margin indicating low condition of CNS when a dark colour

Neuroectodermal tissue – iris muscles are the only other tissues in the body derived from this embryonic tissue, which originated in the frontal lobe of the brain

Neuro optic reflex study – alternative term for iridology, meter of constitutional totality

Neurovascular cramp rings – alternative term for nerve rings

O

Opaque arc – alternative name for arcus senilis

Open lesions – lacunae beginning at ANW and opening out into a field of tissue (also called field lacunae). The easiest lacunae to heal as circulation can get in and elimination can remove wastes

Ophthalmic-somatic analysis – alternative name for iridology
Ophthalmology – branch of medicine concerned with the eye and its diseases

P

Palpabrae – inferior eyelid – often shows liver spots; when white indicates anaemia
Pancreas triad type – pancreas, nasal and bronchial lesions in irides
Pannus – medical term for arcus senilis
Pars iridica retinae – pupil margin, or ruff, reflection of CNS
Pathological polychromia – psoric/drug spots; deposits of various enzymes that are associated with organ cell damage
Pear lacuna – forerunner to asparagus lacuna
Perifocal – outer structure signs, area around lacunae
Peristalsis – wave-like motions of intestine which moves faeces along
Personology – study of personality by shape of face, facial lines, etc.
Peyer's patches – part of lymphatic system in small intestines which activate immune system, raising fevers to kill bacteria, virus, etc.
Phenotypes – generated signs which can be reversed
Physiognomy – the practice of studying or judging a person's character from their facial features
Pigment cells – melanocytes
Pigment ruff – pupillary edge which can indicate assimilation, and state of CNS
Plexus – complex network of nerves, blood vessels or lymphatic vessels
Ponos – Hippocratic word describing the toil of the body to restore normality
Porphyrin destruction – pathological polychromia pigmentation which is the result of a hemalytic/blood destructive condition
Posterior – descriptive term for back of iris (opposite of anterior)
Posterior epithelium layer – layer of iris heavily pigmented with black and brown layers
Posterior marginal layer (of iris) – dilator layer
Posterior membrane – iris dilator layer; thin layer of plain muscle fibre
Posterior pigmented layer – part of 1st layer of iris, the anterior border layer which contains actual iris colour
Profile – light from the side shows depth of contraction furrows or raised reflexive fibres and ANW when reading the iris
Prolapse – the pushing, sinking or falling down of any organ or part from its normal position
Psora – alternative name for drug, pigment or mineral spots, pathological polychromia
Psoric itch spots – alternative name for pathological polychromia
Pterygium – yellow thickened tissue of the white of the eye, which also may cover part of the iris, affecting those areas
Pupil – the dark circular aperture at the centre of the iris of the eye through which light enters the inner eye
Pupillaris majoris – radials from pupil which break through ANW

Pupillaris minores – radials within first zone, from pupillary margin inside ANW

Pupillary margin – alternative term for edge of pupil; assimilation ring

Pupil sugar edge – swelling of pupillary margin indicating diabetes

Pupil tonus – size and shape of pupil gives indication about the nervous system, specific areas of the body, mental and emotional states, ennervation, tension etc.

R

Radial folds – medical term for radii soleris

Radial furrows – radiate out from ANW, less severe than radii soleris

Radial vessels – irritated white reflexive fibre signs radiating singly or in groups, sometimes straight, wavy, curved or zig zag, or transversal or aberrant, indicating pain and irritation

Radii soleris – channels for distribution of toxic material from the pupil digestive system throughout the body, indicating septacaemia and inflammation and a high level of parasite activity

Radii soleris major – radii soleris from the pupil to the ciliary edge

Radii soleris minor – radii soleris from the ANW to the ciliary edge

Rayid method – system of psychological iris analysis created by Denny Johnson which focuses on attraction/repulsion in relationships, right/left brain dynamics and lessons to be learned consciously or unconsciously as we strive for wholeness, love and fulfilment

Reflexive signs – white acute fibre signs or 'radial vessels' (above) of several types, singly, or in groups, indicating irritation

Retina – part of iris. The light sensitive membrane forming the inner lining of the posterior wall of the eyeball composed largely of specialized terminal expansion of the optic nerve

Reversal process – as a person returns to health, disease is reversed and the patient may suffer for a short period, the return of previous symptoms

Rhomboid lesion – diamond-shaped inherent weakness (common in heart area)

S

Sclera – white of eye surrounding iris

Sclerotic rim – alternative term for sodium ring

Sclerosis – the hardening or thickening of organs, tissues, or vessels from chronic inflammation, abnormal growth of fibrous tissue or degeneration of the myelin sheath of nerve fibres

Scurf rim – darkened skin zone due to retention of wastes, suppression and inactivity of the skin, or inherited toxins

Sectoral heterachromia – large area of the eye is a different colour, due to drugs, heavy metal or inorganic substance which has settled

Septicaemia – septic blood, indicated by radii soleris in iris readings

Shingle lacuna – shingle-shaped inherent weakness, pre-cancerous sign

Sigmoid – end of the large intestine bending towards the centre of the body from the bottom of the descending colon, where faeces collect before they are eliminated through rectum and anus

Silver threads - irritation sign inside a lesion indicating spastic etiology

Skin zone - most outward zone, in the ciliary margin, which becomes the scurf rim when darkened

Sodium ring - white, or yellowish-white ring around ciliary edge indicating excess sodium, arteriosclerosis, high cholesterol

Solar plexus - fourth principal ganglion of the sympathetic nervous system supplying nerve fibres to the stomach, liver pancreas, spleen kidneys, adrenal, and upper intestinal viscera

Somatic constitution - alternative for fibre structure

Spastic bowel - tense, cramped bowel area causing constriction and inhibiting movement of faeces

Sphincter pupillae - muscle surrounding the pupil, stomach ring

Splenic flexure - part of large intestine where transverse colon in left side of the body bends down into the descending colon

Step lacunae - squarish lacunae ordered in step fashion, pre-cancerous sign

Stasis - a state or condition in which there is no action or progress; a stagnation in the normal flow of bodily fluids such as lymph, blood and urine

Stomach halo - circular stomach zone around pupil when it becomes white due to hyperactivity

Stomach ring - term for circular stomach area, first zone around pupil in the pupillary zone

Stricture - bowel contracted by tension, inhibiting normal peristalsis and passage of faeces

Stroma - (iris) muscular layer

Subacute - when the acute phase loses strength to complete elimination or it is suppressed, the disease passes to subacute stage where the white acute colour changes to grey, and symptoms subside

Superior - descriptive term for the top of the iris (opposite to inferior)

Suppression - avoidance of and opposite of elimination; conscious or unconscious avoidance of thoughts, or preventing proper function of organs, in their eliminative capacity

Sympatico-tonia - exhaustion of the ANS indicated by a widely dilated pupil

Systemic - conditions where all the body systems are affected

T

Temporal - descriptive term for areas of the iris between superior and inferior; either on medial or lateral side

Texture - iris texture reveals inherent constitution and its strengths and weaknesses (varies from silk to hessian-like textures)

Thermography - a recording process involving the use of heat; measures level of heat in various parts and areas of the body

Tissue regeneration - re-building body tissue through superior nutrition (herbs and special diets) after cleansing of tissues

Tonus (pupil tonus) - size and shape of the pupil give indications of energy level, condition of nervous system and mental, emotional states as well as certain body areas

Tophi (tophus) – flakes, clouds or spots in the iris, from white to yellow, indicate congestion. Usually found in the ciliary zone (especially in the lymph zone). Large white tophi can mean gout, severe uric acid toxicity or sodium deposits

Topolobile – found anywhere

Topostabile – found in specific area; in the same area

Torpedo lacunae – torpedo-shaped lacunae indicate hereditary weaknesses or possible tumours

Toxaemia – level of toxic encumbrance which has caused systemic weakness and disease

Toxic settlements – specific areas, usually inherently weak lesions, have become so encumbered with toxins that they cannot throw them off, and the tissue condition has become chronic or degenerated

Toxins – accumulation of minerals, drugs, chemicals, preservatives, pollutants and body wastes which irritate and weaken specific areas of the body, collect in the blood and lymph and put a stress on all the eliminative channels of the body

Trabeculae – iris fibres especially in a white healing state, healing fibres; structures that bridge a cavity

Transversals – white or vascularized acute reflexive signs which go across the usual fibre direction, indicating acute to chronic irritability; can point to adhesions or indicate varicose veins

Transverse colon – part of the colon which goes across the upper abdomen from the hepatic flexure to the splenic flexure, and which reflect to the brain areas in iridology

Trauma – powerful shock that may have long lasting effects, any bodily injury or wound

Tumour sign – black lacuna or crypt

U

Underacid stomach – see hypoacid stomach

Uric acid – a white odourless tasteless crystalline product of protein metabolism present in the blood or urine

Uvea – part of the eyeball consisting of the iris, ciliary body, and choroid

V

Vagotonia – overstimulation of ANS indicated by an excessively contracted pupil

Vascularized reflexive fibre – a long-term irritated iris fibre becomes red or pink; reflexive sign; a reversible sign, depending on time and proper treatment; iris blood vessel which has become swollen and irritated

Vascular layer – (of iris) tissues containing vessels that conduct and circulate fluids

Venous congestion – bluish coloured ring around ciliary margin on sclera

Vis Mediatrix Naturae – healing power of nature which is the foundation of the principle of homoeostasis and natural therapeutics

Vitality – physical and mental vigour, energy, power or ability to continue in existence, and to live and grow

W

White radial – iris fibres become raised, white and slightly separated so that they appear as radials going from the ANW to the ciliary edge. Can be single or in groups; if inside a lesion this indicates spasms, or irritations

Will – 12 o'clock brain flair area indicating vitality and strength of will

Wisp – European iridologists' term for a particular light type of tophi marking

Wolffian bodies – lymphatic tophi

Courses

Correspondence and seminar lifestyle and professional training is available to students worldwide from the schools founded by Farida Sharan. Diplomas are offered in iridology, herbal medicine and naturopathy. The autho also lectures and travels worldwide. If you are in the USA please send $2.00 to School of Natural Medicine, PO Box 17482, Boulder, Colorado, 80308, USA. If you are in any other country please send an international postage coupon in the value of $5.00 to the school in the U.S.A. The full prospectus with a copy of a recent newsletter will be mailed to you. If you sign up for a course this charge will be refunded. Please deduct from the course fee.

We must decline, however, to respond to personal letters regarding health problems. In England the school maintains a list of graduates which it will forward to you on receipt of a stamped self addressed envelope. Please request a copy of the British Register of Iridologists.

Bibliography

Iridology   Dr Donald Bamer *Applied Iridology and Herbology*, Bi-World Publishers, USA.

Josef Deck *Principles of Iris Diagnosis* 1965, *Differentiation of Iris Markings* 1980, *Institute for Fundamental Research in Iris Diagnosis*.

La Dean Griffin *Eyes: Windows of the Body and Soul, The Essentials of Iridology*, Woodland Books, USA.

Dorothy Hall *Iridology* 1980, Angus & Robertson, UK.

Dr Bernard Jensen Vol. I. *The Science & Practice of Iridology*, Vol. II. *Iridology*, published by author, USA.

Denny Johnson *What the Eye Reveals*, Rayid Publications, USA

Theodore Kriege *Fundamental Basis of Irisdiagnosis*, Fowler & Co. UK

Dr J. H. Kritzer *Textbook of Iridiagnosis: Guide in Treatment* 1924, out of print

Dr Henry Lindlahr *Irisdiagnosis and Other Diagnostic Methods*, (Vol. IV of Natural Therapeutics series), C. W. Daniel, UK

Glenda Schneider *Iris Analysis*, W & G Publishing, USA

Peter J. Thiel *The Diagnosis of Disease by Observation of the Eye*, (1905, out of print) (translation Dr F. W. Collins 1918)

Harri Wolf *Applied Iridology*, Vol. I NIRA, USA

Herbal Medicine   Dr John Raymond Christopher *Childhood Diseases, School of Natural Healing, Every Woman's Herbal*, Christopher Publications, USA

Juliette de Bairacli Levy *Illustrated Herbal Handbook, Natural Rearing of Children, Herbal Handbook for Farm and Stable, Complete Herbal Book for the Dog, Herbal Handbook for Everyone, Traveller's Joy* Faber & Faber Ltd, UK

Dr Shook *Elementary Treatise of Herbology, Advanced Treatise of Herbology*

David Hoffman *Holistic Herbal*, Findhorn Press, UK

Farida Sharan *Herbs of Grace* (published by author)

Virgil Vogel *American Indian Medicine*, Norman, USA

R. S. Clymer, MD *Nature's Healing Agents*, Humanitarian Society, USA

Robert Thomason *Natural Medicine*, Wildwood House, UK

Barbara Griggs *Green Pharmacy*
Jeannine Parvati *Hygeia – A Woman's Herbal*, Wildwood House, UK
Alma Hutchins *Indian Herbology of North America*, Merco, Canada
John Heinerman *Science of Herbal Medicine*
Ann Wigmore *Be Your Own Doctor*
Maria Treben *Health From God's Garden*, Thorsons, UK
Michael Tierra *Way of Herbs*, Washington Square Press, USA

Dr Henry Lindlahr, MD *Natural Therapeutics, Vol. I, II, III, A Doctor's View of Nature Care*, C. W. Daniel, UK **Naturopathy**
Roger Newman Turner *Naturopathic Medicine*, Thorsons, UK 1984
E. K. Lederman, MD *Natural Therapy*, Watts & Co., UK 1953, *Good Health Through Natural Therapy*, Wheaton & Co., UK 1976
James C. Thomson *An Introduction to Nature Care*, C. W. Daniel, UK 1930
Sebastian Kneipp *My Water Cure, Thus Shalt Thou Live, My Will, The Codicill to My Will, Baby Kneipp Cure*, Health Research, USA
J. W. Armstrong *The Water of Life*, Health Science Press, UK 1971
Robert Gray *Colon Health Handbook*, Rockbridge Publishing Co.
Bernard Jensen *Tissue Cleansing Through Bowel Management*, (published by author)
Gerhard Leibold *Practical Hydrotherapy, Common Sense Diet and Health*, Botanica Press 1986
Jethro Kloss *Back to Eden*

John H. Clarke, MD *Constitutional Medicine – The Three Constitutions of Von Grauvogl*, Jain Publ. Co., India **Homeopathy**
James Tyler Kent *Repertory of the Homeopathic Materia Medica*, Homeopathic Book Service 1986
Samuel Hahnemann, *Organon of Medicine*, Gollancz, UK 1986

Dr Edward Bach *Heal Thyself*, C. W. Daniel, UK **Bach Flower**
Gregory Vlamis *Flowers to the Rescue*, Thorsons, UK **Remedies**
Nora Weeks *Medical Discoveries of Edward Bach, Physician*, C. W. Daniel, UK
Collected Writings of Edward Bach, Bach Educational Programme
Chandler *Handbook of the Bach Flower Remedies*

Dr Saul Miller *Food for Thought*, Prentice Hall, USA **Nutrition**
Dr Bernard Jensen *Vibrant Health From Your Kitchen*, (published by author)

Catherine Ponder *The Healing Secret of the Ages*, Parker Publishing, USA **Miscellaneous**
J. D. Ratcliff, *I Am Joe's Body* Berkley, USA, 1987

Index

Further Information

Slides, drawings and further information on the case studies in the book can be obtained for $35.00 US or $17.00 sterling by writing to The School of Natural Medicine, P.O. Box 7369, Boulder, Colorado 80306–7369, USA, or telephone 303–443–4882. Payment must be made by Visa/Mastercard in US dollars or pounds sterling, by US check, or by International Money Order at the current exchange rate.